HORSE CONFORMATION

HORSE CONFORMATION

Structure, Soundness, and Performance

EQUINE RESEARCH

Veterinary Editor
JULIET HEDGE, DVM

Editor
DON WAGONER

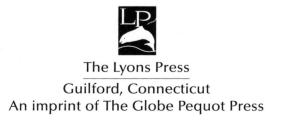

The Lyons Press
Guilford, Connecticut
An imprint of The Globe Pequot Press

Copyright © 1999 by Equine Research, Inc.

First Lyons Press edition, 2004

The Lyons Press is an imprint of The Globe Pequot Press.

10 9 8 7 6 5 4

Printed in the United States of America

ISBN 978-1-59228-487-0

Library of Congress Cataloging-in-Publication Data is available on file.

Disclaimer
Every effort has been made in the writing of this book to present quality information based on the best available and most reliable sources. Neither the author, editors, consultant, nor the publisher assumes any responsibility for, nor makes any warranty with respect to results that may be obtained from the procedures described herein. Neither the author, editors, consultant, nor the publisher shall be liable to anyone for damages resulting from reliance on any information contained in this book whether with respect to conformational examination procedures, feeding, care, treatments, drug usages, or by reason of any misstatement or inadvertent error contained herein.

Foreword

The relationship between conformation and performance in the horse has been studied and appreciated for at least as long as there has been a relationship between horses and humans. Conformation is the key to why—the racehorse runs fast, the jumper jumps high, and the barrel horse does gymnastics. But, what is conformation, really? Conformation is the outer covering of the internal working structures—the Anatomy. Conformation is the horse we see—Anatomy is the horse that actually performs. Good conformation is a reflection of the structural integrity of the skeleton as it is enhanced and modified by the muscles, tendons, ligaments, and fascia, and supplied by nerves and blood vessels.

The beauty of this book is that it walks you through the conformation and allows the reader to evaluate what is visible to the eye. Then it takes that next all-important step and reveals the unseen—the internal beauty of structural anatomy of the horse as it relates to that conformation, and ultimately performance.

The text is highly readable and the pictures and illustrations very demonstrative. As a reference text both novice and professional alike will find many uses. As a Veterinarian, it is particularly delightful to see this project come to fruition. It will give horsepeople everywhere a better understanding in their continuing relationship with horses.

Juliet Hedge, DVM

Contents

5

6

7

8

9

10

1

INTRODUCTION TO
CONFORMATION & ANATOMY

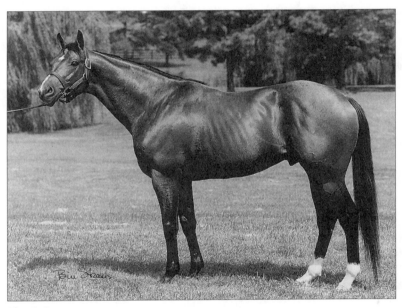

Fig. 1–1.

CONFORMATION

A horse's *conformation* is its overall body shape or form. Conformation has also been described as the relationship between form
and function. It ultimately determines how a horse moves and with-
stands impact-related stress. This in turn affects not only the horse's
beauty and presence, but its health and soundness. A horse with
good conformation is more comfortable to ride and easier to train.

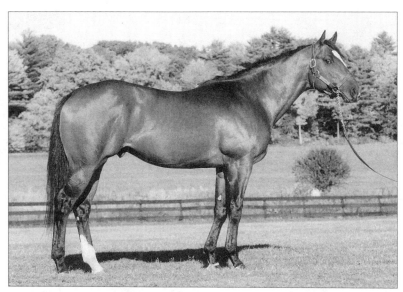

Fig. 1–2. A Thoroughbred with good conformation.

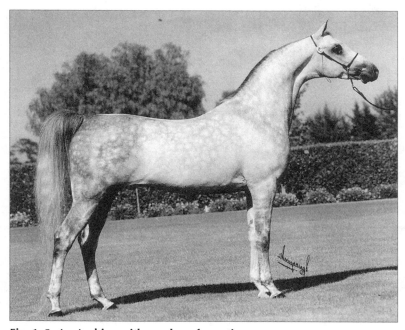

Fig. 1–3. An Arabian with good conformation.

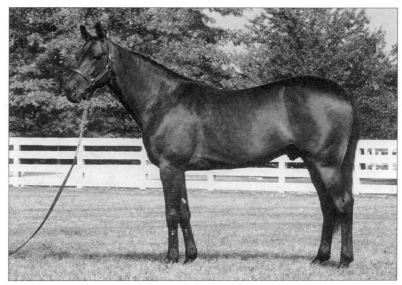

Fig. 1–4. A racing-type Standardbred with good conformation.

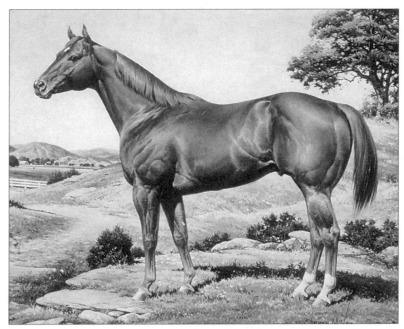

Fig. 1–5. The Orren Mixer painting shows ideal Quarter Horse conformation.

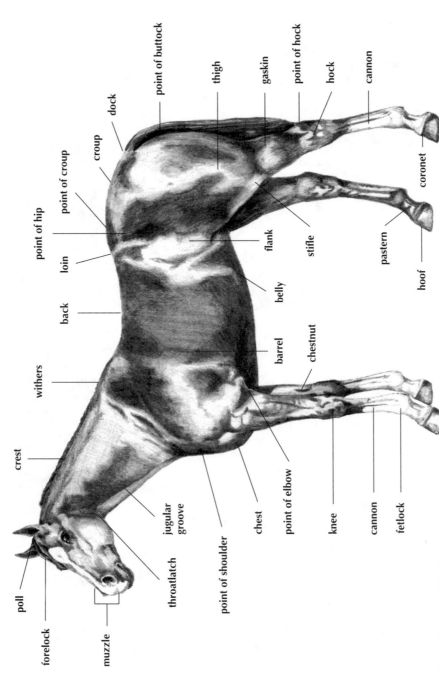

Fig. 1–6. Parts of the horse.

poll

forelock

muzzle

crest

throatlatch

jugular groove

point of shoulder

chest

point of elbow

knee

cannon

fetlock

withers

back

barrel

chestnut

point of hip

loin

point of croup

point of croup

croup

dock

point of buttock

thigh

gaskin

point of hock

hock

cannon

flank

stifle

belly

pastern

coronet

hoof

4

Conformation has two facets:
1. The skeleton.
2. The muscles and deposits of fat.

A horse that has a fundamentally correct skeleton can be fed and conditioned properly until the muscles are approximately correct. On the other hand, muscle development and excess fat deposits can obscure skeletal problems.

While conditioning can help to compensate for skeletal problems, it cannot eliminate them. Using the points of the horse *(point of the shoulder, point of the hip; See Figure 1–2)* will help to accurately evaluate conformation, because these skeletal points do not change with feeding or conditioning.

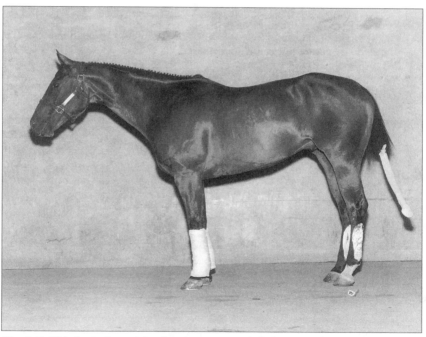

Fig. 1–7. This horse has a nice head. However, it has an overly long neck, an upright shoulder, and is slab-sided. It also has disproportionately small hindquarters and is camped under behind.

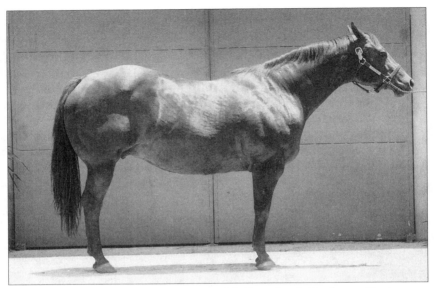

Fig. 1–8. This aged broodmare was a World Champion halter horse. She has good conformation but is not conditioned.

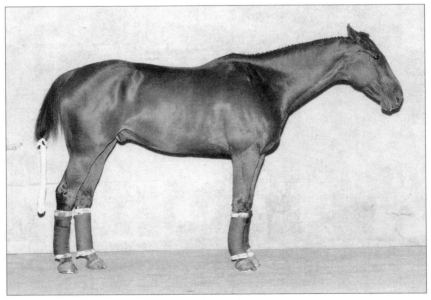

Fig. 1–9. This horse is conditioned but its conformational faults are apparant.

Common Conformational Traits

Although concepts of "perfect conformation" vary among breeds, all breed registries agree that the overall quality and balance of a horse's build should be symmetrical. There are slight differences, but researchers have found that the musculoskeletal systems of great performance horses of all breeds are surprisingly similar. A superb Quarter Horse and a superb Standardbred have different overall dimensions, yet they possess many common conformational traits.

"Balance" means that each part is proportional to all the others. To illustrate this concept, a well-conformed horse's body should be roughly divisible into thirds:

I   the point of the shoulder to the withers
II   the withers to the point of the hip
III   the point of the hip to the point of the buttock

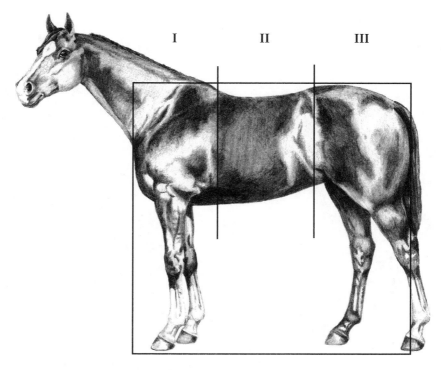

Fig. 1–10. Good horses are generally "balanced."

Although there are no absolutes, most breed registries will agree on these conformational traits:

- The neck should be long for grace and flexibility, the topline should be short and smooth for strength, and the underline should be long for freedom of movement.

- The peak of the withers should be the same height or higher than the point of the croup.

- The shoulder should be long, sloping forward and downward.

- The forelegs, measured from the elbow to the fetlock, should be about the same length as the depth of the body, measured from girth area to withers.

- From the elbow to the fetlock, the legs should be straight so that concussion is evenly distributed up the leg.

- The pastern and hoof wall should slope toward the ground at the same angle as the shoulder to help the foreleg absorb shock.

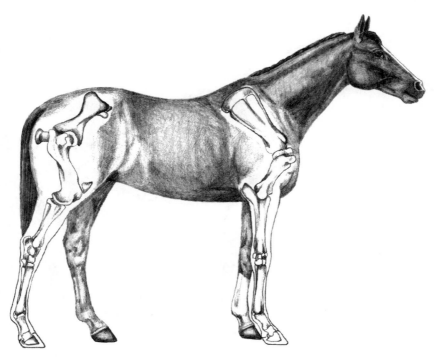

Fig. 1–11. The angled column of bones is a system designed to absorb shock and to distribute concussion evenly throughout each leg.

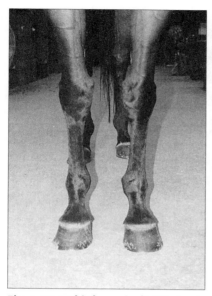 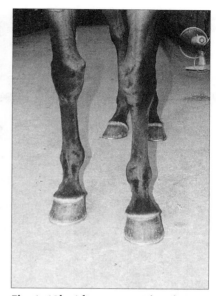

Fig. 1–12a. This horse is slightly toed-out in both front feet.

Fig. 1–12b. After proper trimming the horse's feet look almost normal.

It is essential that the horse's feet are proportional to its body size. They should be round at the toes and broad at the heels, with the coronet even all the way around. The hoof wall should slope at the same angle as the pastern.

The feet should also be balanced properly. Trimming and shoeing can significantly change the appearance of a horse's feet—for better or for worse. Improper trimming can make a normal horse look toed-out. On the other hand, a truly toed-out horse can be skillfully trimmed to look almost normal. (See Chapter 9, *Feet.*)

Analysis vs. Criticism

The word "analysis" indicates an examination of the horse's conformational characteristics; it is not the same as criticism. No horse has perfect conformation. Guidelines are flexible—their purpose is to guide, not to dictate the choice of a horse. A horse can have conformational faults and still be acceptable for many purposes. Of course, in show horses, overall excellence of conformation is a primary consideration. But in performance or pleasure horses, specific good traits may outweigh less desirable traits. For example, strong

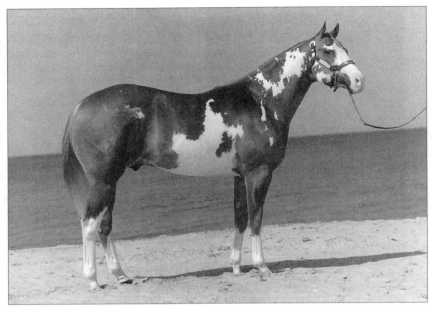

Fig. 1–13. This well-conditioned Paint horse has good conformation.

hindquarters and sturdy, straight legs in a racing Quarter Horse might outweigh a shorter-than-ideal neck.

Sometimes compensatory devices are built in. For example, a horse with upright shoulders (which absorb little impact and make for a rough gait) might have long pasterns. The pasterns compensate for the shoulders by absorbing more shock than shorter pasterns, providing an acceptably smoother ride.

Another compensatory device might be seen in a horse with a wide chest. Such a horse might turn its toes inward. This stance helps to balance the forehand weight more evenly than if the horse stood wide (and placed excess weight on the inside wall of the hooves). It also helps the horse keep a foot under each structural corner of its body. In turn, the horse will usually develop a gait abnormality to compensate for being toed-in: it will paddle (swing its forelegs in outward arcs as it moves), to keep its legs from interfering.

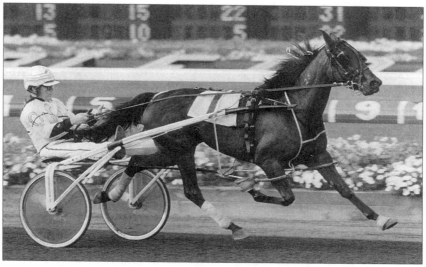

Fig. 1–14. Several top pacers have raced well despite toeing-out.

Conformational Analysis

To begin an analysis, square the horse up on a level surface. Thoroughly examine the horse from all angles, both up close and at a distance. It helps to run a hand over the horse, especially the legs, feeling for bumps, swellings, etc. After assessing conformation from each angle, judge the animal in motion, particularly at the walk and trot. This overall picture is important: a horse with a slight conformational defect should not be excluded from consideration if it performs acceptably.

Conformation is one of the major factors in determining the potential soundness of the horse's legs. Stress, strain, and/or concussion forces cause most lameness. Poor conformation causes extra stress on specific areas of the leg. For example, base wide conformation places extra stress on the inside of the legs, causing these horses to be susceptible to injuries on the inside of the leg.

A casual visual inspection can be misleading because many conformational defects that lead to unsoundness are not so obvious.

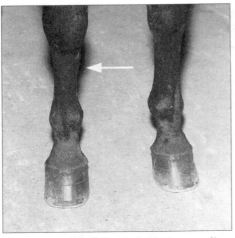

Fig. 1–15. This base wide horse has a splint on the inside of the right leg.

At first glance, a horse may seem acceptable. However, it could have some conformational defect that would prevent it from performing up to standards. That is why a veterinarian is relied upon to conduct a prepurchase examination. A veterinarian may distinguish between blemishes and unsoundness, and detect hidden faults that may lead to problems. (For more information, read *Equine Lameness,* published by Equine Research, Inc.)

Conformation and Heredity

Athletic ability and breeding potential depend largely upon basic conformational factors. By knowing what factors constitute good conformation and what injuries are likely to occur with specific inherited faults, selecting horses that are capable of producing winning offspring is made easier. Also, a better training program can be planned for the individual.

Conformation is highly heritable, passed down from both sire and dam. If sound conformation is not given sufficient consideration when selecting breeding stock, problems are perpetuated in subsequent generations. Heritable conformational defects may include parrot mouth/bulldog mouth, ewe neck, flat feet, and abnormal leg structure, such as:

- base narrow/base wide
- knock knees/bow legs
- bench knees
- camped out/camped under
- cow hocks/bow legs

- toed-in/toed-out
- calf knees/buck knees
- tied in below the knees
- straight behind
- sickle hocks

Most inherited conformational defects are not characteristic of any one breed, but common throughout the equine population.

Although conformational defects can be due to a variety of causes, environmental as well as hereditary, there is a proven relationship

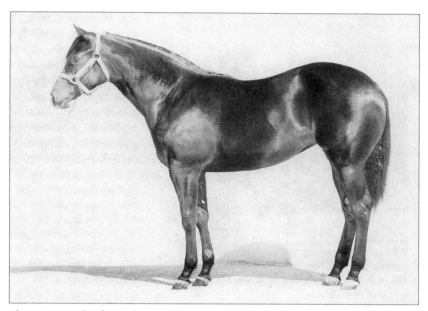

Fig. 1–16. A nice horse in many respects, but the croup is higher than the withers, the hocks are high, and the cannons are thin. Also, the hind pasterns are overly straight.

between conformation and lameness. An effort should be made to determine whether a conformational defect is inherited or acquired. If it is inherited, it is best to eliminate the defect in future foals by modifying the breeding program. Studying pedigrees, breeding records, and the conformation of close relatives will indicate whether a specific defect is inherited.

Conformation and Size

The height of a horse is traditionally measured from the ground to the peak of the withers. The unit of measurement used is *"hands"*: each hand is equal to 4 inches. Any horse under 14.2 hands (58 inches) is considered to be a pony.

Different sized people naturally prefer different sized horses, but size can be important in determining how a horse will perform. A racehorse with determination and a will to run can overcome deficiencies in size and achieve victories over larger horses. But generally, sizable horses that are long in the forearm and gaskin make the best racehorses because they have longer strides. In hunting, large

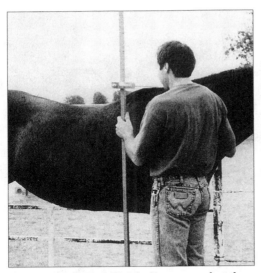

Fig. 1–17. A horse's height is measured at the peak of the withers.

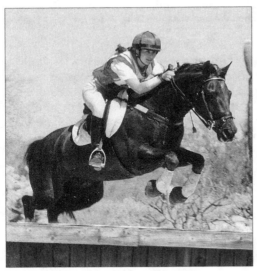

Fig. 1–18. Smaller horses, such as this Morgan, may have a more difficult time on hunt courses.

horses often have an advantage over smaller horses because hunt courses are designed for horses with long strides.

Each person must decide if size will be a limiting factor. Is a yearling with outstanding conformation passed over because it is a few inches shorter than average yearlings of the breed? While such a lack of size might limit a racehorse, hunter, or jumper, it might be preferred in a pleasure horse.

On the other hand, it is important to remember that individual horses mature at different rates. A colt that is comparatively small as a yearling might be larger than horses of his same age as a two-year-old. Larger horses may not reach full physical maturity until age six or perhaps even age seven.

Also, certain breeds are known for slower development. The very beautiful and graceful Lipizzans are sometimes awkward-looking until they are four or five years of age.

ANATOMY

To accurately assess a horse's conformation, it is important to be familiar with its *anatomy*—the underlying structures that determine conformation. Also, it is easier to understand and deal with injuries or diseases when one understands how the horse's body functions.

This section describes the musculoskeletal system of the horse, generally defining bones, muscles, joints, tendons, and ligaments. Chapter 14, *Body Systems,* addresses other systems, including the digestive, respiratory, circulatory, nervous, and reproductive systems.

While it is necessary to divide the horse's musculoskeletal system into parts, and to discuss them separately, it is better to think of them as an interdependent whole. For example, locomotion occurs when a muscle contracts, activating its tendons and moving the bones at their joints, which are held together by ligaments.

Bones

Bones make up the skeletal framework of the horse: the scaffolding from which tendons, muscles, and vital organs are suspended or encased. The *skeleton* supports and protects these soft tissues, and individual bones act as levers for the muscles, creating movement.

There are 205 bones in the horse's skeleton:

Vertebrae in the spinal column	54
Ribs	36
Sternum, or breastbone	1
Skull, including those of the inner ear	34
Forelegs, or thoracic limbs	40
Hindlegs, or pelvic limbs	40

The bones also serve as the body's major storage sites for important minerals such as calcium and phosphorus. Sometimes bone is dense, which means it contains greater amounts of these minerals. Sometimes it is more spongy, and therefore less dense.

Bones can be divided into one of the following categories:

Long bones—long, cylinder-shaped bones, including the ribs, humerus, radius, femur, tibia, and cannon bone. They act as levers and supports.

Cuboidal bones—block-shaped bones of the knee and hock. They absorb concussion.

Flat bones—thin, flat bones of the skull, scapula, and pelvis. They provide scaffolding for body muscle attachments and leg formation. They also form cavities to protect the brain and other vital organs.

Pneumatic bones—contain air spaces, including the frontal bones and maxillary bones of the skull, housing the nasal passages.

Sesamoid bones—accompany other bones in a joint to reduce friction or act as pulleys for tendons, including the sesamoid bones of the fetlock (proximal sesamoids), navicular bone in the foot (distal sesamoid), and patella.

Irregular bones—oddly shaped, unpaired bones, including the vertebrae, short pastern bone, coffin bone, accessory carpal (knee) bone, and larger tarsal (hock) bones.

TYPES OF BONES			
Type	**Description**	**Example**	**Function**
Long	long, cylinder-shaped	cannon bone, radius, humerus, tibia, femur	as levers and supports
Cuboidal	block-shaped	knee/hock bones	absorb concussion
Flat	thin, flattened	skull, scapula, pelvis	scaffold for muscles and leg formation; protect organs
Pneumatic	contain air spaces	frontal, maxillary	house nasal passages
Sesamoid	accompany other bones in a joint	proximal sesamoids, navicular, patella	reduce friction or act as pulleys for tendons
Irregular	oddly shaped, unpaired	vertebrae, short pastern, coffin, accessory carpal, larger hock bones	various

Fig. 1–19. Bones can be categorized based on their shape and function.

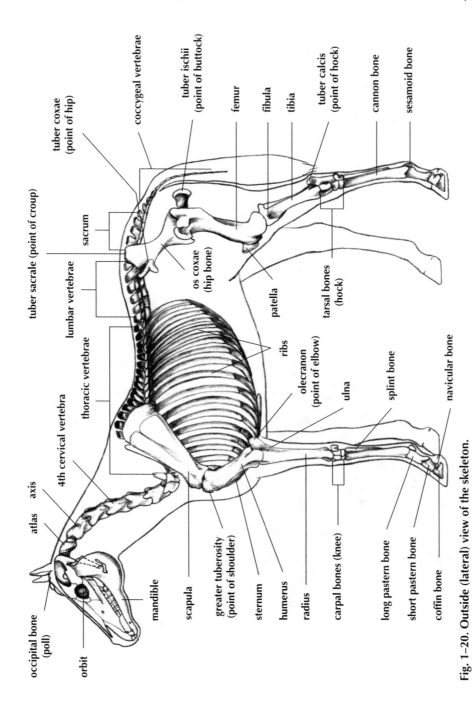

Fig. 1–20. Outside (lateral) view of the skeleton.

Bone Structure

Bone is living tissue. It constantly renews itself, and stores or releases minerals depending on the body's needs. In the process, it changes its shape and density to accommodate the stresses it is under. Conformation, exercise, and nutrition (both before and after birth) can affect both the thickness and density of a bone.

Some bones fuse with maturity or aging. For example, the bones of the skull are joined by cartilage at birth, but fuse with bone as the horse matures. The splint bones fuse to the cannon bones. And sometimes the hock bones fuse together, to stabilize that joint.

Each bone has a thin, strong membrane covering its surface, called the *periosteum.* Under the periosteum is the bone's *cortex:* an outer layer of dense bone that gives the bone strength. The center of the bone consists of *cancellous bone* that absorbs concussion.

The long bones of the legs and ribs also have a *medullary cavity* in their center. In young horses this cavity contains red bone marrow where red and white blood cells are manufactured. In mature horses the red bone marrow is gradually replaced with fat, and blood cells are produced instead in the spleen.

Each bone has unique surface features. These features resemble ridges, hills, and hollows. For example, a *"tuberosity"* is a protrusion on a bone. It is usually a site of muscle attachment. A projection, or *process,* functions as a pulley for the muscles that run over it. A hollow, or *fossa,* sometimes gives an overlying muscle more room to move. One example is in the scapula (shoulder blade), where two muscles lie in hollows on either side of a ridge. Sometimes a fossa contains an organ such as a gland. Or it may accommodate another bony

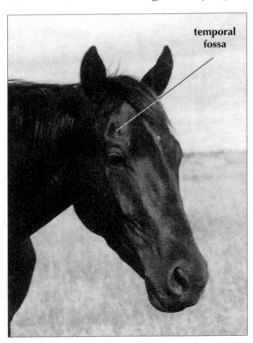

temporal fossa

Fig. 1–21. The temporal fossa over this horse's eye is clearly visible.

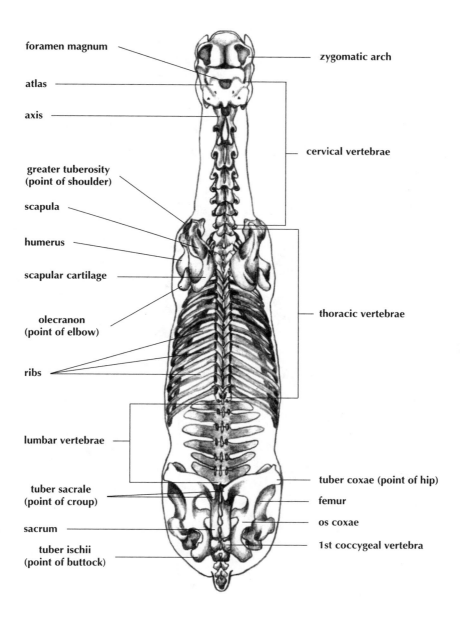

foramen magnum

zygomatic arch

atlas

axis

cervical vertebrae

greater tuberosity
(point of shoulder)

scapula

humerus

scapular cartilage

olecranon
(point of elbow)

thoracic vertebrae

ribs

lumbar vertebrae

tuber coxae (point of hip)

tuber sacrale
(point of croup)

femur

os coxae

sacrum

1st coccygeal vertebra

tuber ischii
(point of buttock)

Fig. 1–22. Top (dorsal) view of the skeleton.

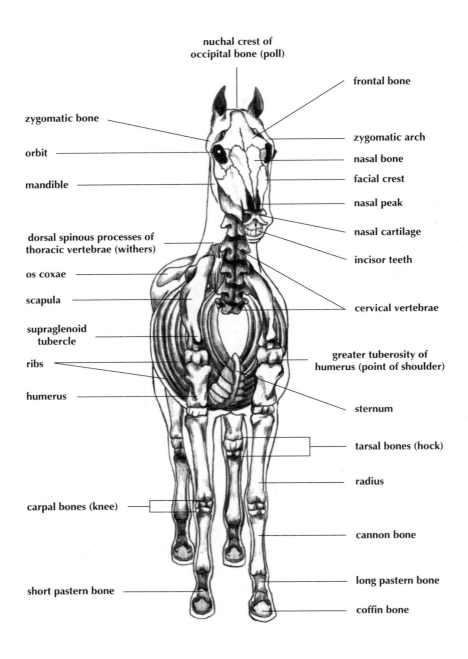

nuchal crest of
occipital bone (poll)

frontal bone

zygomatic bone

zygomatic arch

orbit

nasal bone

facial crest

mandible

nasal peak

nasal cartilage

dorsal spinous processes of
thoracic vertebrae (withers)

incisor teeth

os coxae

scapula

cervical vertebrae

supraglenoid
tubercle

greater tuberosity of
humerus (point of shoulder)

ribs

humerus

sternum

tarsal bones (hock)

radius

carpal bones (knee)

cannon bone

short pastern bone

long pastern bone

coffin bone

Fig. 1–23. Front (cranial) view of the skeleton.

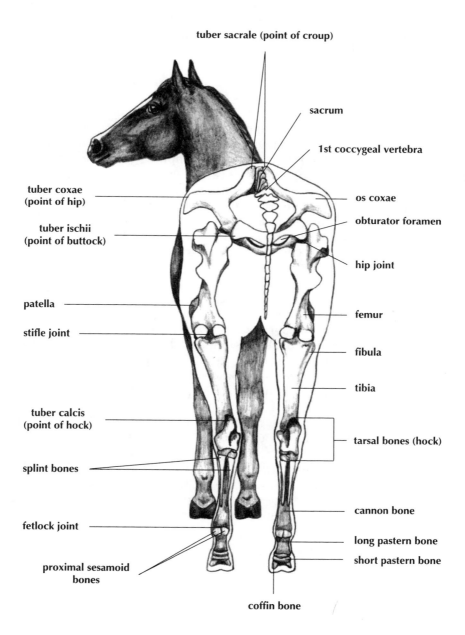

tuber sacrale (point of croup)

sacrum

1st coccygeal vertebra

tuber coxae
(point of hip)

os coxae

obturator foramen

tuber ischii
(point of buttock)

hip joint

patella

femur

stifle joint

fibula

tibia

tuber calcis
(point of hock)

tarsal bones (hock)

splint bones

cannon bone

fetlock joint

long pastern bone

short pastern bone

proximal sesamoid
bones

coffin bone

Fig. 1–24. Rear (caudal) view of the skeleton.

structure, such as the temporal fossa in the skull accommodates the coronoid process of the mandible (jawbone). Movement of the coronoid process (covered by a pad of fat) in the temporal fossa can be seen when the horse chews.

Cartilage

In addition to bone, the horse's skeleton contains *cartilage*. Cartilage is a special kind of tough, yet elastic body tissue. It does not have a blood supply, so the cartilage cells receive nutrients from surrounding body fluids via diffusion. Examples include the cartilages that shape the external ear, the scapular cartilage at the top of the scapula, and the five joined cartilages that create the larynx.

There is a special type of cartilage, called *growth cartilage* at the ends of a foal's long bones. As the foal matures, the growth cartilage gradually changes into bone. At maturity, only a thin layer of *articular cartilage,* which covers the joint surfaces of a bone, remains.

Joints

A *joint* is a point of contact between two bones. It may be immovable, slightly movable, or freely movable. Immovable joints include the sutures between the bones of the skull. Slightly movable joints include the joints between the vertebrae or between the cannon and splint bones. Freely movable joints are also called true joints—their purpose is to allow locomotion. Examples of true joints include the shoulder, hip, knee, hock, and fetlock.

The articular cartilage covering the joint surfaces of each bone absorbs concussion and reduces friction. In true joints, a *joint capsule* surrounds the joint. Lining the inside of the joint capsule is the synovium, which secretes *synovial fluid* into the joint space. Synovial fluid nourishes and lubricates the joint.

Most joints have ligaments—very strong, inelastic bands—around them or even within them. The ligaments are responsible for holding the bones together.

True joints can move in one or more of the following ways:

Flexion—bending

Extension—straightening

Rotation—twisting around the axis

Adduction—moving toward the midline of the body

Abduction—moving outward from the midline of the body

JOINT MOTION		
Type	**Description**	**Example**
Flexion	bending	A jumper folding its forelegs has its knees flexed.
Extension	straightening	A racehorse reaching forward has at least one knee extended.
Rotation	twisting around the axis	A polo pony turning quickly to follow the ball rotates on one forefoot.
Adduction	moving toward the midline of the body	A dressage horse performing a side-pass crosses the left foot over the right to adduct the left leg...
Abduction	moving away from the midline of the body	...and when it lands, the right foot reaches out sideways for the next step, abducting the right leg.

Fig. 1–25.

Soft Tissues

Soft tissues are fascia, ligaments, tendons, bursae, muscles, etc. Although the bones provide the framework, it is the soft tissues that are directly responsible for movement. (Specific structures are discussed in the Anatomy section of each chapter.)

Fascia

Fascia is the body's connective tissue. Arranged in layers of sheets or bands, it is thin, fibrous, and strong. Superficial fascia lies just under the skin and holds the skin to the underlying structures. It is also called subcutaneous tissue. Beneath the superficial fascia lies the deep fascia, also called aponeurotic fascia. In addition to covering much of the muscle mass, deep fascia serves as a point of attachment to some muscles. It can cover joints and merge with ligaments.

The deep fascia of the horse's barrel helps to support the weight of the internal organs. The deep fascia of the legs attaches to the bones, muscles, tendons, and ligaments, helping to give them definition and direction. *(See Figure 1–26.)*

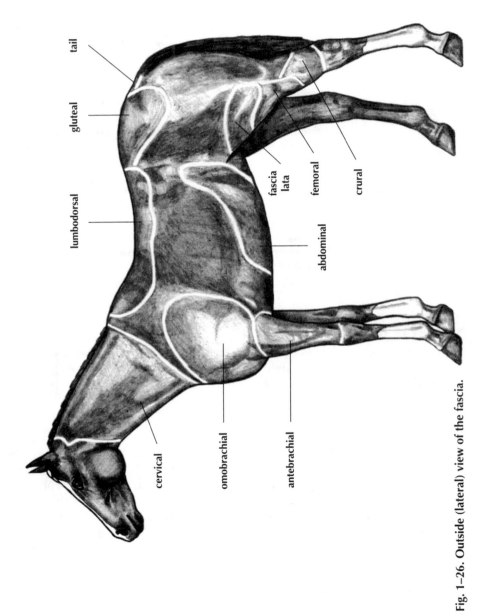

Fig. 1–26. Outside (lateral) view of the fascia.

tail

gluteal

lumbodorsal

fascia
lata

femoral

crural

abdominal

cervical

omobrachial

antebrachial

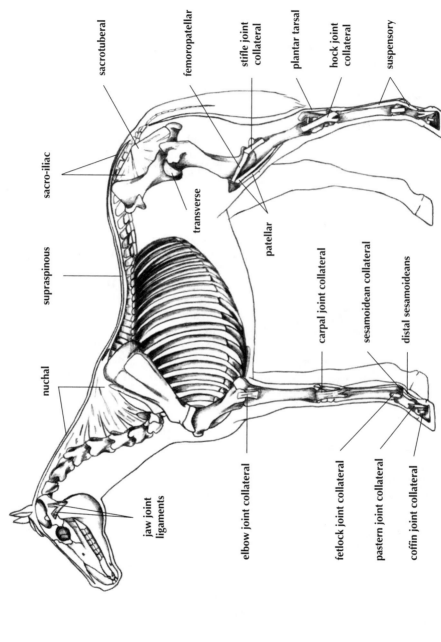

Fig. 1-27. Outside (lateral) view of the ligaments.

sacrotuberal

femoropatellar

stifle joint collateral

plantar tarsal

hock joint collateral

suspensory

sacro-iliac

transverse

patellar

supraspinous

carpal joint collateral

sesamoidean collateral

distal sesamoideans

nuchal

jaw joint ligaments

elbow joint collateral

fetlock joint collateral

pastern joint collateral

coffin joint collateral

Ligaments

A *ligament* is a strong, fibrous band that connects two bones. Many joints have *collateral ligaments*—ligaments on either side of the joint—that hold the bones together. A few joints, such as the stifle and hip, have ligaments on the inside *(intra-articular ligaments)*. A special type of ligament, called a *check ligament,* connects a bone to a tendon. Its function is to limit the action of the tendon, preventing injury due to overstretching. Another special type of ligament is called an *annular ligament.* The word "annular" means ring-shaped. Such ligaments run horizontally across a joint and serve to bind the nearby tendons close to the joint. *(See Figure 1–27.)*

Tendons

Cord-like *tendons* connect a muscle to a bone, transmitting the energy generated by muscle contraction to the bone, which creates movement. Some tendons attach to more than one bone, and act on several joints simultaneously with one contraction.

Tendons are made of collagen fibers arranged lengthwise. They are stronger, but less elastic, than muscle tissue. If a tendon must travel over a joint, it is protected by a *tendon sheath.* The lining of the sheath produces synovial fluid, which reduces friction.

Tendons are named for their accompanying muscle. For example, the radial carpal extensor tendon connects the radial carpal extensor muscle to the radius and cannon bone. *(See Figures 1–29 and 1–30.)*

Bursae

A *bursa* (plural = bursae) is a fluid-filled sac. It lies between two structures, and its function is to protect both structures from friction. For example, the navicular bursa in the foot lies between the deep digital flexor tendon and the navicular bone, ensuring that the tendon glides easily over the bone without being damaged.

Muscles

A *muscle* is a bundle of elastic fibers surrounded by a membrane of fascia. It may be named for its function, location, shape, or attachments. The deep digital flexor muscle is a good example. It is deep within the forearm, closer to the bone than its companion, the superficial digital flexor muscle. Via its long tendon, this muscle activates the digit (the fetlock, pastern, and coffin joints). And more specifically, it acts to flex, or bend the digit.

A muscle might be voluntary or involuntary. *Involuntary muscles* are those which the horse does not control. They include the muscles of the circulatory system (including the heart itself), digestive tract, and reproductive system. The horse does have control over the *voluntary muscles*. They include the cutaneous (skin) muscles, locomotor muscles, and the muscles of the nostrils, mouth, eyes, ears, tail, anus, and vulva.

The *cutaneous muscle* is a sheet of tissue between the superficial and deep fascia. It is mostly attached to the skin, connecting to the skeleton at only a few places. This is the muscle that flicks a fly off the horse's skin.

The *locomotor muscles*—responsible for movement—are usually shaped like bands. Each has a body, sometimes called the muscle belly, and two ends. Each end of the muscle becomes a tendon before it attaches to a bone. (Some muscles attach to other muscles, fascia, or skin.) When it is stimulated by a nerve impulse, the muscle contracts, pulling on the bone and causing movement. Most of the locomotor muscles come in pairs: one on each side of the body. They can act together to produce one movement, or independently to produce a very different movement.

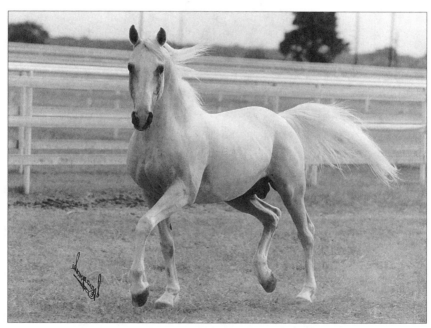

Fig. 1–28. The deep digital flexor muscle bends the joints of the lower foreleg.

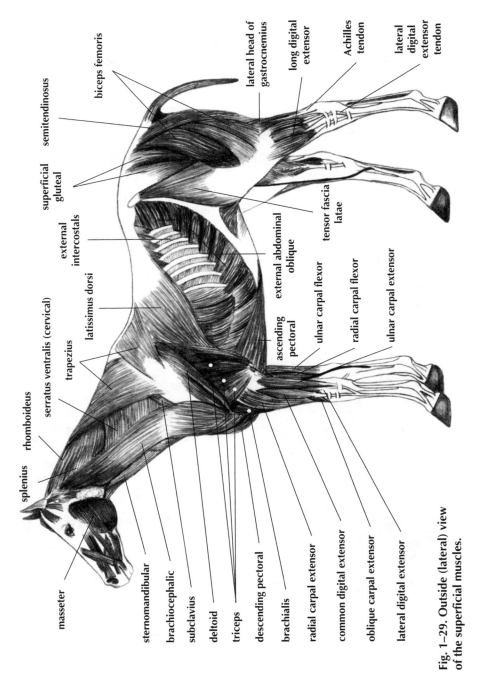

masseter

splenius

rhomboideus

serratus ventralis (cervical)

trapezius

latissimus dorsi

external intercostals

superficial gluteal

semitendinosus

biceps femoris

lateral head of gastrocnemius

long digital extensor

Achilles tendon

lateral digital extensor tendon

tensor fascia latae

external abdominal oblique

ulnar carpal flexor

radial carpal flexor

ulnar carpal extensor

ascending pectoral

sternomandibular

brachiocephalic

subclavius

deltoid

triceps

descending pectoral

brachialis

radial carpal extensor

common digital extensor

oblique carpal extensor

lateral digital extensor

Fig. 1–29. Outside (lateral) view
of the superficial muscles.

28

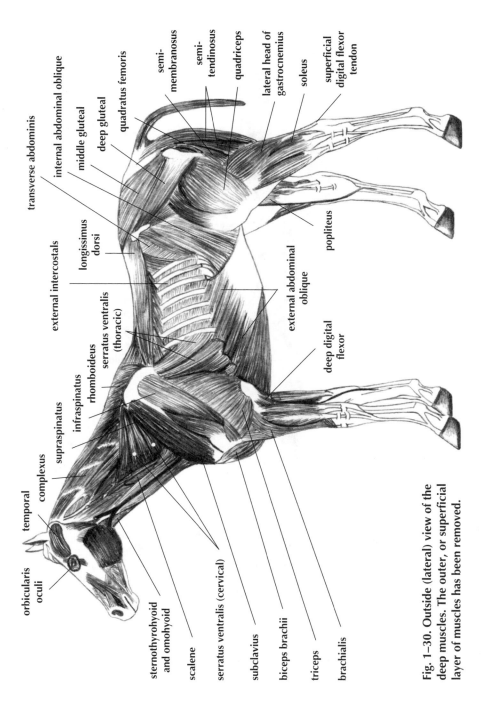

Fig. 1–30. Outside (lateral) view of the deep muscles. The outer, or superficial layer of muscles has been removed.

29

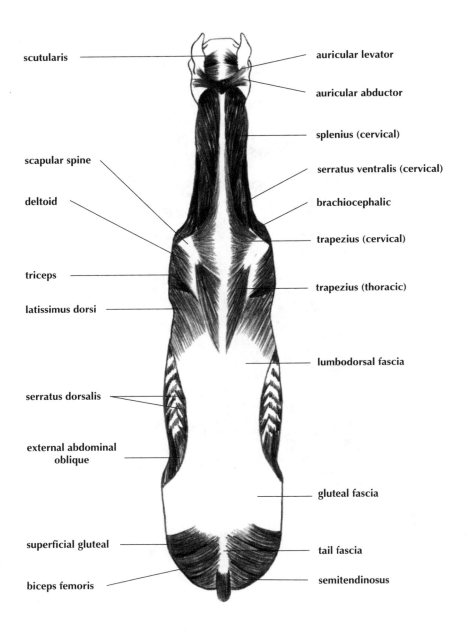

scutularis

auricular levator

auricular abductor

splenius (cervical)

serratus ventralis (cervical)

scapular spine

brachiocephalic

deltoid

trapezius (cervical)

triceps

trapezius (thoracic)

latissimus dorsi

lumbodorsal fascia

serratus dorsalis

external abdominal
oblique

gluteal fascia

superficial gluteal

tail fascia

biceps femoris

semitendinosus

Fig. 1–31. Top (dorsal) view of the superficial muscles.

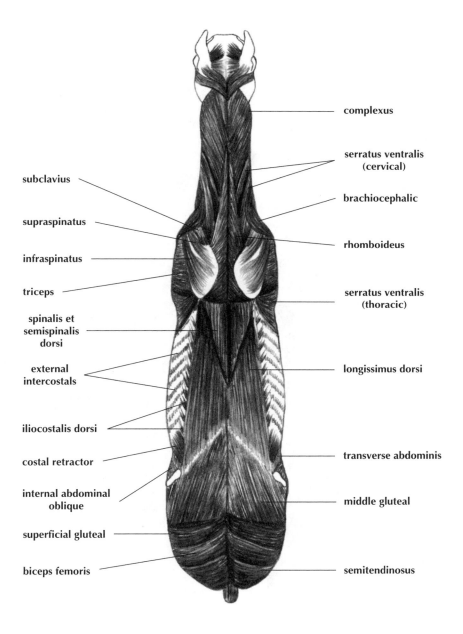

Fig. 1–32. Top (dorsal) view of the deep muscles. The outer, or superficial layer of muscles has been removed.

complexus

serratus ventralis (cervical)

brachiocephalic

rhomboideus

serratus ventralis (thoracic)

longissimus dorsi

transverse abdominis

middle gluteal

semitendinosus

subclavius

supraspinatus

infraspinatus

triceps

spinalis et semispinalis dorsi

external intercostals

iliocostalis dorsi

costal retractor

internal abdominal oblique

superficial gluteal

biceps femoris

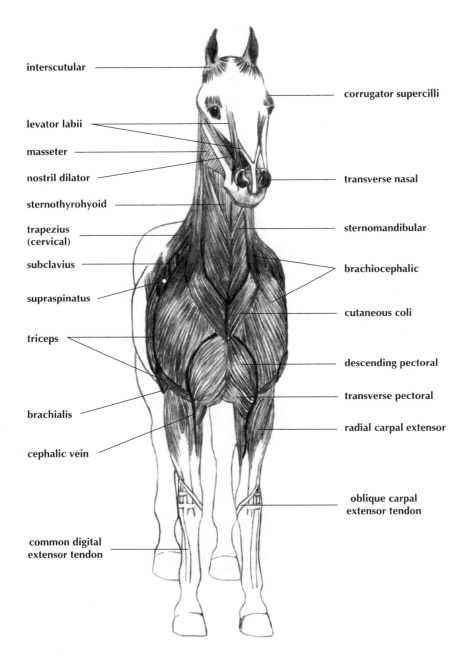

interscutular

corrugator supercilli

levator labii

masseter

nostril dilator

transverse nasal

sternothyrohyoid

trapezius
(cervical)

sternomandibular

subclavius

brachiocephalic

supraspinatus

cutaneous coli

triceps

descending pectoral

transverse pectoral

brachialis

radial carpal extensor

cephalic vein

oblique carpal
extensor tendon

common digital
extensor tendon

Fig. 1–33. Front (cranial) view of the muscles.

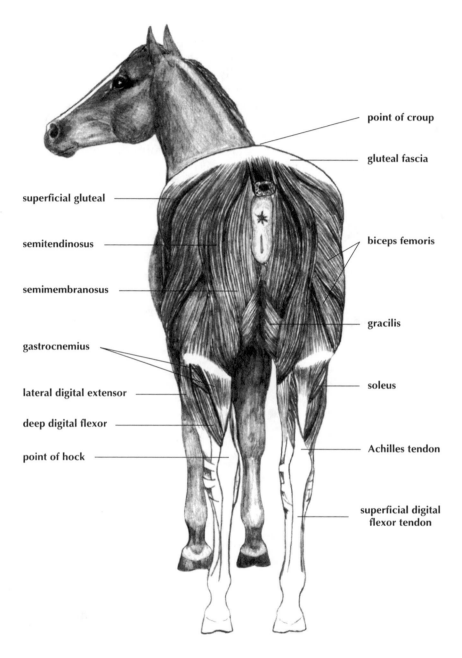

point of croup

gluteal fascia

superficial gluteal

semitendinosus

semimembranosus

biceps femoris

gracilis

gastrocnemius

lateral digital extensor

deep digital flexor

point of hock

soleus

Achilles tendon

superficial digital
flexor tendon

Fig. 1–34. Rear (caudal) view of the muscles.

One end of the muscle is called its *origin*, and the other is its *insertion*. The origin is usually on the less movable side. Also, the origin is usually attached to its bone more firmly than the insertion. In the legs, the origin of a muscle is generally closer to the trunk of the body.

In addition to causing movement, muscles are also responsible for limiting or preventing movement. For example, the same muscles that act to pull the forearm in toward the body also prevent it from being pulled too far out from the body. Other muscles have the sole function of supporting a joint, limiting the joint movement to within the normal range of motion.

(See Figures 1–29 through 1–34 for illustrations of the muscles of the horse from all views.)

2

HEAD

It is natural to look first at the horse's head. The head is the focal point of the horse's body, and generally reveals its intelligence, character, and physical condition. Also, the characteristics that define a breed are often evident in the head. For these reasons, the conformation of the horse's head is given a great deal of attention. But as long as the head is proportional in size to the body, a plain-looking head will function just as well as a beautiful one.

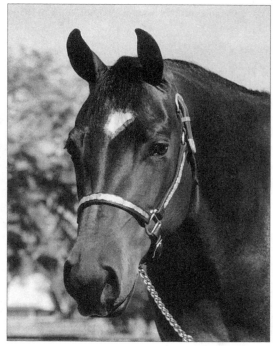

Fig. 2–1.

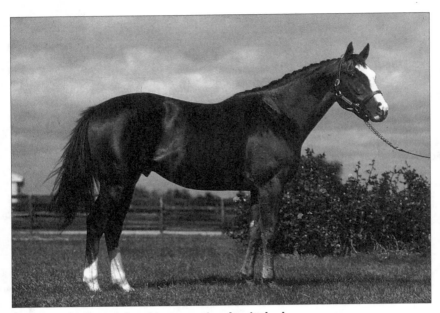

Fig. 2–2. This horse's head is proportional to its body.

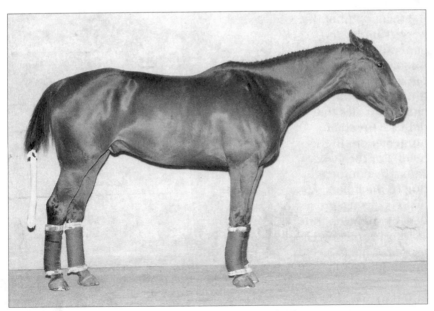

Fig. 2–3. This horse's head is relatively large for its body.

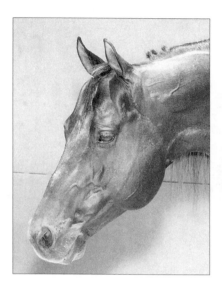

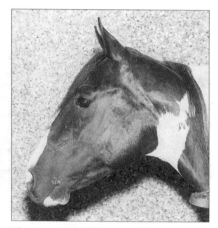

Fig. 2–4. Left: Clean-cut features. Right: An acceptable, though not beautiful head.

CONFORMATION OF THE HEAD

It is important in any breed that the size of the horse's head be proportional to the size of its body. The features should be clean-cut or chiseled; that is, the bones, muscles, and blood vessels should be well defined. The head should be long enough to provide room for large, clear nasal passages and strong, well-placed teeth.

More specific characteristics are based on standards of appearance for different breeds. Thoroughbred standards demand that the profile show a straight line from ears to muzzle, and prefer a head that is long. Arabian owners value a concave profile, or one that has a bulging forehead and a *"dish"* below the eyes. The trait is considered a sign of refinement and good breeding, even though breeders of other horses may select against it. However, even an Arabian may have too much dish to its face, or have the dish in the wrong place. Both Arabians and Quarter Horses have relatively short heads.

Many excellent draft horses have a *Roman nose;* in fact in some of these breeds it is a desirable trait. A Roman nose occurs when the profile bulges slightly outward from the eyes down. (This trait is not to be confused with a *"bull head,"* where only the forehead bulges outward.) A Roman nose is considered undesirable in other breeds because it can interfere with vision and indicates coarseness.

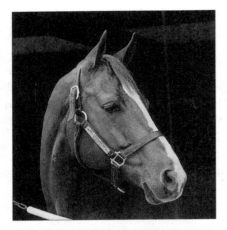

Fig. 2–5. Straight profile.

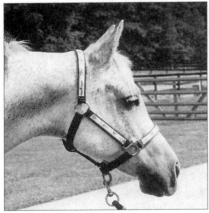

Fig. 2–6. Concave profile.

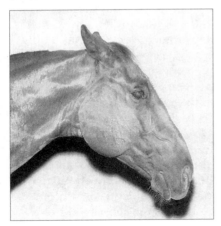

Fig. 2–7. Convex profile,
or Roman nose.

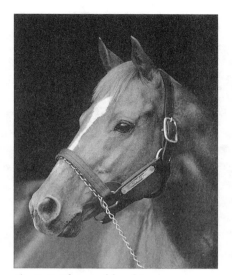

Fig. 2–8. Thoroughbred type.

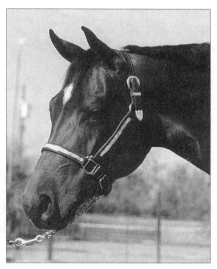

Fig. 2–9. Quarter Horse type.

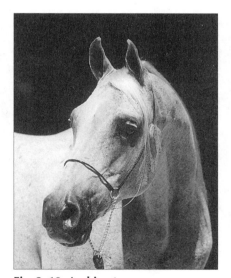

Fig. 2–10. Arabian type.

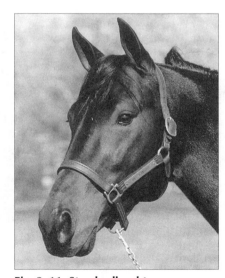

Fig. 2–11. Standardbred type.

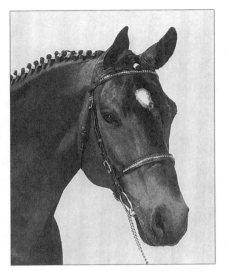

Fig. 2–12. Warmblood type.

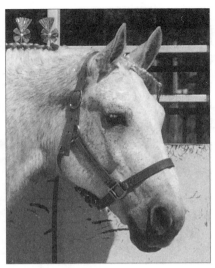

Fig. 2–13. Draft type.

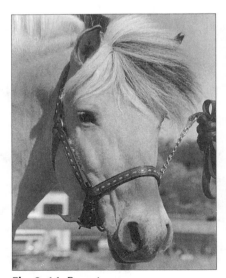

Fig. 2–14. Pony type.

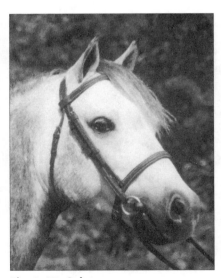

Fig. 2–15. Cob type.

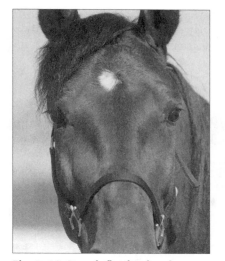

Fig. 2–16. Broad, flat forehead.

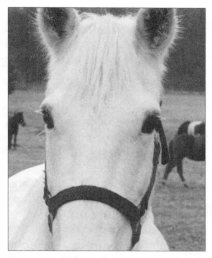

Fig. 2–17. Relatively narrow forehead.

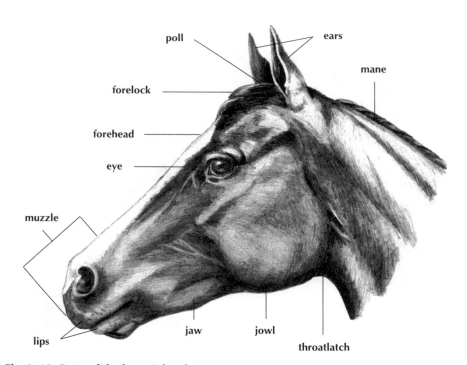

Fig. 2–18. Parts of the horse's head.

A front view of the head should reveal a broad, flat *forehead* in proportion to the size of the *poll* and nostrils. A broad forehead indicates that the cranium (bones that encase the brain) is large enough to provide adequate brain space.

Eyes

"Intelligent" *eyes* are bright, clear, and alert. They should be large, round, and prominent without bulging. Warm, dark brown eyes are generally preferred, because blue or glass-eyed horses tend to be more sensitive to light. Most people also prefer dark *sclera* rather than white sclera (in humans, the sclera is the "white of the eye"). However, for Appaloosa fanciers, white sclera are attractive because they look "human."

Widely-spaced eyes, placed on the corners of the forehead, offer a proper range of vision. However, hunters, jumpers, and racehorses can be excepted from this general rule. These horses need excellent forward vision and may perform better when their eyes are placed slightly closer together.

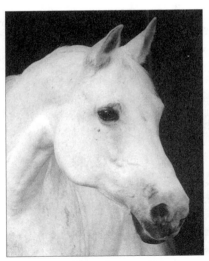

Fig. 2–19. Bright, clear, and alert eye.

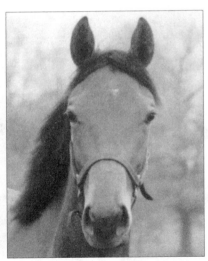

Fig. 2–20. Widely-spaced eyes placed on the corners of the forehead.

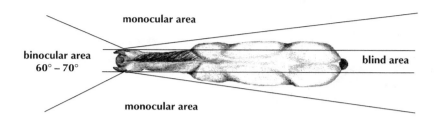

monocular area

binocular area
60° – 70°

blind area

monocular area

Fig. 2–21. The horse has both monocular and binocular vision. When facing forward, the horse has two blind spots: directly in front and directly behind.

The horse can see almost 360° around itself because each eye operates independently and sees a different picture. This is called *monocular vision*. There is an overlapping field of about 60° – 70° in front of the horse where its vision becomes *binocular*. The horse has poor depth perception, because it is accurate only in the overlapping field. It has two blind spots: directly behind, and directly in front and below the muzzle, to about four feet ahead. The horse must turn its head to see these spots.

Conformational Faults of the Eyes

An overly wide forehead and a deep eye socket decrease the degree of binocular vision. This may cause the horse to be nervous and apprehensive. (Horses with good dispositions have been known to have sudden changes in temperament when they begin to experience vision problems.)

Too small an eye is called a *"pig-eye."* Such eyes are usually set too far back and have thick eyelids. Not only is a pig-eye unattractive, it limits the horse's field of vision. Interestingly, the size of the eyeball itself varies little in horses. It is the bone structure that makes the eye appear large or small.

A *"gotch-eye"* is improperly positioned as compared to the other eye. The eyeball may be turned too far outward, turned downward, or turned upward and outward. These problems can cause the horse to shy at odd times or to bump into things. *Crossed eyes* cause the horse to see two objects instead of one. The horse is unsure of its footing, and afraid of bridges, railroad tracks, etc.

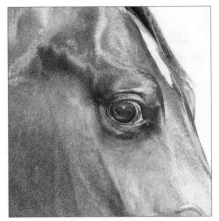

Fig. 2–22. The whites of the eyes are showing because the horse is worried.

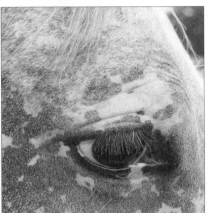

Fig. 2–23. The whites of the eyes are showing because the horse naturally has white sclera—this is an Appaloosa.

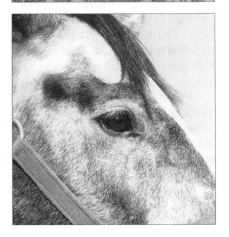

Fig. 2–24. The eyes are too small.

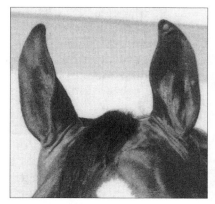

Fig. 2–25. Refined ears.

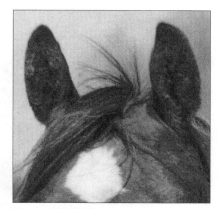

Fig. 2–26. Thick, coarse ears.

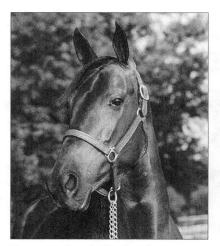

Fig. 2–27. Ears indicating interest.

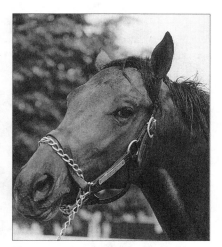

Fig. 2–28. Ears indicating irritation.

Ears

Ears should be refined (rather than thick), slightly arched, and active. The ears usually face whereever the horse is looking. An attentive, inquisitive horse has erect, alert ears. The ears should be placed close together, just below the poll, over a wide forehead.

The ears should be medium-sized. Mares tend to have slightly larger ears than stallions, but the ears are no less refined. Although it is not always achieved, the Quarter Horse community prefers small,

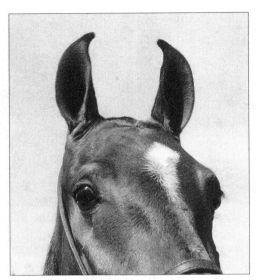

Fig. 2–29. Curly ears placed close together.

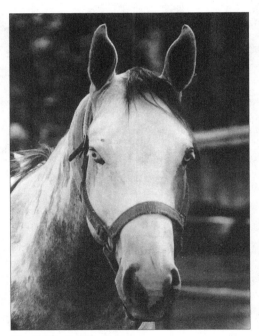

Fig. 2–30. Relatively large ears.

triangular, "fox-like" ears. Thoroughbreds tend to be thin-skinned and often have more delicate ears than Standardbreds or Quarter Horses.

Conformational Faults of the Ears

An ill-tempered animal may frequently pin its ears back. A horse with droopy ears is ill or uninterested. A horse with overactive, twitchy ears may be nervous or may have vision or hearing problems.

Ears that are too large or too small can make a face appear disproportionately large or small. Ears that are too long are called *"mule" ears*. Droopy ears placed too far apart are called *"lopped" ears*. But most people consider this to be only a minor fault.

Jaw

The horse's *jaws* should be strong and broad, and they should meet evenly. Ample width between the jaws means that there is more space in the throat, which allows the horse to withstand the heavy breathing associated with hard work. To measure jaw width, place an up-right fist under the horse's *throatlatch,* and slide it forward between the branches of the mandible (jawbone). The throatlatch should accommodate all four knuckles of an average-sized hand. Both tradition and equine science indicate that there is a correlation between jaw width and good respiratory health.

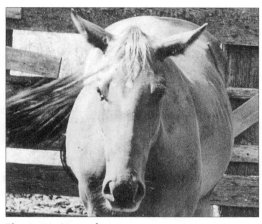

Fig. 2–31. Lopped ears.

As well as the usual up-and-down motion, the joints of the jaw need good side-to-side motion to properly grind food.

Conformational Faults of the Jaw

A horse with an overbite is said to have a *parrot mouth.* A horse with an underbite is said to have a *bulldog mouth.* Parrot mouth and bulldog mouth seem to be inherited characteristics, and should be selected against because they interfere with the horse's eating efficiency. If the incisors do not meet properly, it could be that the cheek teeth are also offset. The cheek teeth must be correctly aligned

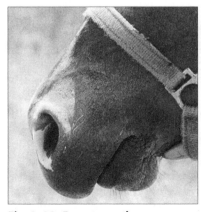

Fig. 2–32. Parrot mouth.

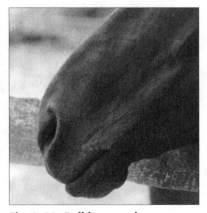

Fig. 2–33. Bulldog mouth.

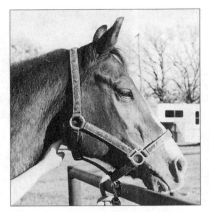

Fig. 2–34. Using a closed fist to measure the width of the jaws.

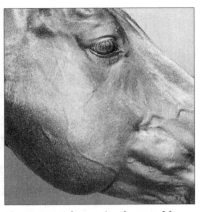

Fig. 2–35. A heavy jawbone adds weight to the head.

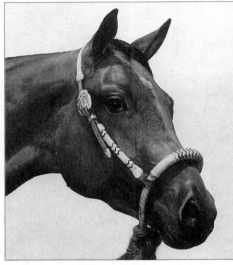

Fig. 2–36. Stallions have larger jowls than mares.

to grind food well and to wear evenly.

A horse with narrow jaws may also have a narrow throatlatch (see Chapter 3, *Neck*). This characteristic makes the horse more susceptible to roaring or other respiratory problems.

Stallions usually have larger *jowls* than mares. In some types, heavy jowls are a fairly severe fault. They add weight to the head and reduce flexion at the poll. In other types they are acceptable as long as the horse's throatlatch is not overly thick.

Muzzle

The face should taper to a relatively small *muzzle*. A horse can only breathe through its nose, so the *nostrils* should be large, open, and thin-walled, capable of handling large quantities of oxygen. This fea-

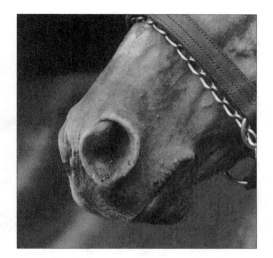

Fig. 2–37. A small muzzle with open, generous nostrils.

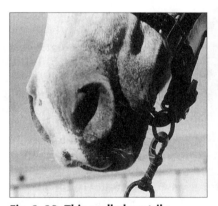

Fig. 2–38. Thin-walled nostrils.

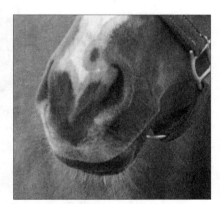

Fig. 2–39. Thick-walled nostrils.

ture is especially important for any equine athlete. A deeply dished face pinches the nostrils and nasal passages, reducing oxygen intake. The *lips* should be firm and muscular because the horse uses them to select and grasp food.

The Head and Locomotion

The head and neck affect the horse's movement and locomotion. This is similar in principle to that of a weight, lever, and fulcrum. That is, a small weight at one end of a lever can be used to balance a much

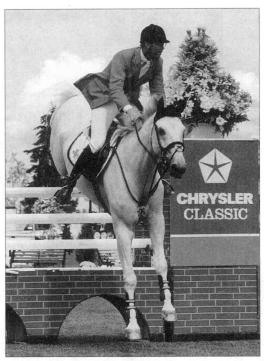

Fig. 2–40. This jumper's head and neck are raised to balance the hindquarters, pulling them underneath the body in preparation for landing.

larger weight at the opposite end as it rotates around a fixed point or fulcrum. The horse's head acts as a weight that is raised or lowered on one end of the lever (the neck).

The point of the fulcrum in the horse is located over the center of gravity—below the withers at the level of the spinal cord and formed by the angle of the scapula (shoulder blade) and the sternum (breast bone). As it rotates around the fulcrum, the lever allows the heavier hindquarters to be balanced by the much lighter weight of the head.

A galloping horse demonstrates this principle well. As the horse's hindlegs move forward and impact the ground, the body is propelled forward as well. The forelegs are extended in the air with the head and neck raised. As the forelegs impact the ground, the horse's weight is shifted forward over the forelegs, the neck is lowered, and the head now acts as a counterbalance to the elevating hindquarters. With the hindquarters raised, the horse can collect its hindlegs for another powerful thrust. As the hindlegs impact the ground, the horse's weight is shifted backward, the head and neck are raised for balance as the forelegs come forward off the ground, and the cycle begins again.

Because of the head's function as a weight on a lever, there is an interaction between head size and weight, neck length, body length, and the ability to elevate the hindquarters. A horse with a head that is too big or too small for its body size is usually not a good mover because it cannot properly counterbalance the heavier hindquarters.

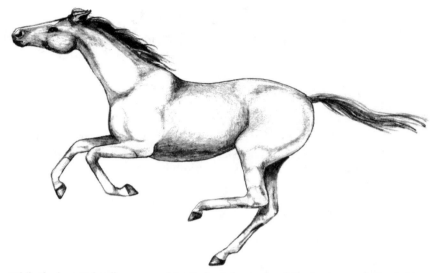

While the horse's hindlegs are pushing its body forward and the forelegs are extended in the air, its head and neck are raised.

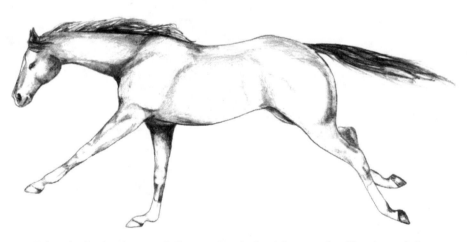

When the forelegs impact, the horse swings its head downward, pulling the neck down to shift its weight forward over the forelegs and raise the hindquarters.

Fig. 2–41. The horse in motion at the gallop.

ANATOMY OF THE HEAD

The skin over the horse's head is fairly thin. Surface features such as ridges of bone, blood vessels, and nerves can easily be seen or felt.

Bones of the Head

Skull

The *skull* is a complex of 34 bones. The flat bones are joined by cartilage at birth. As the horse matures, the cartilage is replaced by bone. This process is usually complete by the time the horse is eight years old.

For purposes of description, the skull is divided into two areas: the cranium and the face.

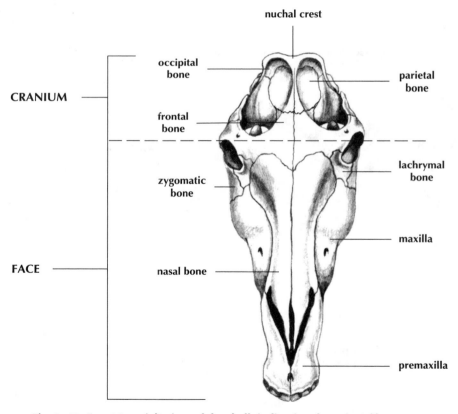

Fig. 2–42. Front (cranial) view of the skull, indicating the pairs of bones.

Cranium

The functions of the *cranium* (or cranial bones) are to enclose the brain and to form part of the cavities for the eyes and nasal passages. The poll is formed by the peak of the *occipital bone,* called the *nuchal crest.* (The spinal cord enters the base of the skull through an opening in the back of the occipital bone called the *foramen magnum.* See Chapter 3, *Neck,* for an illustration.)

The roof of the cranium is formed by flat pairs of bones. The largest of these are the *parietal bones.* The forehead is formed by the *frontal bones.* These bones also form the *supraorbital processes* (or ridges) immediately above the *orbits*—the cavities in which the eyeballs lie. As each supraorbital process arches away from the eye, it joins the cranium at a *temporal bone.* The "bar" this forms is called the *zygomatic arch.* Above the orbit is the *temporal fossa,* seen externally as a rounded hollow above the horse's eye. The temporal fossa deepens as the horse ages.

The temporal bone provides the "canal" or opening into the skull that leads to the middle and inner ear. It also creates the *glenoid fossa,* which forms a joint with the mandible, or jawbone.

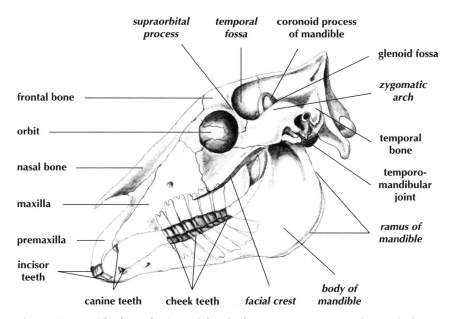

Fig. 2–43. Outside (lateral) view of the skull. Compare parts in italics with those of Figure 2–44.

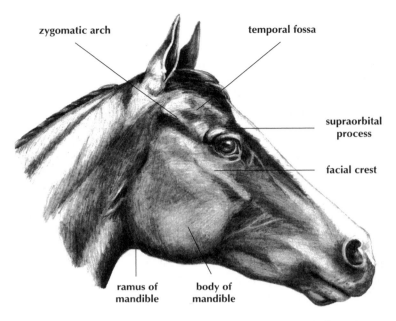

zygomatic arch

temporal fossa

supraorbital process

facial crest

ramus of mandible

body of mandible

Fig. 2–44. Many of the ridges and hollows of the horse's skull can be seen or felt on the surface.

Face

The face of the horse includes the lower part of the frontal bones, the *nasal bones,* and the *maxilla.* The maxilla and *premaxilla* form the *hard palate* (roof of the mouth), which contains the upper teeth. The face also houses the nasal passages.

Mandible

The *mandible,* or lower jawbone is the largest bone in the horse's head. It has two halves that are fused together. The fused area forms a flat, horizontal surface, the front of which contains the lower *incisor* and *canine teeth.* The middle of the jawbone contains the lower *cheek teeth.* Each *ramus* (plural = *rami*) of the mandible forms a jowl at the back of the jaw. The mandible joins the skull at the *temporomandibular joint* under the zygomatic arch. This joint is between the glenoid fossa in the temporal bone and the *coronoid process* of the mandible. The movement of the coronoid process (covered by a pad of fat) can be seen in the temporal fossa when the horse chews.

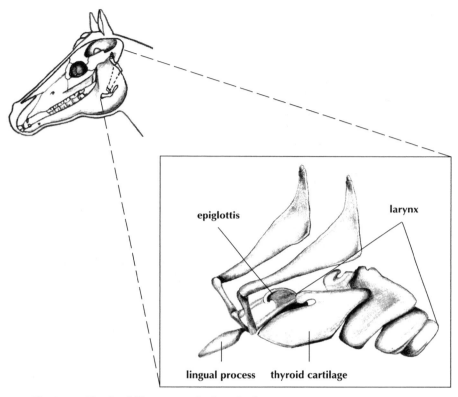

Fig. 2–45. The hyoid bone attached to the larynx.

Hyoid Bone

The *hyoid bone* functions to support the root of the tongue, pharynx, and larynx (discussed later). It looks much like a small jawbone, and is situated between the two rami of the mandible. The upper end of the hyoid bone attaches to the temporal bone; its lower end attaches to the *thyroid cartilage* of the larynx. Jutting out of the lower end is a bony spine called the *lingual process,* which imbeds in and supports the root of the tongue.

Nasal Passages

The *nasal passages* are pathways conducting outside air to the horse's throat. Other vital functions of the nasal passages include warming and moistening the air, and filtering out small foreign particles. The openings of the nasal passages are the *nostrils* (or nares).

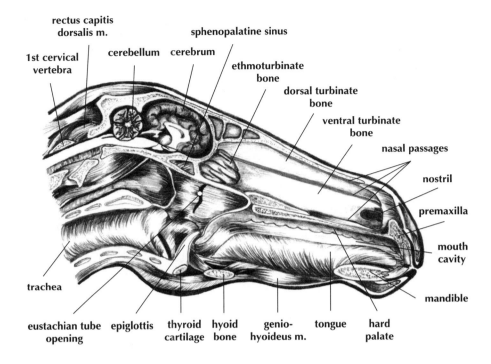

Fig. 2–46. A cross-section of the head.

The nostrils are built around crescent-shaped cartilages. These cartilages may be expanded, or flared, to take in more air during exercise. The left and right nasal passages are separated by a strip of cartilage called the *nasal septum*.

Each nostril contains three delicate bones called *turbinates*. These bones are covered by a thick, soft, mucous membrane. The upper (dorsal) and lower (ventral) turbinates are long. They are rolled into the shape of a scroll, and penetrated by many holes, like a sieve. Together with the mucous membrane, these features contribute to the accuracy of the horse's sense of smell because they provide a broad surface area. The third bone is the *ethmoturbinate*. This structure is actually a group of plate-like projections in the back of the nasal cavity. The surface of the mucous membrane that covers this structure is penetrated by olfactory nerves, which transmit "scent" messages to the horse's brain.

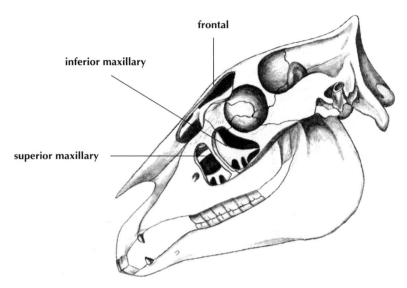

Fig. 2–47. The sinuses within the skull.

Sinuses

Each side of the nasal cavity is connected, directly or indirectly, to four air-sinuses:

- *frontal sinus*
- *inferior maxillary sinus*
- *superior maxillary sinus*
- *sphenopalatine sinus*

(**Note:** The sphenopalatine sinus is deeper than the other three sinuses. It is illustrated in Figure 2–46.) These pockets in the bone lie just beneath most of the surface bones of the forehead and occupy some space under the facial bones, immediately beneath the eyes. Sinuses serve no evident purpose beyond giving the horse's face a smooth appearance and shaping it without adding weight. In addition, the superior maxillary sinus houses the upper cheek teeth.

Muscles of the Head

Motion of the head is controlled mainly by the neck muscles. There are a few tiny, deep muscles between the skull and the first two cervical vertebrae that assist in head movement. The most important of these muscles is the *rectus capitis dorsalis (see Figure 2–46)*. It helps to extend the horse's head outward.

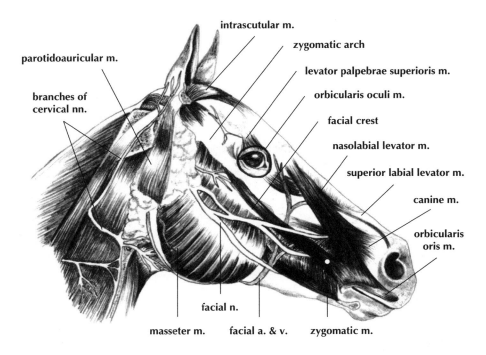

intrascutular m.

zygomatic arch

parotidoauricular m.

levator palpebrae superioris m.

branches of
cervical nn.

orbicularis oculi m.

facial crest

nasolabial levator m.

superior labial levator m.

canine m.

orbicularis
oris m.

facial n.

masseter m.   facial a. & v.   zygomatic m.

Fig. 2–48. The muscles (m.), blood vessels (a. & v.), and nerves (n.) of the head.

The superficial muscles within the head give the horse expression, allowing movement of the lips, nostrils, external ears, eyelids, and jaw. Most of these muscles originate on the frontal, nasal, and maxilla bones. Some muscles have more than one function.

The lips are closed by, among other muscles, the *orbicularis oris*, which encircles them and acts as a sphincter (ring-like muscle). Beginning just below each eye and running down the face to the upper lip are paired muscles called the *superior labial levators*. The tendons of these muscles join between the nostrils and the common tendon continues down to the upper lip. These muscles dilate the nostril and raise the upper lip (for example, the flehmen response of a stallion to a mare in heat).

Each ear is moved by 17 muscles in a complex fashion resembling ball-and-socket joint movement. Each set of eyelids is acted upon by 4 muscles. The *orbicularis oculi* muscle encircles the eye and closes the upper and lower eyelids, and the *levator palpebrae superioris* muscle (and others) opens the eyelids.

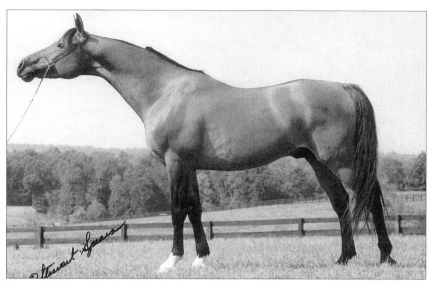

Fig. 2–49. Movement of this Arabian's head is controlled mostly by the neck muscles.

The lower jaw is moved by six muscles. The largest and strongest of these muscles is the *masseter*, which functions to bring the jaws together. The masseter covers the jowls, originating on the *facial crest* and zygomatic arch, and inserting onto the outer curve of the mandible. It helps to determine the size of the horse's jowls.

The hyoid bone is acted upon by eight muscles, some of which also move the tongue. The *genio-hyoideus* muscle *(see Figure 2–46)*, for instance, draws both the hyoid bone and the tongue forward.

Other Structures in the Head
Brain

The brain is surrounded and protected by the cranium. The *cerebrum* at the front is the largest part of the brain. Intelligence, memory, and emotion are directly controlled by the cerebrum, as well as the senses. It may also have secondary control over other parts of the central nervous system (see Chapter 14, *Body Systems*).

The *cerebellum* is located slightly behind and beneath the cerebrum. It is responsible for muscle coordination and balance.

(See Figure 2–46 for an illustration of the cerebrum and cerebellum.)

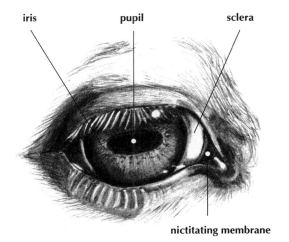

iris   pupil   sclera

nictitating membrane

Fig. 2–50. The parts of the horse's eye.

Eye

The eyeball lies inside the orbit of the skull on either corner of the forehead. Like the human eye, the equine eye is lubricated by lacrimal fluid secreted from the *lacrimal gland*. The *lacrimal caruncle* is the pea-sized prominence at the inside corner of the eyelid. There are two tiny holes near the caruncle. They come together to form a tear duct about 12 inches long that opens into the nasal cavity just above the nostril. This is called the *nasolacrimal duct*. It allows excess fluid to drain from the eye down into the lower nose.

The horse's eye has a third eyelid, or *nictitating membrane*. It consists of a curved, roughly triangular plate of cartilage that is surrounded by mucous membrane. The third eyelid is positioned at the inside corner of the eye where it protects the eye and "wipes" away any foreign objects.

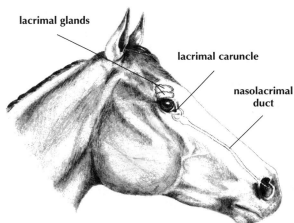

lacrimal glands

lacrimal caruncle

nasolacrimal duct

Fig. 2–51. The nasolacrimal apparatus.

Ear

Sound is collected by the *auricle*, or *external ear*. The auricle is formed and supported by several cartilages. These cartilages are also attachment sites for many of the auricle muscles that move the external ears.

The *middle ear* lies behind the tympanic membrane, or *eardrum.* Within the middle ear are three small bones called the *malleus, incus, and stapes* (the common names are *hammer, anvil,* and *stirrup*). These bones transmit vibrations from the eardrum to the membrane covering the inner ear. The fluid-filled *inner ear* contains the *cochlea,* which house the receptors of the *auditory nerve.* The auditory nerve then transmits the sound messages to the horse's brain.

On each side of the head, the horse has a *eustachian tube* that connects the middle ear to the *pharynx.* The eustachian tube is normally closed, except when the horse swallows. At this time, the tube opens into the pharynx. The resulting flow of air into the middle ear ensures that the air pressure on the inside of the eardrum is equal to the air pressure on the outside.

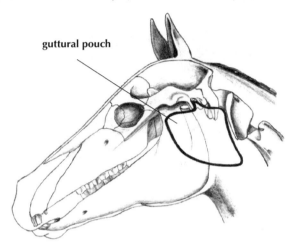

Fig. 2–52. The approximate location and size of a guttural pouch.

Unlike other domestic animals, equids (horses, zebras, and donkeys) have additional structures of the eustachian tube called the *guttural pouches (see Figures 2–52 and 2–55).* These are blind sacs (open on only one end) extending from each eustachian tube to the trachea. Air moves in and out of each pouch during respiration.

Mouth

The mouth is bounded in front by the lips, on the sides by the cheeks, above by the hard palate, and below by the *tongue* and the mucous membranes beneath it. The tongue is a muscular organ supported by the hyoid bone and mandible. The *soft palate* extends backward from the hard palate, acting as a tube to allow food and water to pass from the mouth to the pharynx (but not from the pharynx into the mouth).

The lips pick up loose food and pass it back into the mouth with the help of the tongue. The incisor teeth are used to grasp and nip food when grazing. The molar or cheek teeth grind the food into small particles while it is mixed with saliva.

Pharynx

The *pharynx* is a muscular passage that separates the mouth from the *esophagus*. The pharynx also provides an air passage between the nostrils and the larynx. Seen from the side, the pharynx is shaped roughly like a funnel. The large end of the funnel leads to the nasal passages. The small end leads to the larynx. It is built on a framework of cartilage held together by

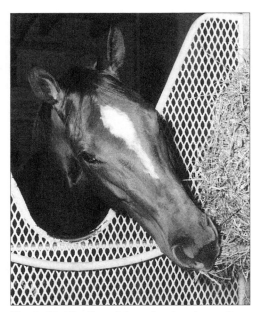

Fig. 2–53. The lips pick up food and pass it back to the tongue and teeth.

ligaments, and is moved by muscles. The bottom slope of the funnel is formed by the soft palate. Its other side is at the back of the mouth.

At the bottom of the soft palate, the pharynx is overlapped by a soft flap of cartilage called the *epiglottis*, which is part of the larynx. Most of the time this overlapping effectively separates the mouth from the pharynx and allows the free flow of air into the larynx. When the horse swallows, however, the epiglottis flips over the opening of the larynx, the soft palate moves up, and food is admitted into the pharynx and down the esophagus to the stomach.

The side walls of the pharynx are furnished with small slits that are openings of the eustachian tubes.

Larynx

The *larynx* is the gateway from the horse's nasal passages to the *trachea* and then the lungs. It is essentially a hollow "shell" made of nine joined cartilages. It is suspended from the back of the skull by the hyoid bone, and fits over the top end of the trachea. Most of it is covered with a mucous membrane. Two strong ligaments are

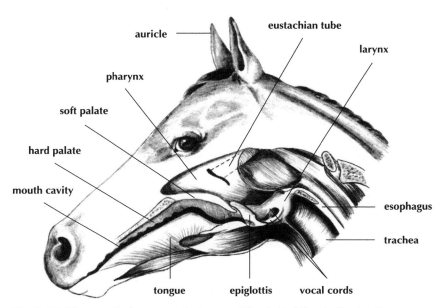

Fig. 2–54. The mouth, larynx, and pharynx. The dotted line indicates the location of the eustachian tube.

stretched over the opening of the larynx—these are the *vocal cords.* The epiglottis closes the larynx during swallowing, preventing the horse from inhaling food.

The larynx can be felt between the jowls, closest to the horse's neck. (The veterinarian can make the horse cough by gently pinching the top of the trachea.)

Salivary Glands and Lymph Nodes

Three main pairs of salivary glands secrete saliva into the mouth: the parotid, mandibular, and sublingual. The *parotid glands* are the largest and are located below each ear and behind the jaw. The *mandibular glands* are located, one on each side, partly under the parotid gland and partly inside the mandible. The *sublingual glands are* beneath the tongue and can be felt just beneath the skin under the jaw.

Also in this area are the *mandibular lymph nodes.* This pair of nodes are joined at the center and can be felt between the jowls. These are the structures that commonly swell, and sometimes burst, when the horse has a strangles infection. (Other lymph nodes can also be affected.)

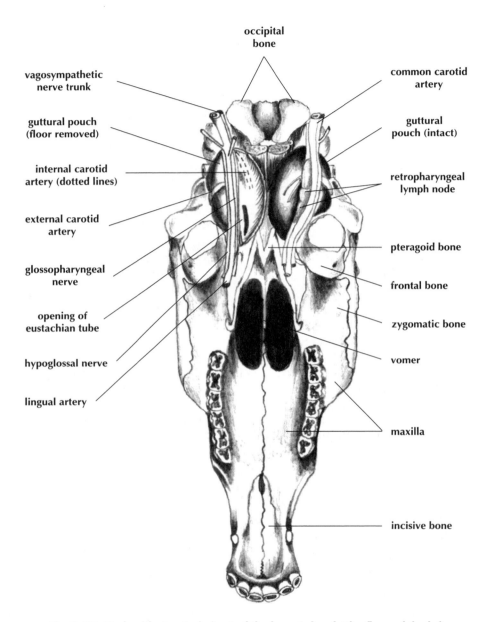

occipital
bone

common carotid
artery

vagosympathetic
nerve trunk

guttural
pouch (intact)

guttural pouch
(floor removed)

retropharyngeal
lymph node

internal carotid
artery (dotted lines)

external carotid
artery

pteragoid bone

frontal bone

glossopharyngeal
nerve

zygomatic bone

opening of
eustachian tube

vomer

hypoglossal nerve

lingual artery

maxilla

incisive bone

Fig. 2–55. Underside (ventral view) of the horse's head. The floor of the left guttural pouch has been removed to reveal the structures inside.

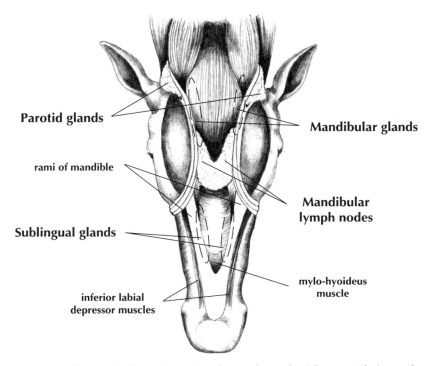

Parotid glands

Mandibular glands

rami of mandible

Mandibular lymph nodes

Sublingual glands

mylo-hyoideus muscle

inferior labial depressor muscles

Fig. 2–56. Salivary glands and lymph nodes on the underside (ventral view) of the throat. The mandibular and sublingual salivary glands lie deep to the jaw and tongue muscles.

Blood Vessels and Nerves

The *facial artery* and *facial vein* cross the mandible just in front of the masseter muscle. It is possible to take the horse's pulse by pressing the facial artery against the underside of the jaw. The *facial nerve* runs parallel to the jaw, across the horse's cheek and over the masseter muscle. Its branches supply the facial muscles. It can be seen in thin-skinned horses. *(See Figure 2–49 for an illustration of these structures.)*

3

NECK

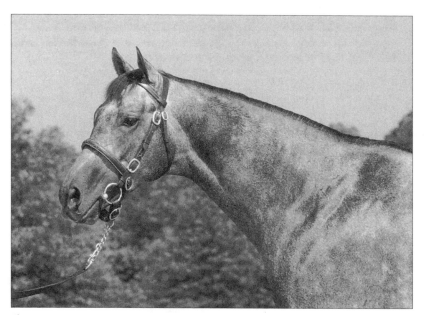

Fig. 3–1.

An attractive, graceful neck improves a horse's appearance and figures very prominently in its movement. The different breed associations have various preferences in neck length and shoulder attachment, but there are some general characteristics of a good neck that are always desirable.

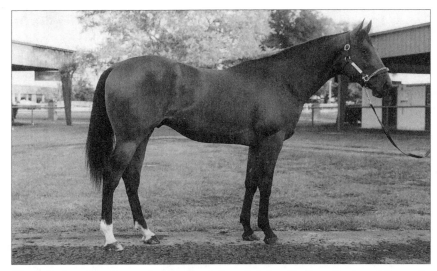

Fig. 3–2. An attractive neck. The clean throatlatch will allow flexion at the poll. It is long, but less than 1 1/2 times the length of the back.

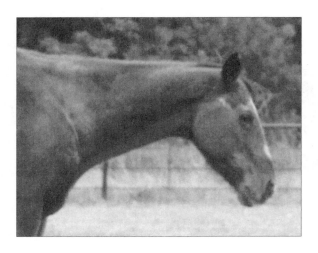

Fig. 3–3. The shape and muscling of this horse's neck could be improved with conditioning, but it is a good length and has a clean throatlatch.

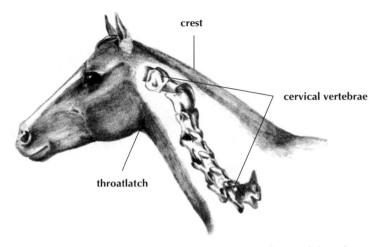

Fig. 3–4. The lengths of the seven cervical vertebrae determine neck length.

CONFORMATION OF THE NECK

The neck should be fairly long and slender with a slightly arched *topline*, a fine *throatlatch*, and a straight underline. Neck length is determined by the lengths of the seven *cervical vertebrae*. Ample length gives the horse maneuverability, balance, and good carriage. The neck should have some *crest*, especially in the stallion, but not excessively so. The topline should flow smoothly into the withers and shoulders. On the underside, a good throatlatch is free of excess fat and muscling. The base of the neck should be set on at the point of the shoulder or higher.

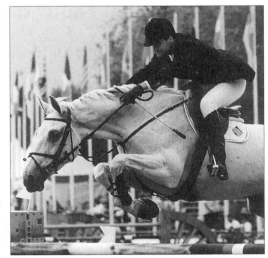

Fig. 3–5. A well-conformed neck gives an equine athlete maneuverability and balance.

69

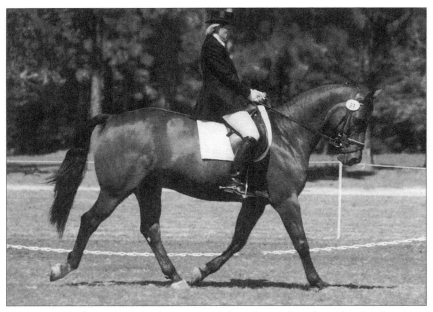

Fig. 3–6. This dressage horse has a graceful neck and fine throatlatch, allowing the flexibility that is essential for proper balance and collection.

Conformational Faults of the Neck

Thick Throatlatch

All of the things that keep a horse going—air, food, blood, the total nerve supply—pass through the throatlatch. When a horse with a thick throatlatch tucks its head, these supplies are severely limited.

Another term sometimes used is a *"close-coupled" neck.* It may indicate jowls that are too large or a throatlatch that is too thick. Either fault prevents the neck from arching properly.

Short Neck

A short, thick, *"pony" neck* or *"bull" neck* and a thick throatlatch are undesirable because they limit flexion, both at the poll and side-to-side. The ability to flex and bend is essential for proper balance and collection. A short, heavy neck also adds weight to the front of the horse, reducing rapid maneuverability. Overly crested necks pose the same problems. If the crest is so large and heavy that it hangs to one side, it is called a *"broken crest."*

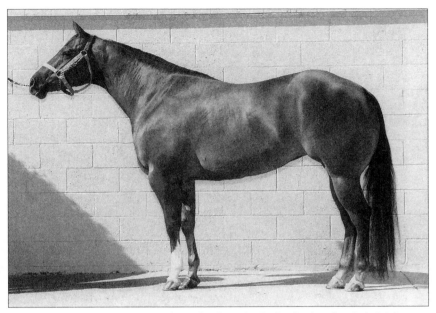

Fig. 3–7. This horse's neck is relatively short for its body size, but it is fairly well-shaped.

A short neck contributes to a choppy stride, for two reasons. First, neck muscles are the means by which a horse moves its shoulder and forelegs forward to produce stride. Because these muscles can only contract two-thirds of their natural length, a short-necked horse has a short stride. Second, a short neck usually ties in to a short, straight shoulder, which also limits stride length. (See Chapter 6, *Forelegs*, for more information.)

Depending on the activity, a short, thick neck is not necessarily a major fault if it is well-shaped. Indeed, some width in the lower neck is necessary to safely encase the internal structures (trachea, jugular vein, carotid artery, etc.).

Long Neck

Ideally, the neck should have enough length and refinement to allow the horse to respond readily to the bit, and to collect and balance itself for difficult maneuvers. However, a neck can be too long, reducing its effectiveness. The neck should be no longer than about 1½ times the length of the horse's back.

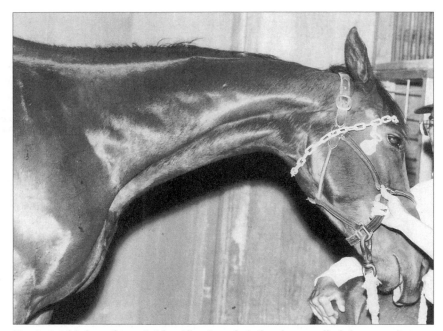

Fig. 3–8. This broodmare's identification chain has been pulled down to show that she has a thin neck.

Thin Neck

A thin neck may be properly arched, but it lacks muscling and is therefore weak. If it is also too long, the horse is predisposed to upper airway disease.

Ewe Neck and Swan Neck

A common conformational fault is the *ewe neck.* This term indicates that both the upper and lower sides of the neck arch downward. In a *swan neck,* the top third arches upward properly, but the bottom third is concave. In these horses, the neck is set too low on the chest: below the point of the shoulder. Ewe-necked and swan-necked horses tend to carry their heads high. Such "stargazing" interferes with the horse's vision and does not allow proper bit contact and control.

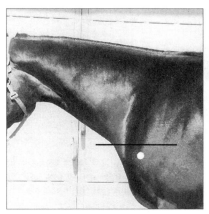

Fig. 3–9. The base of the neck is set on above the point of the shoulder.

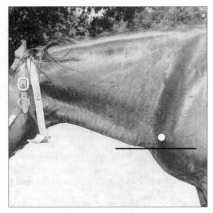

Fig. 3–10. The base of the neck is set on below the point of the shoulder.

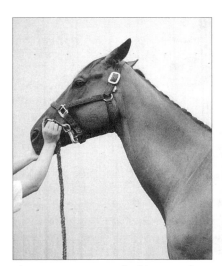

Fig. 3–11. A ewe-necked horse—the topline and underline are concave.

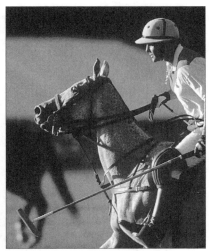

Fig. 3–12. A ewe neck creates a high head carriage and "stargazing."

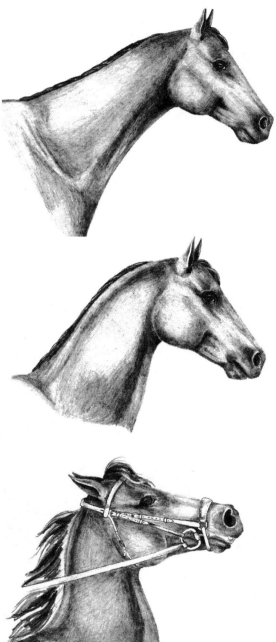

Fig. 3–13a. A ewe-necked horse: the upper and lower sides of the neck are concave.

Fig. 3–13b. A swan-necked horse: the lower third of the neck is concave.

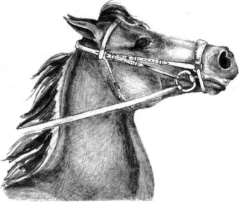

Fig. 3–13c. "Stargazing" interferes with the horse's vision and does not allow proper bit contact and control.

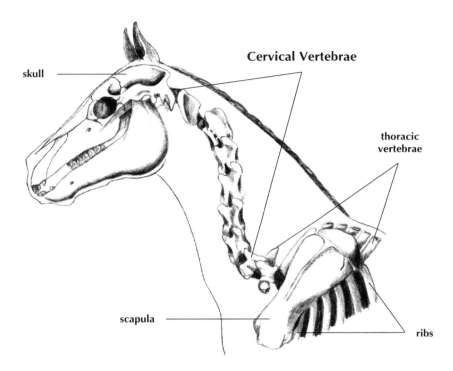

Fig. 3–14. Outside (lateral) view of the bones of the horse's neck. Note that the topline does not follow the cervical vertebrae.

ANATOMY OF THE NECK
Bones

The seven bones of the neck are called *cervical vertebrae.* They are constructed and woven together in such a way as to make the horse's neck extremely flexible. The joints between the cervical vertebrae allow the horse to bend its neck from side to side, arch its neck upward, lower its head for grazing, and slightly rotate its head and neck.

Viewed from the side, the cervical vertebrae make an elongated "S." However, the crest of the neck does not follow the vertebrae. The lower curve of the "S" is located within the bottom third of the neck.

The first and second vertebrae are known respectively as the *atlas* and the *axis.* The atlas forms the *atlanto-occipital joint* with the skull's *occipital bone,* which has two hook-like projections called *occipital processes* for that purpose. On the bottom surface of the

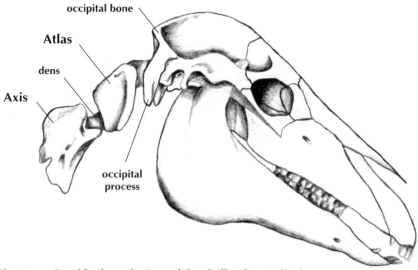

Fig. 3–15. Outside (lateral) view of the skull, atlas, and axis.

atlas, two deep, oval pockets called the *anterior articular cavities* receive the occipital processes. Formed this way, the joint allows the head to move up and down independently. The atlas is wide and short, and the upper surface of its lower (ventral) arch forms the *fovea dentis*, a wide, slightly concave articular surface. On this surface rests the *odontoid process (dens)* of the axis.

The axis is the second cervical vertebra. It is the longest of the vertebrae, and is characterized by the presence of the dens, a process that has a profile resembling a thumb. On either side of the dens are anterior articular surfaces. The *atlanto-axial*

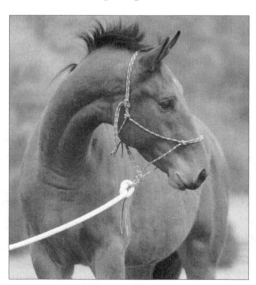

Fig. 3–16. A horse's neck is extremely flexible.

joint formed by the fovea dentis and the dens allows the horse's head to move independently from side to side. It also allows the head to rotate a little.

The third, fourth, and fifth cervical vertebrae are very similar to each other in design and function. Each is large compared to other vertebrae, and each has an opening *(foramen)* for the spinal cord to pass through. The "floor" of the foramen is formed by the *body*, the "ceiling" by the *arch*. The *dorsal spinous process* is

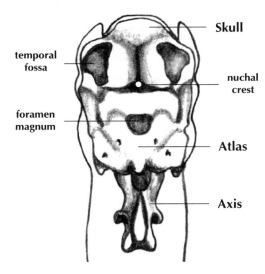

Fig. 3–17. Top (dorsal) view of the skull, atlas, and axis.

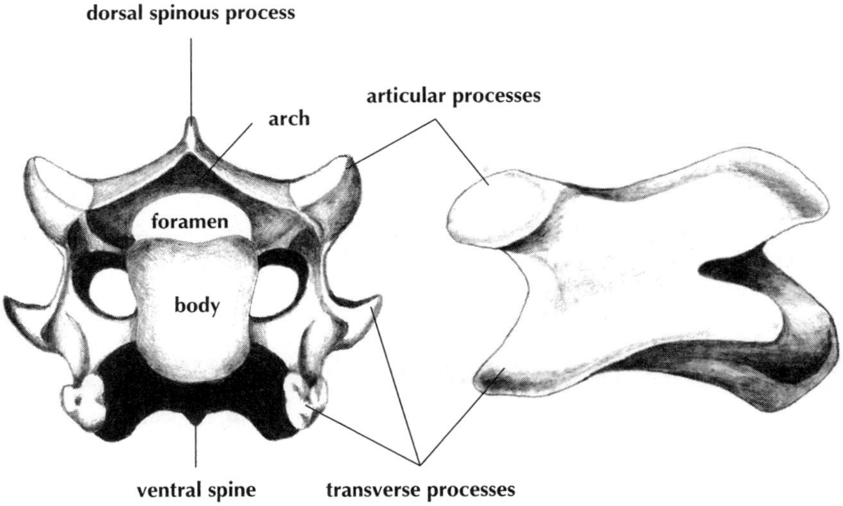

on the upper surface, the *ventral spine* on the lower surface. There are two *transverse processes* projecting out from each side and slightly downward. These transverse processes are sites of muscle

Fig. 3–18. Parts of a cervical vertebra. Left: Front (cranial) view. Right: Side (lateral) view.

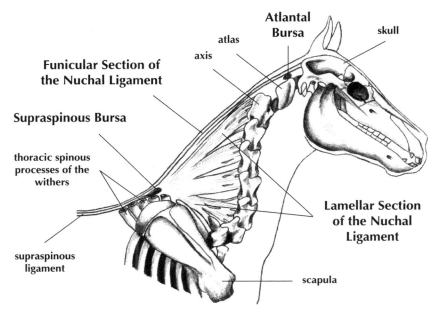

Atlantal Bursa

atlas

Funicular Section of the Nuchal Ligament

axis

skull

Supraspinous Bursa

thoracic spinous processes of the withers

Lamellar Section of the Nuchal Ligament

supraspinous ligament

scapula

Fig. 3–19. The nuchal ligament and associated bursae.

attachment. They can sometimes be felt in about the center of the neck. There are also two *articular processes* projecting upward and outward. Viewed from the side, the articular processes of each vertebra slope backward, and form a joint with the articular process of the next vertebra. Each vertebra also has an articular surface immediately below the vertebral foramen, in the front and back.

The sixth vertebra is like the others in design. But it is shorter and wider than the preceding vertebrae and its dorsal spinous process is taller. The seventh vertebra is again shorter and wider, and has a dorsal spinous process about twice as tall as that of the sixth vertebra. Unlike any other cervical vertebra, it has two facets on the back of the body, which partly form a joint with the first rib.

Ligaments of the Neck

The head and neck are supported by a strong, elastic ligament called the *nuchal ligament*. Its main function is to assist the extensor muscles of the head and neck. The ligament has two parts, which differ strikingly from each other. The first part is the funicular section. It resembles a cord, and is strung between the poll and the peak of the withers. The cord is heavy, flat, and thick where it is attached to the skull, but it becomes smaller in diameter (about ½ inch) on the back of the neck. The *atlantal bursa* (a fluid-filled sac) protects the cord where it rubs against the atlas. The cord flattens and becomes 5 – 6 inches wide over the top of the withers. The *supraspinous bursa* lies between it and the bones of the withers, protecting the ligament from friction.

The other part of the nuchal ligament is the lamellar section. It consists of two layers of slender fibers. The fibers are strung loosely between the cervical vertebrae, and the thoracic spines and funicular part of the ligament.

From the withers, the ligament becomes the *supraspinous ligament*. It covers the horse's back all the way to the loins.

Muscles of the Neck

The horse's neck is acted upon by 24 pairs (one on each side) of muscles, in several layers. They function to arch, straighten, lift, bend, and rotate the head and neck. The heavy weight of the neck muscles is also an efficient counterbalance for the weight of the body. The most influential muscles are described below. They are listed from relatively superficial to relatively deep.

(Some muscles in the middle layers appear on both Figure 3–19 and 3–20. This is done for perspective.)

Trapezius—There are two parts to this muscle: a cervical part in the neck and a thoracic part over the withers. It originates along the nuchal ligament from the second cervical vertebrae through the tenth thoracic vertebrae. The cervical part of the trapezius inserts along the entire scapular spine (a ridge down the middle of the shoulder blade). This muscle elevates the shoulder by lifting the scapula up and forward. It is also considered a shoulder muscle.

Rhomboideus—This muscle also has two parts: a cervical part in the neck and a thoracic part over the withers. The cervical part follows the topline of the neck. It originates at the back of the skull and inserts along the inside surface of the scapula. It lifts the scapula up and forward, elevating the shoulder. For this reason, it is also considered a shoulder muscle.

Brachiocephalic—This long, flat muscle originates on the skull between and behind the ear and also on the atlas. It runs diagonally down the side of the neck as it widens, runs over the shoulder joint, and then inserts onto the lower front of the humerus (upper arm bone). The brachiocephalic flexes the neck sideways. It also extends

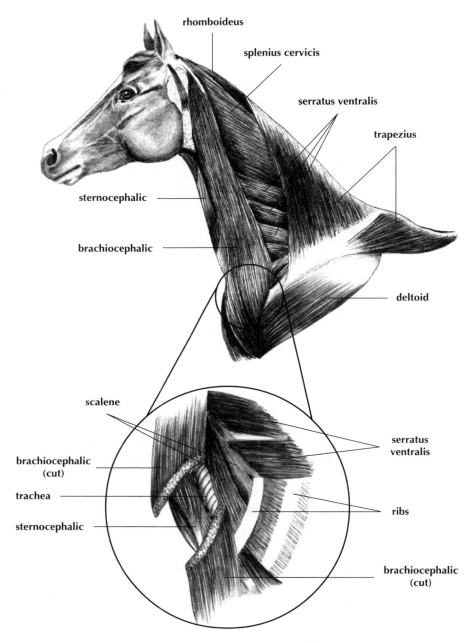

Fig. 3–20. Outside (lateral) view of the superficial neck muscles.
Inset: The brachiocephalic has been reflected to reveal the scalene muscle.

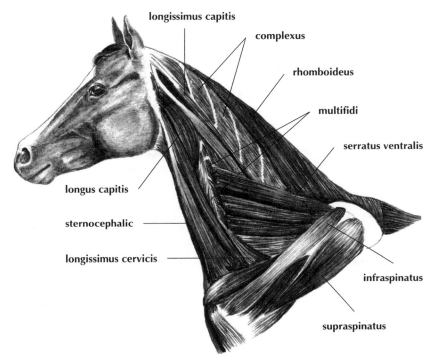

longissimus capitis

complexus

rhomboideus

multifidi

serratus ventralis

longus capitis

sternocephalic

longissimus cervicis

infraspinatus

supraspinatus

Fig. 3–21. Outside (lateral) view of the deep neck muscles.

the shoulder joint and pulls the forearm forward. For this reason, it is also considered a shoulder muscle.

Serratus ventralis—The cervical portion of this muscle originates on the last five cervical vertebrae. It fans out from the withers over the neck and shoulder area, although it lies underneath the scapula. It attaches to the inside surface of the scapula. The serratus ventralis supports the body like a sling, but is also considered a foreleg muscle.

Scalene—This neck muscle has two parts: a small upper part and a larger lower part. However, they are usually described together. They originate at the first rib and insert onto the last four cervical vertebrae. The scalene act to raise the base of the neck higher when flexed together, an action that is essential in proper collection. Acting independently, each muscle inclines the neck to that side.

Splenius cervicis—This flexor muscle is wide and flat. The splenius cervicis originates at the first three or four thoracic vertebrae. It

MUSCLES OF THE NECK			
Name	**Origin**	**Insertion**	**Function**
Trapezius	CV 2 – TV 10 along nuchal ligament	scapular spine	lift scapula up and forward
Rhomboideus	back of skull	inside surface of scapula	lifts scapula up and forward
Brachiocephalic	skull between and behind ears; also atlas (CV 1)	lower front of humerus	bend neck sideways; pull forearm forward
Serratus ventralis	CV 3 – CV 7	inside surface of scapula	support the body like a sling
Scalene	first rib	CV 4 – CV 7	pair: raise base of neck; single: incline neck to that side
Splenius cervicis	TV 1 – TV 3 or 4	top of skull – CV 5	pair: raise head and neck; single: bend neck to that side
Longissimus capitis	TV 1 – TV 3	temporal bone of skull	pair: extend head and neck outward; single: bend neck to that side
Longus capitus	TV 3, 4, 5	occipital bone of skull	pair: flex head; single: turn head
Longissimus cervicis	humerus	CV 1 – CV 7	extend neck; flex spine laterally

Fig. 3–22. Neck muscles, part 1. CV = cervical vertebra. TV = thoracic vertebra.

MUSCLES OF THE NECK, cont.			
Name	Origin	Insertion	Function
Complexus	CV – TV	top of skull	pair: extend head; single: incline head
Multifidi	CV 2 – CV 7; TV 1	CV 1 – CV 7	pair: extend neck; single: bend neck, rotate neck
Sternocephalic	top of sternum	mandible	pair: flex head and neck; single: turn head

Fig. 3–23. Neck muscles, part 2. CV = cervical vertebra. TV = thoracic vertebra.

inserts from the top of the skull through the fifth cervical vertebrae. When the splenius cervicis muscles on each side contract together, they elevate the head and neck. If one contracts independently, it bends the neck, turning the head to that side.

Longissimus capitis—This muscle originates on the first few thoracic vertebrae and inserts on the temporal bone in the skull. When both muscles function together, they extend the head and neck outward. When one contracts independently, it flexes the neck sideways.

Longus capitis—This muscle originates on the third, fourth, and fifth thoracic vertebrae and inserts on the occipital bone in the skull. When both muscles function together, they flex the head. When one contracts independently, it turns the head sideways. In some older texts it is called the rectus capitis ventralis major.

Longissimus cervicis—This is the cervical portion of the *longissimus dorsi* muscle. It runs from the humerus to the cervical vertebrae. It helps to extend the neck and flex the spine from side to side.

Complexus—Actually the lower half of the *semispinalis capitis* muscle, the complexus originates along the length of the cervical and thoracic vertebrae, inserting on the top of the skull. The pair of complexus muscles is the chief extensor of the head when operating together. When operating independently, each muscle inclines the head to that side.

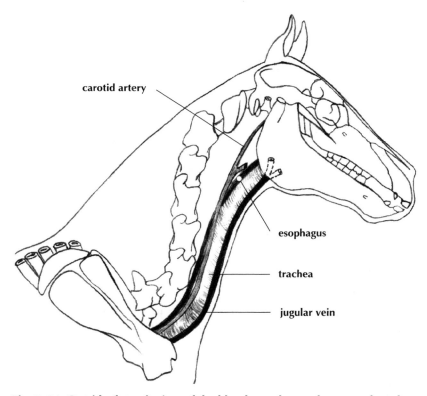

carotid artery

esophagus

trachea

jugular vein

Fig. 3–24. Outside (lateral) view of the blood vessels, esophagus, and trachea within the neck.

Multifidi—This deep muscle is made of many short bands that weave the vertebrae together. In the neck, it originates on the second through seventh cervical and first thoracic vertebrae, and inserts on all of the cervical vertebrae. Acting together, the pair extends the neck. Acting independently, it flexes the neck sideways and rotates the neck to the opposite side. (See Chapter 7, *Body*, for more information.)

Sternocephalic—It is a long, narrow muscle that lies along the underside of the neck, just below the jugular groove. It originates at the top of the sternum (breastbone) and inserts on the mandible, on the back of the jowl. Acting together, the pair flexes the head and neck. Acting independently, each muscle turns the head to that side.

Rectus capitis dorsalis—This muscle extends the head outward. It is discussed and illustrated in Chapter 2, *Head.*

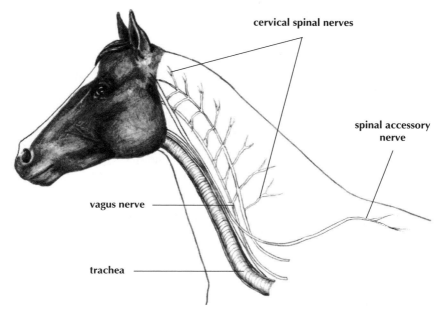

Fig. 3–25. Outside (lateral) view of the major nerves in the neck.

Blood Vessels of the Neck

The *jugular vein* and *carotid artery* are the major blood vessels in the neck, running on each side of the neck along the jugular groove. The jugular vein carries blood from the head back to the heart. The carotid artery carries blood to the head from the heart. Of the two, the jugular vein is closer to the skin surface; the carotid artery is deeper within the horse's neck.

Nerves of the Neck

There are eight pairs of *cervical nerves* branching off of the spinal cord. The first pair emerges from the first cervical vertebra. The second pair emerges from between the first and second cervical vertebrae. Likewise, the remaining pairs of nerves also emerge from between sets of vertebrae. These cervical nerves supply the neck muscles.

In addition to these cervical nerves, two cranial nerves (which originate from the brain) travel down the neck. One is called the *spinal accessory nerve*. It travels from the head and down across the splenius muscle to end near the withers, and supplies the muscles of the neck.

The other cranial nerve in the neck is the *vagus nerve*. Its branches are responsible for:

- sensation in the ear, pharynx, and larynx
- movement of the pharynx, larynx, and esophagus
- supplying many internal organs in the thorax and abdomen

This nerve travels with the cervical part of the *sympathetic trunk*. Together, the vagus nerve and the sympathetic trunk are called the *vagosympathetic trunk*. (See Chapter 14, *Body Systems,* for more information about the sympathetic nervous system.)

Other Structures Within the Neck

Esophagus

The *esophagus* is a tube about 5 feet long that connects the pharynx (see Chapter 2, *Head*) to the stomach. It can be seen in the groove along the lower left side of the neck by watching as a horse swallows food or water. The esophagus is the structure down which a nasogastric tube (stomach tube) is passed. *(See Figure 3–24.)*

Trachea

The *trachea* connects the larynx (see Chapter 2, *Head*) to the lungs. It is a tube that is reinforced by rings of cartilage along its length. The trachea is lined with a mucous membrane. *(See Figure 3–24.)*

4

WITHERS

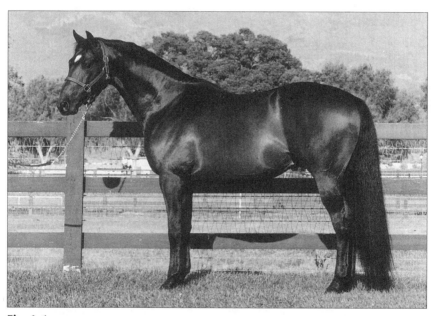

Fig. 4–1.

CONFORMATION OF THE WITHERS

The prominent area that is the meeting point of the neck, back, and peak of the shoulders is called the withers. The withers are an important part of a horse's structure. They should be well defined and muscular, and slope smoothly into the back. There should be no dents or bumps.

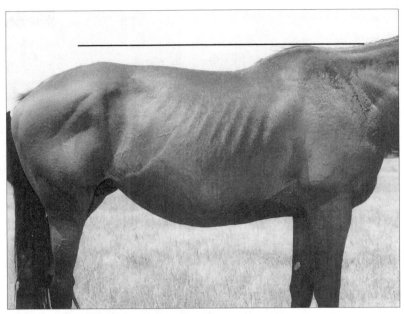

Fig. 4–2. The withers are higher than the croup.

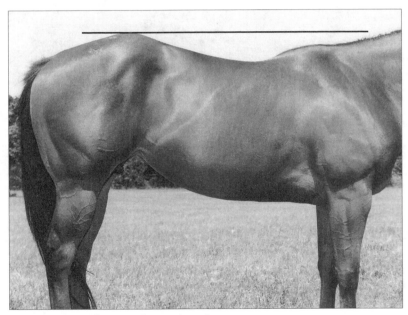

Fig. 4–3. The withers are lower than the croup.

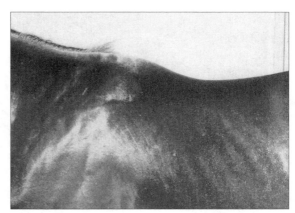

Fig. 4–4. Good, medium-
high withers.

Good definition of the withers helps to anchor a saddle, and muscularity provides padding. The withers should be level with or very
slightly higher than the croup. Some draft and Quarter Horses are
lower at the withers than at the croup, and although this is not necessarily desirable, it is not a major fault.

Medium high, sloping withers are often accompanied by long,
sloping shoulders and longer muscles. These traits allow greater
foreleg extension and freer movement both in front and behind.

Conformational Faults of the Withers

Withers that are very low and thick are not desirable because a
saddle depends on some prominence to help hold it in place. Also,
such horses often have loaded (overly thick) shoulders and thick

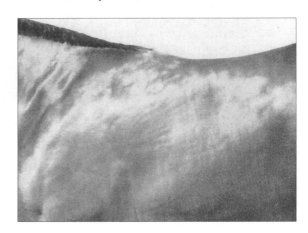

Fig. 4–5. Low withers.

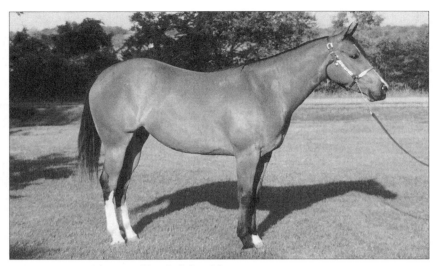

Fig. 4–6. Low withers and loaded shoulders.

necks, each of which impairs agility in the forehand. Very high withers are also undesirable because they are subject to injury by a saddle riding against the top of them.

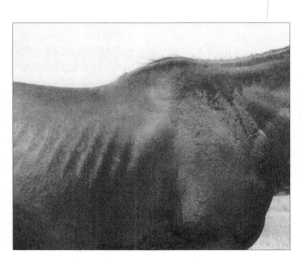

Fig. 4–7. High withers are subject to injury by a saddle. Care should be taken to ensure that the padding is adequate and the saddle fits properly.

ANATOMY OF THE WITHERS
Bones

The dorsal spinous processes of the first 10 or so *thoracic vertebrae* form the upper skeletal outline of the withers. (The thoracic vertebrae are the second "set" of bones in the spinal column after the cervical vertebrae of the neck.) The highest point of the of the withers is formed by the third and fourth thoracic vertebrae. The top edge of the scapula (shoulder blade) gives the withers breadth.

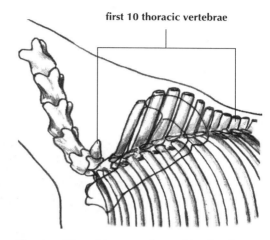

first 10 thoracic vertebrae

Fig. 4–8. The withers are formed by the dorsal spinous processes of the first 10 or so thoracic vertebrae.

Ligaments

The major ligament in the neck is the strong *nuchal ligament.* It begins at the horse's poll and runs straight down the topline. It ends by attaching to the withers. From this point it merges with the *supraspinous ligament,* which runs down the back to the loins. The nuchal ligament assists the extensor muscles of the head and neck.

There are also many small ligaments between and around the dorsal spinous processes. These ligaments stabilize the vertebrae.

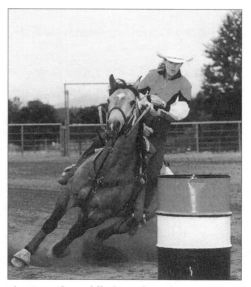

Fig. 4–9. If a saddle is anchored by medium-high, broad withers it will not slip during sharp turns.

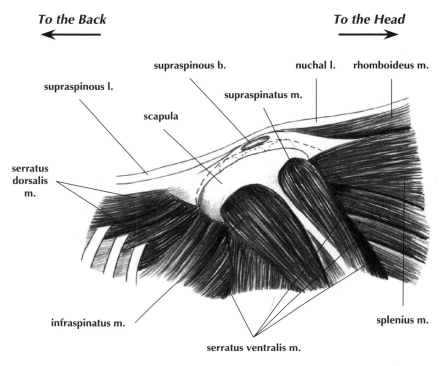

To the Back ←

To the Head →

supraspinous b.

nuchal l.

rhomboideus m.

supraspinous l.

supraspinatus m.

scapula

serratus
dorsalis
m.

infraspinatus m.

splenius m.

serratus ventralis m.

Fig. 4–10. Outside (lateral) view of the muscles (m.), ligaments (l.), and bursa (b.) over the withers.

Bursae of the Withers

Several bursae (lubricating sacs) are found in the area of the withers. The most important one is called the *supraspinous bursa*. It covers the tops of the first three to five thoracic spinous processes, and protects the nuchal ligament and the vertebrae. Each thoracic spinous process located behind the major bursa has a small bursa of its own.

Muscles of the Withers

Because the withers is a meeting point between the neck, shoulder, and back, several of the muscles activating these three areas attach to the skeletal outline of the withers and contribute to its mass. *(See Figures 4–10 through 4–12.)*

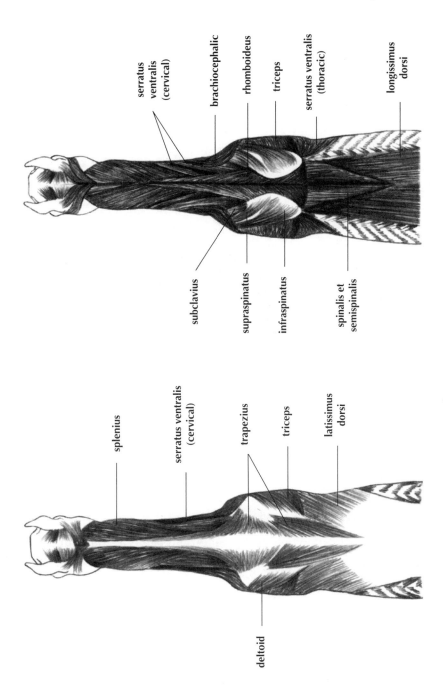

Fig. 4–11. Top (dorsal) view of the muscles over the withers. Left: Superficial muscles. Right: Deep muscles.

serratus ventralis (cervical)

brachiocephalic

rhomboideus

triceps

serratus ventralis (thoracic)

longissimus dorsi

subclavius

supraspinatus

infraspinatus

spinalis et semispinalis

splenius

serratus ventralis (cervical)

trapezius

triceps

latissimus dorsi

deltoid

93

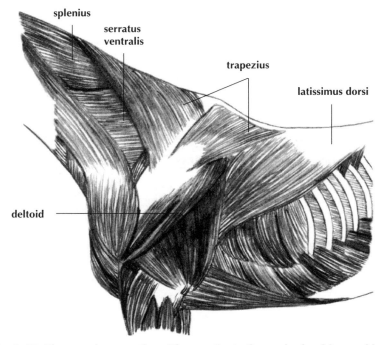

Fig. 4–12. The muscles over the withers activate the neck, shoulder, and back.

Neck Muscles
- trapezius (cervical part)
- rhomboideus (cervical part)
- serratus ventralis (cervical part)
- spinalis et semispinalis

Shoulder Muscles
- supraspinatus and infraspinatus
- latissimus dorsi
- serratus ventralis (thoracic part)
- trapezius (thoracic part)
- rhomboideus (thoracic part)

Back Muscles
- longissimus dorsi
- multifidi

The origins, insertions, and functions of these muscles are discussed in the relevant chapters.

5

CHEST

The horse's chest runs from the bottom of the neck down to the bottom of the barrel and tops of the forelegs, as viewed from the front of the horse. Some people call this area the breast, and use the term, "chest" for the heartgirth area behind the shoulders and forelegs. In this book, that area is addressed in the Barrel section of Chapter 7, *Body*.

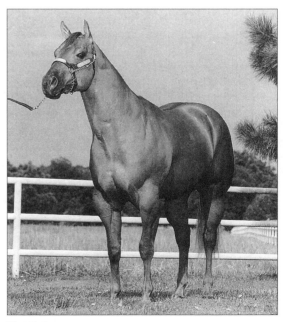

Fig. 5–1.

CONFORMATION OF THE CHEST

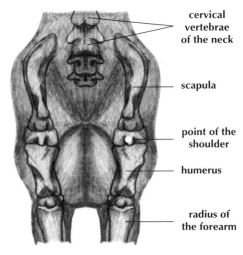

cervical vertebrae of the neck

scapula

point of the shoulder

humerus

radius of the forearm

Fig. 5–2. The chest is only as wide as the bones that form it.

The chest should be well defined (not blending into the neck) and fairly wide. A wide chest displays a large gap between the two forelegs.

It is important not to be fooled by muscle development or obesity in the chest. Both characteristics can make the chest appear wide. In reality, the chest is only as wide as the bones that form it—the *scapula* and *humerus* on each side. To evaluate chest width precisely, it is important to locate and reference the *points of the shoulders.*

Conformational Faults

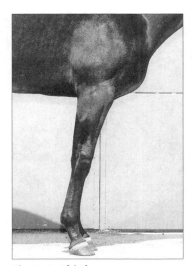

Fig. 5–3. This horse appears to be "bosomy" because it is camped under in front.

There are different opinions on good chest width, but in general, either extreme should be avoided. A narrow chest lacks power and causes the forelegs to be too close together. An overly wide chest causes the horse to roll from side to side in action. Also, these horses are often *"camped under"* as seen from the side. Of all the breeds, draft horses and working Quarter Horses are minor exceptions. Advocates of both breeds prefer a wider chest and excellent muscle development for the horse to perform its intended work.

From the side, it should be possible to see the bulge of the pectoral muscles, but the horse should not look too *"bosomy."*

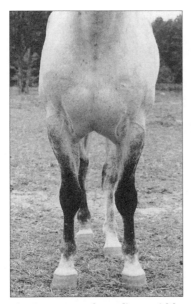

Fig. 5–4. A good, medium-width, muscular chest.

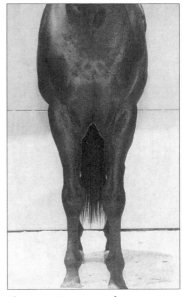

Fig. 5–5. A narrow chest.

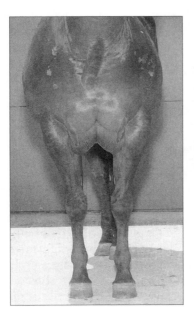

Fig. 5–6. An overly wide chest may cause the horse to roll from side to side in action.

ANATOMY OF THE CHEST

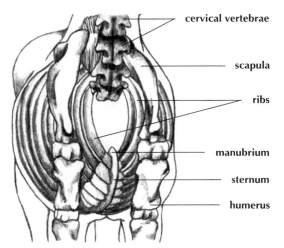

Fig. 5–7. Front view of the bones of the chest.

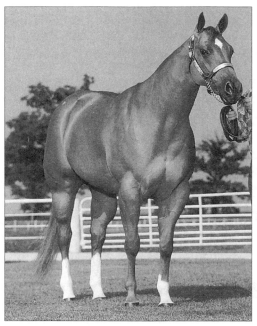

Fig. 5–8. The pectoral muscles of the chest form the inverted "V" shape in front.

Bones

The horse's chest is formed by a humerus on each side, the *sternum* (breastbone), and the *ribs*. The humerus is the upper arm bone between the shoulder joint and the elbow joint. Viewed from the front, these two bones are located on either side of the horse's chest.

The sternum runs down the center of the chest and between the forelegs. The sternum is the bone to which the lower ends of the first eight ribs are attached. It is vaguely canoe-shaped, and consists of eight joined segments called *sternebrae*. The uppermost part of the sternum is called the *manubrium*.

Muscles

There are many muscles in this area, some of which are also considered neck or shoulder muscles. The substance of the horse's chest is shaped by the *pectoral muscles*—large paired muscles forming the inverted "V" shape in front. Their function is to move the foreleg in toward the midline of the body (adduction). They also advance the body when the leg is planted on the ground. These muscles are divided into superficial pectoral muscles and deep pectoral muscles.

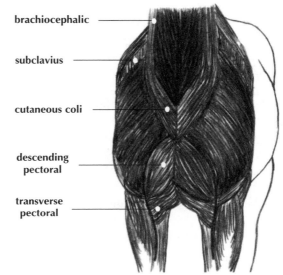

Fig. 5–9. Front (cranial) view of the superficial pectoral muscles.

Superficial Pectoral Muscles

Descending pectoral— This muscle originates on the manubrium and the ribs next to it. It travels downward between the forelegs and then inserts onto the upper inside surface of the humerus. This muscle is also called the cranial superficial pectoral.

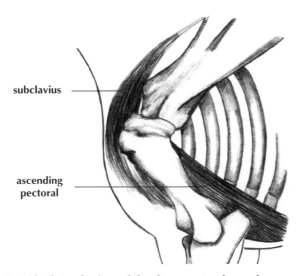

Fig. 5–10. Outside (lateral) view of the deep pectoral muscles.

MUSCLES OF THE CHEST			
Name	**Origin**	**Insertion**	**Function**
Descending pectoral	manubrium & nearby ribs	upper inside of humerus	adduct and advance foreleg
Transverse pectoral	lower half of sternum & nearby ribs	inside surface of humerus	adduct the foreleg
Subclavius	sternum	front edge of scapula	extend and support shoulder
Ascending pectoral	sternum	inside surface of top of humerus	adduct and draw foreleg backward

Fig. 5–11.

Transverse pectoral —This muscle runs side-to-side between the horse's forelegs, just underneath the chest. It originates on the lower half of the sternum and the ribs next to it. It inserts on the inside surface of the humerus. This muscle is also called the caudal superficial pectoral.

Deep Pectoral Muscles

Subclavius— This large muscle begins at the sternum and runs upward over the front of the shoulder. It inserts onto the front edge of the scapula and nearby soft tissues. The function of the subclavius is to extend the shoulder. It also acts as a support structure, holding the shoulder joint together. Another name for this muscle is the cranial deep pectoral.

Ascending pectoral —This muscle originates on most of the sternum, and inserts onto the upper inside surface of the humerus. In addition to its function as an adductor, it draws the foreleg backward. It is also called the caudal deep pectoral.

6

FORELEGS

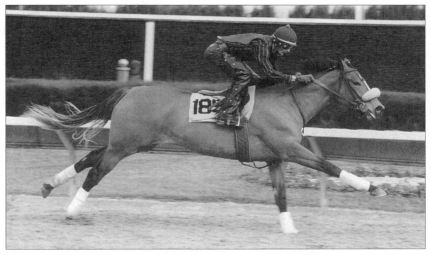

Fig. 6–1.

The forelegs carry about 65% of the horse's total body weight. Since they support this weight, propel the body, and absorb the shock of impact, the forelegs are susceptible to injury if not correctly conformed. Proper sloping and angling of the bones, from the shoulder to the foot, help the forelegs to absorb concussion upon impact because they allow give-and-take at the joints. This is a major reason that people look for long, sloping shoulders.

The forelegs are angled where the shoulder meets the upper arm, and the upper arm meets the forearm. But from the elbow to the fetlock, the forelegs must be straight, because crooked legs cause weight to be unevenly distributed. This results in excess pressure on a certain bone or joint, or excess pull on a muscle, tendon, or ligament.

CONFORMATION OF THE FORELEG
From the Front

To determine straightness of the forelegs from the front of the horse, an imaginary line dropped from the point of the shoulder to the center of the foot should bisect the knee, cannon, and fetlock. If the leg is not straight, stress falls on the out-of-line area and causes problems such as splints, sidebone, and windpuffs.

"Toed in" and *"toed out"* are conformational faults that are visible from the front. The feet of a toed in, or "pigeon-toed" horse point inward. The legs may be crooked anywhere from the elbow to the fetlock. The feet of a toed out, or "splay-footed" horse turn outward because the legs are turned too far outward, usually from the elbow.

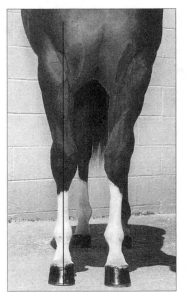

A. Straight forelegs.

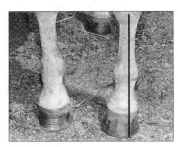

B. Toeing-in.

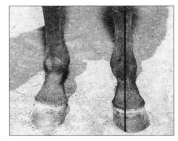

C. Toeing-out.

Fig. 6–2. A line dropped from the point of the shoulder to the center of the foot should bisect the knee, cannon, fetlock, and toe.

From the Side

Viewed from the side, the foreleg from the elbow to the fetlock should be perpendicular to the ground. At the fetlock the foreleg angles again, with the pastern sloping forward and down into the hoof. The shoulder, pastern, and hoof wall angles should match for effective shock-absorption.

An imaginary line running up from just behind the foot and bisecting the leg should also bisect the shoulder, ending well in front of the withers. If the line ends in the middle of the withers, the forelegs are set too far back, the horse will be heavy on the forehand, and probably has an upright shoulder.

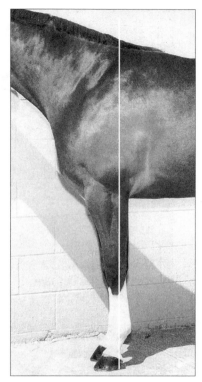

Fig. 6–3. Good foreleg conformation from the side.

Shoulder

"Ideal" *shoulder* conformation varies to an extent, depending upon the horse's breed and activity. However, certain characteristics are desirable in all situations. Well-developed, smooth, symmetrical muscling of the shoulder, best fitting the purpose of the horse, is important. The shoulder should be fairly long, about as long as the neck from the poll to the front of the withers.

Shoulder Length and Action

The shoulder forms the foreleg's main point of attachment to the rest of the body. The foreleg is not connected to the spinal column by bones but by sheets of muscles. A longer shoulder provides more area for muscle attachment, resulting in greater support and smoother movement.

The length and slope of the shoulder determine its range of motion. A horse with a long, sloping

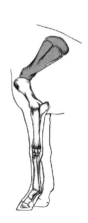

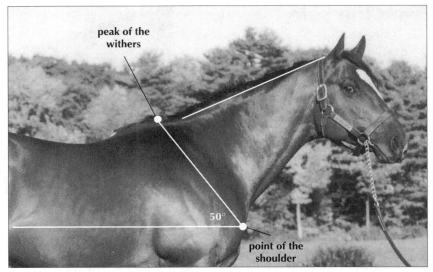

Fig. 6–4. The shoulder should be about as long as the neck from the poll to the front of the withers.

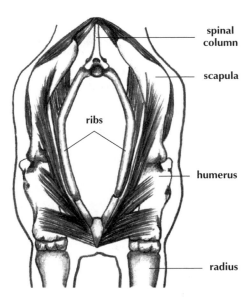

Fig. 6–5. Front (cranial) view of the chest. The foreleg is attached to the spine by sheets of muscles.

shoulder has a greater range of motion than a horse with a relatively short, upright shoulder and correspondingly short humerus (upper arm bone). For example, this conformation allows the galloping horse to extend its foreleg out further, increasing its stride length.

The range of motion of the foreleg is also influenced by the flexibility of the shoulder muscles. A horse with a short, upright shoulder and humerus absorbs more concussion upon impact, straining the shoulder muscles and tendons. Excessive strain causes these tissues to become overdeveloped and fibrous, stiffening the shoulder. On the other hand, a longer shoulder distributes concussion over a larger area, sparing the shoulder muscles and tendons much strain. The stride length is therefore increased because the muscles remain flexible.

Shoulder Angle and Action

Measuring the Shoulder Angle

To measure the angle of the shoulder, draw a line parallel to the ground from the *point of the shoulder* to the rump. Next, draw a line from the *peak of the withers* to the point of the shoulder. The angle created by this juncture should be about 50°. An angle that is more open than 50° tends toward an upright shoulder.

Visually drawing a line from the peak of the withers to the point of the shoulder is a handy reference, and usually accurate. However, the slope

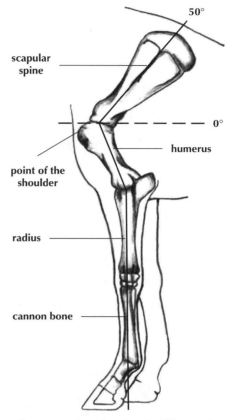

Fig. 6–6. Measuring the shoulder angle using the scapular spine.

of the shoulder is actually determined by the *scapular spine,* which is a ridge bisecting the scapula (shoulder blade). Some horses have an upright shoulder that is set so far forward on the body that the eye is deceived. In this case, if the point of the shoulder is used as the reference, the shoulder appears more sloping than it is. It is best to follow the scapular spine.

Sloping Shoulder (Closed Angle)

In addition to increased stride length, a more closed angle between the scapula and humerus allows the horse more room to tuck its legs when jumping over fences. As a horse prepares to jump, the muscles at the back of the scapula pull it backward and down, toward a more

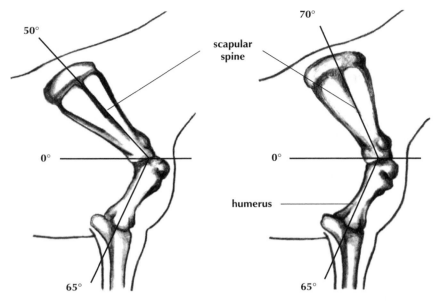

Fig. 6–7. Angle of the shoulder. The sloping shoulder on the left allows smoother action and greater range of motion than the upright shoulder on the right.

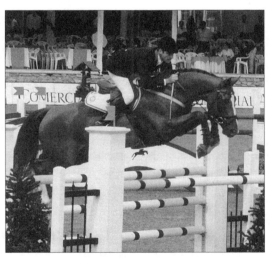

Fig. 6–8. A sloping shoulder and long humerus increase the horse's ability to tightly tuck its legs.

horizontal position. This action allows the horse to lift its forelegs. The more horizontal the scapula becomes, the greater the range of motion, increasing the horse's ability to tightly tuck its forelegs.

A horse with a long, sloping shoulder is suited to almost any performance activity, including eventing, jumping, dressage, cutting, and flat, harness, or endurance-type racing.

Conformational Faults of the Shoulder
Upright Shoulder (Open Angle)

A relatively upright shoulder has a much more open angle between the scapula and humerus. This shorter, more upright positioning restricts foreleg swing and stride length, resulting in high knee action and a choppy stride. It also decreases shock absorption capacity. The forelegs will hit the ground more times to cover the same distance as a horse with a sloping shoulder. The result is a foreleg that is subject to both increased frequency *and* intensity of concussion, and is therefore at greater risk for unsoundness.

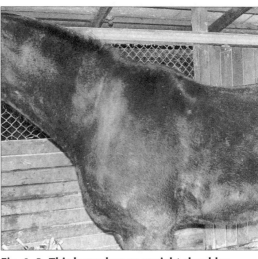

Fig. 6–9. This horse has an upright shoulder.

An open angle occasionally results from a shoulder that is *too* long. This conformation lowers the point of the shoulder, creating an excessively steep angle between the scapula and humerus.

A horse with a more upright shoulder is suited to activities where stride length is not as important as quick turnover, such as roping and Quarter Horse racing. Also, the greater knee action associated with a fairly upright shoulder can make for a pleasing, flashy effect for gaited or parade horses.

Upper Arm

The *upper arm* is often overlooked when discussing conformation, but it is important because its structure and angle influence the horse's motion. The upper arm bone, or humerus, connects the point of the shoulder to the elbow. The humerus is heavily muscled, and serves as a lever for muscles attaching near the elbow. Ample length adds power

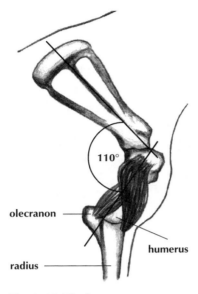

Fig. 6–10. The humerus serves as a lever for muscles attaching near the elbow.

to the action of these muscles. A long humerus also increases the range of motion of the foreleg, but it should be in balance with the rest of the body.

The angle between the scapular spine and the humerus should be 105° – 120° in the normal standing position. An upright humerus opens this angle. It allows a show jumper to tuck its forelegs well over a jump, or a cutting horse to crouch down to head a calf.

Conformational Faults of the Upper Arm

A short *humerus* creates a choppy gait. And, a horizontal humerus closes the angle between the scapula and humerus. This limits elbow movement, and can cause

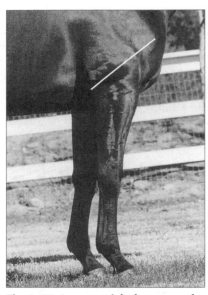

Fig. 6–11. Long, upright humerus of a Warmblood.

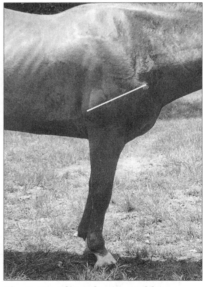

Fig. 6–12. Short, horizontal humerus of a stock horse.

the horse to stand "camped under," where the forelegs are set too far underneath the body. A horizontal humerus (common in stock horses) may result from breeding for long, sloping shoulders.

Elbow

The *elbow* should have a clean appearance and be in balance with the horse's entire body. The *point of the elbow* should be in front of the peak of the withers. The elbow should turn very slightly outward (to point the toes forward and ensure a straight, free stride) and blend into a long, smoothly muscled forearm.

Conformational Faults of the Elbow

The elbow should not be angled too far out nor tied in, because both restrict movement to a certain degree. An elbow that is angled too far out will probably cause the horse to toe in. An elbow that is tied-in does not allow the forearm to be pulled as far forward, which shortens the horse's stride. A *tied-in elbow* is determined by the pectoral muscles that run from the scapula to the humerus (see Chapter 5, *Chest*). These muscles are responsible for holding the foreleg in toward the body. The lower they attach on the humerus, the tighter the elbow is held in.

The elbow joint is high up on the foreleg. Therefore, improper positioning of the attachment of the foreleg at the elbow results in poor total

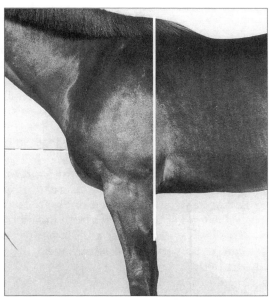

Fig. 6–13. The point of the elbow should be in front of the peak of the withers.

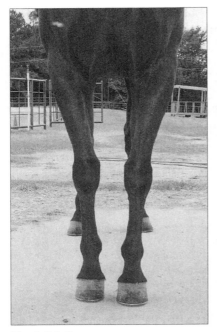
Fig. 6–14. Base narrow.

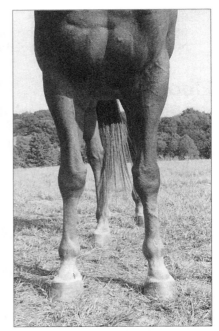
Fig. 6–15. Base wide.

leg conformation. For example, a *base narrow* horse has a greater distance between the forearms than between the feet. Base narrow conformation places more strain on the outside of the legs, so these horses are prone to problems on the outside of the leg. In the opposite situation, a *base wide* horse has a smaller distance between the forearms than between the feet. Base wide conformation places excess stress on the inside of the legs, so these horses are susceptible to injuries on the inside of the leg.

"Camped under" in front and *"camped out"* in front are both faults that result when the forelegs are improperly directed from their origin at the elbow. Camped under in front means that the forelegs do not extend straight down from the elbow, but angle under the body. This fault is also called standing under or pigeon-breasted. With camped out in front conformation, the forelegs angle out away from the body.

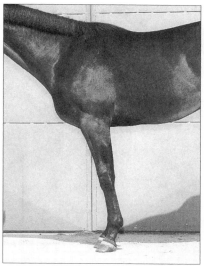
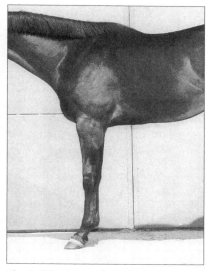

Fig. 6–16. Camped under in front.   **Fig. 6–17. Camped out in front.**

Forearm

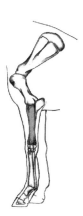

The *forearm* connects the elbow to the knee. A forearm with good conformation is well directed, long, and wide. "Well-directed" means that the forearm is straight in line with the knee and cannon from all views. The major bone of the forearm is the radius. A long radius creates a long forearm, which provides the horse with a greater stride length. At the back of the elbow is another bone, the ulna, which fuses with the radius about half way down the forearm. The top of the ulna forms the point of the elbow. The width of the radius and ulna determines the width of the forearm, as viewed from the side. Good forearm width, when in balance with the horse's body, is desirable because major muscles for strength of propulsion attach here.

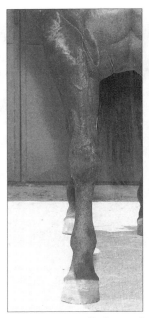
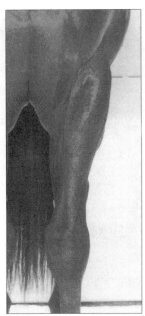
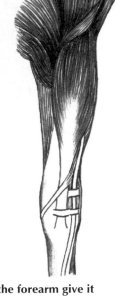

Fig. 6–18. A well-directed forearm.

Fig. 6–19. The muscles of the forearm give it shape.

Because very little body fat is deposited in this area, the amount of forearm muscling is a good indicator of the degree of muscling throughout the horse's body. Viewed from the front, the forearm

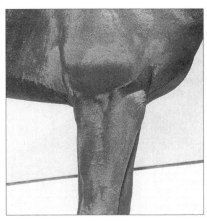
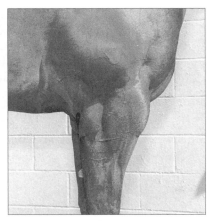

Fig. 6–20. Typical Thoroughbred forearm muscling.

Fig. 6–21. Typical Quarter Horse forearm muscling.

should appear thick and strong due to the underlying muscles. Forearm muscling is most concentrated at the top, becoming tendinous and slimmer at the bottom. The actual amount of muscling varies among breeds (for example, Quarter Horses are typically heavily muscled here). In any case, the muscles should be smooth and lengthy rather than bunchy and short.

A short forearm contributes to a short, choppy stride, and increased knee action. This action is desirable for gaited, show, and parade horses, and does not greatly hinder horses in events such as reining, roping, and cutting.

Knee

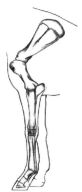

The *knee* (carpus) joins the forearm to the cannon and should be straight and placed squarely on the leg. From all directions the knee should correspond with the line formed by the forearm and the cannon with no deviation in any direction.

The knee should be of adequate size in proportion with the horse, well balanced, and well defined. It should not be round-looking, especially at the front. A flattened front of the knee provides a

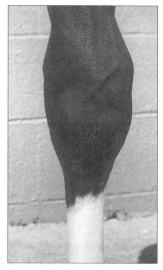

Fig. 6–22. Correct, smooth knee.

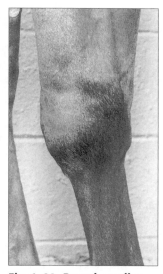

Fig. 6–23. Round, swollen knee due to an old injury.

113

smooth surface for the up and down actions of the extensor tendons, which straighten the knee.

Viewed from the side, the knee should be wide from front to back and exhibit a clean look. A knee that is deep, thick, and wide provides good cushioning for the leg. An excessively large or swollen knee could indicate an old injury, poor conformation, and a lack of adequate flexibility.

Conformational Faults of the Knee

Poor knee conformation affects the weight-bearing efficiency of the entire foreleg. With any conformational fault of the knee, concussion is not spread equally over the bones of the leg. Some parts of the leg are subjected to greater stress while others receive lighter stress. This uneven stress predisposes the horse to injuries involving the knee and lower leg, particularly the fetlock joint.

Front View

Viewed from the front, there are several conformational faults that may be seen. *"Knock knees,"* or *"in at the knees"* is an example. In this case the knees deviate toward each other. The opposite condition is *"bow legs,"* where the knees deviate away from each other.

Also noticeable from the front is the defect called *"bench knees,"* or *"offset knees."* In this situation, the cannon bone is offset to the outside of the knee. A horse with this fault is very prone to breaking down under hard work.

In each of these cases, the horse is particularly vulnerable to injuries of the foreleg. Splints and "popped knee" are two of the most common lamenesses due to improperly aligned bones.

Side View

Viewed from the side, there are a few other conformational faults that may be present. *"Calf knees"* or "back at the knee" is where the foreleg bends back at the knee. Tendons and check ligaments in particular are prone to injury as a result of this conformational fault. Sports in which the foreleg is exposed to excess stress, such as racing, jumping, barrel racing, and reining make the horse more vulnerable to unsoundness.

"Bucked knees" (also called "sprung knees" or "over at the knees") is the opposite conformational fault, with the foreleg appearing to arc forward at the knee. The horse may be born with this fault, or it may be the result of injury to the structures of the back of the knee. It

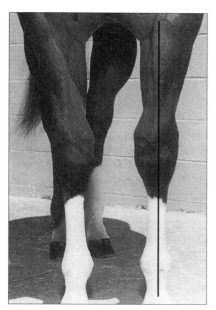

Fig. 6–24. Good, straight knees.

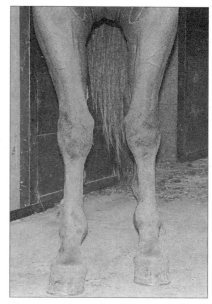

Fig. 6–25. Knock knees.

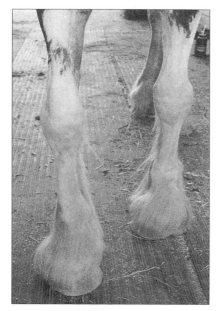

Fig. 6–26. Bow legs.

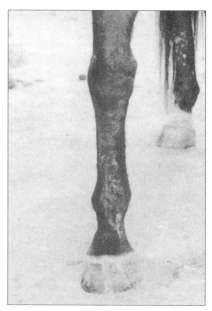

Fig. 6–27. Bench knee.

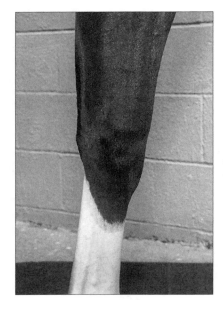

Fig. 6–28. Side view of a good knee. The knee should be wide from front to back and exhibit a clean look. This knee will provide effective shock absorption.

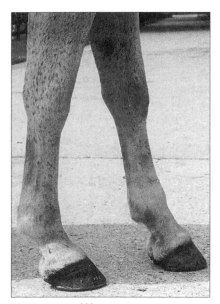

Fig. 6–29. Calf knees.

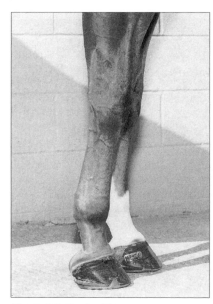

Fig. 6–30. Bucked knees.

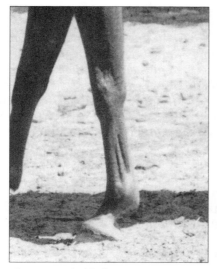

Fig. 6–31. Tied in knees.

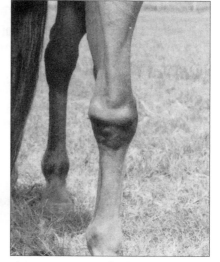

Fig. 6–32. Severe physitis.

is not considered to be as serious as calf knees. However, the horse is still predisposed to injury, especially at the front of the fetlock, back of the knee, suspensory ligament, and sesamoid bones. As with calf knees, a horse with this conformational defect will likely remain sound if used in lighter, non-speed activities.

A horse is *"tied in at the knees"* when the flexor tendons appear to be too close to the cannon bone just below the knee. In this case the tendons are too small and not adequate to support the horse under stress. Sometimes the cannon bone is also too small. Tied in knees inhibit free movement; the degree of movement lost depends upon the severity of the defect. *"Cut out under the knees"* means that there is a dent, or cut out appearance, just below the knee on the front of the cannon bone.

Also apparent from the side are *"open knees,"* although in severe cases it can be seen from the front. In this situation, the profile of the knee is irregular due to the swelling at the lower end of the radius. This problem, clinically called *physitis,* usually becomes less obvious with proper treatment and maturity.

Cannon

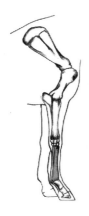

Between the knee and the fetlock is the *cannon* area. The cannon should be short and straight. Short cannons are usually accompanied by long forearms, correspondingly increasing the horse's stride length. The cannon should be narrow when viewed from the front and wide when viewed from the side. Width indicates solidity that reduces susceptibility to splints and fractures.

Part of the reason the cannon looks flat and wide from the side is due to the presence of the flexor tendons and suspensory ligament at the back. These structures should be well defined: the superficial digital flexor tendon is set well away from the cannon bone. Thin skin and sparse connective tissue make the bone, ligaments, tendons, and blood vessels stand out in relief. They can be easily felt and individually identified.

To determine if the horse has "good bone," measure the circumference (the distance around) of the horse's cannon just below the knee. A horse with good bone has at least 7 inches of bone per 1,000 pounds of body weight. (However, the bone's mineral content has just as much influence on its strength as the circumference.)

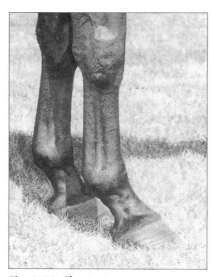

Fig. 6–33. Short, strong cannons.

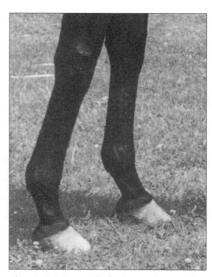

Fig. 6–34. Long, light-boned cannons.

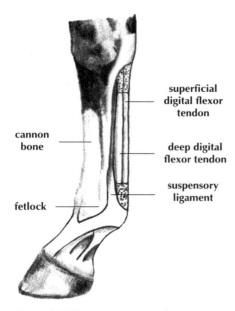

superficial
digital flexor
tendon

cannon
bone

deep digital
flexor tendon

suspensory
ligament

fetlock

Fig. 6–35. The structures at the
back of the cannon give it width.

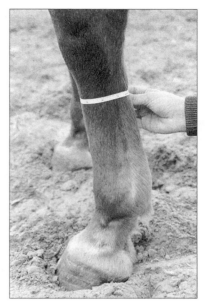

Fig. 6–36. Measuring the circumference of the cannon.

Fetlock

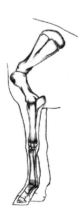

The cannon should blend into a flat, wide *fetlock*. The fetlock should be smooth and wide to allow for strong attachments of the ligaments supporting the joint. There also needs to be enough room for the tendons to pass around and between the sesamoid bones at the back of the joint. The fetlock should angle adequately for maximum use of tendons and ligaments in propulsion, shock absorption, and weight bearing. Most horses have a fetlock angle from the front of about 140° in the foreleg, and 145° in the hindleg. Marks or small scars on the fetlock may indicate that the horse interferes while in motion. Puffy, swollen-looking fetlocks may indicate lameness, and should be viewed with suspicion.

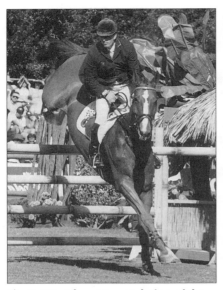

Fig. 6–37. Adequate angulation of the fetlock is vital to shock absorption.

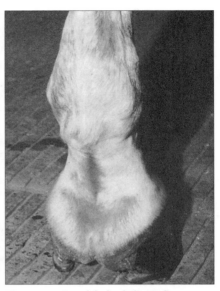

Fig. 6–38. Good fetlock from the rear.

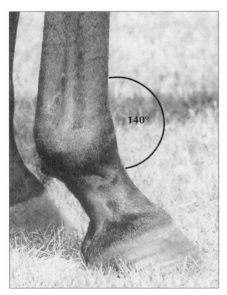

Fig. 6–39a. Good front fetlock, viewed from the side.

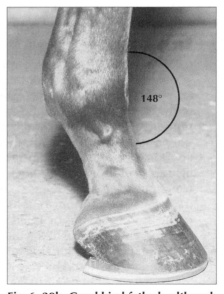

Fig. 6–39b. Good hind fetlock, although the pastern is a little long.

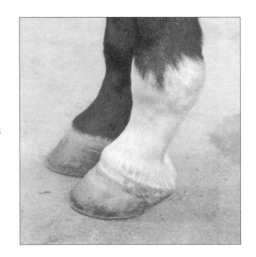

Fig. 6–40. Swollen-looking fetlocks may indicate previous or current lameness.

Pastern

The *pastern*, which lies between the fetlock and the coronet, should be fairly long and slope downward in a continuous line with the hoof wall. Good conformation of the pastern centers around the *pastern axis.* This axis is an imaginary line running through the core of the pastern. The pastern axis should be exactly the same angle as the foot axis.

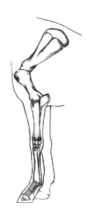

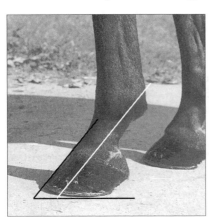

Fig. 6–41. The pastern axis should be the same angle as the foot axis.

This results in a straight, unbroken line through the pastern and foot. If the line is "broken forward" or "broken backward" the bones, joints, tendons, and ligaments are subjected to greater than normal stress. The two pastern bones are relatively small, but function to absorb and dissipate

121

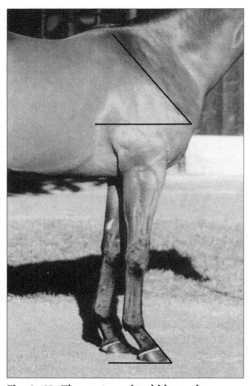

much of the force from concussion.

For most horses, the slope of the pastern and foot is 47° – 54° in the foreleg (49° – 56° in the hindleg). In length, the pastern should be ½ – ¾ the length of the cannon.

To help the leg absorb shock, the pastern and the hoof wall should slope toward the ground at about the same angle as the shoulder. This slope can differ from the "ideal" and still be effective in shock absorption. It is the angled stacking of the leg bones that allows the joints to absorb much of the shock of impact. The result is a much smoother gait than bones stacked end-on-end can provide.

Fig. 6–42. The pastern should have the same angle as the shoulder.

Conformational Faults of the Pastern

Horses with short, upright pasterns tend to have rough, choppy gaits. Even worse are upright pasterns combined with straight shoulders. Upright pasterns greatly increase concussion to all of the bones in the leg. This is because they lack the natural shock-absorbing quality ("springiness") of sloping pasterns. Therefore, pasterns that are too upright predispose a horse to bone injuries of the lower leg such as ringbone, navicular syndrome, and fetlock joint arthritis. One advantage of short pasterns is that they allow for quick acceleration.

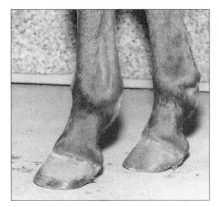
Fig. 6–43. Short, upright pastern.

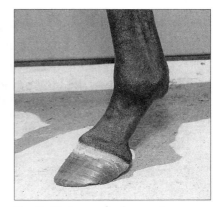
Fig. 6–44. Long, sloping pastern.

Some people are also critical of horses with excessively long pasterns. Although these horses have a smooth gait, their tendons and ligaments are subject to excess strain, and they may break down more easily from increased stress on the sesamoid bones. Bowed tendons, suspensory ligament injuries, and sesamoiditis are very common in horses with long, sloping pasterns.

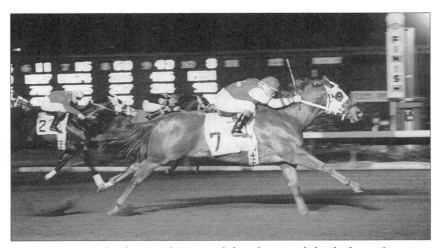
Fig. 6–45. Proper foreleg angulation, and therefore good shock absorption, helps to prevent injuries in athletic horses.

ANATOMY OF THE FORELEG
Shoulder and Upper Arm

The shoulders' main function is to move the forelegs. Large shoulder muscles pull the bones of the shoulder and upper arm forward. The length and slope of the bones determine the length of the forearm swing. Long, sloping shoulders help to decrease concussion, support weight, and permit the foreleg to extend farther, lengthening the stride.

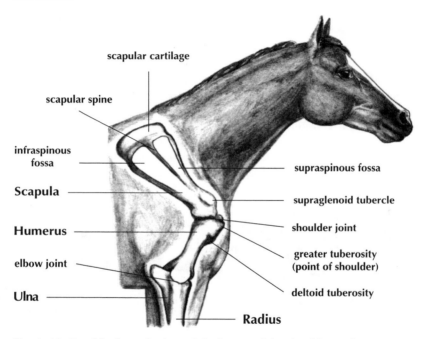

Fig. 6–46. Outside (lateral) view of the bones of the shoulder and upper arm.

Bones

The underlying bone in the horse's shoulder is the shoulder blade, or *scapula*. The scapula is a flat, triangular-shaped bone that overlies the first six to seven ribs. Its function is to attach the foreleg to the body and transmit motion to the body. The top curve of the scapula is made of cartilage instead of bone—this is called the *scapular cartilage*. The scapula's outer (lateral) surface has a ridge, called the *scapular spine*, extending from the top to almost the lower edge of

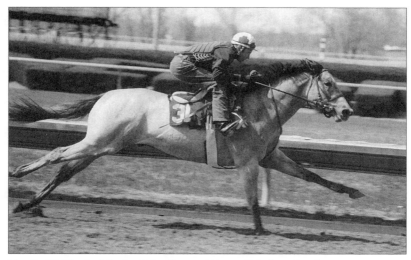

Fig. 6–47. The inside shoulder (toward the rail) is in extension.

the bone. On each side of the spine is a hollow, depressed area called a fossa. The upper front fossa is called the *supraspinous fossa,* and the lower rear is called the *infraspinous fossa.* There is also a large depression called the *subscapular fossa* on the inner (medial) surface of the scapula. Most of the muscles that attach the foreleg to the body attach to this inner surface of the scapula.

The shoulder joint, called the *scapulo-humeral joint,* is a ball and socket joint formed by the scapula and the humerus. The *humerus* is the bone in the upper arm. The upper end of the humerus is the "ball" of the shoulder joint. On the lower end of the scapula is the cup-shaped "socket" called the *glenoid cavity.*

The humerus is a very strong and relatively short bone. It has many irregular tuberosities that serve as sites of muscle attachment. The point of the shoulder is formed by a protrusion at the upper end of the humerus called the *greater tuberosity.* The *deltoid tuberosity* is located on the outside of the shaft of the humerus, and can be felt almost halfway down. The *teres tuberosity* is located on the inside (medial) surface of the humerus, about halfway down. At the lower end of the humerus are the *lateral* and *medial condyles.* The condyles are rounded projections, shaped to form the elbow joint with the radius and ulna of the forearm.

The normal standing position creates an angle between the scapula and the humerus of about 105° – 120°. When the horse reaches the

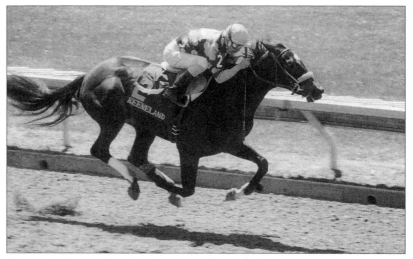

Fig. 6–48. The outside shoulder (away from the rail) is in flexion.

foreleg forward during maximum extension, the angle increases to about 145°. When the foreleg is reaching backward in full flexion, the angle reduces to about 80°.

An extensive joint capsule encloses the shoulder joint. The ligaments that bind the joint together are weak and poorly developed—the shoulder is the only leg joint that has no collateral ligaments on each side. Therefore, some of the muscles surrounding the shoulder joint function as ligaments to support it. Because muscles are more flexible than ligaments, this gives a greater range of motion to the joint. However, the heavy muscular arrangement in this area also limits the direction of joint action, making flexion and extension the primary movements of the shoulder joint.

Muscles of the Shoulder and Upper Arm

There are many strong muscles—over, under, and around the scapula—that function to support the shoulder joint, or move the scapula and humerus. Because of their locations and multiple functions, some muscles may also be listed in other sections.

Shoulder Girdle

There is a group of large muscles that forms the shoulder girdle (or pectoral girdle). It includes the trapezius, rhomboideus, latissimus dorsi, brachiocephalic, pectorals, and serratus ventralis muscles.

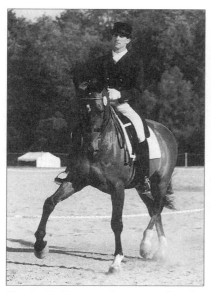 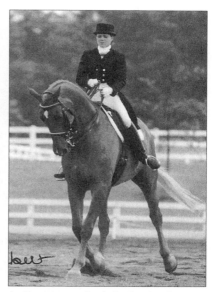

Fig. 6–49. Dressage horses performing the half-pass. On the left, the forelegs are in abduction. On the right, the forelegs are in adduction. The spine is not flexing laterally very much, if at all.

Together they encircle the chest to attach and support the forelegs. In the horse there is no bony connection (joint) of the scapula to the trunk of the body, so these muscles are extremely important and strong. The large muscles also help to absorb concussion forces traveling up the leg. These two factors reduce impact on the spinal column.

Aside from holding the scapula in place and absorbing concussion, the muscles of the shoulder girdle also aid in its movement. They permit the scapula to move back and forth. At a gallop, this enables the horse to extend the forelegs further. Therefore, the horse can run very fast, despite a relatively rigid spine.

The girdle arrangement also allows the horse's barrel to move independent of the forelegs. The body can move up and down, which changes the horse's center of gravity.

The shoulder girdle also enables the horse to adduct/abduct the forelegs, moving them in toward and away from the body's midline, respectively. This ability allows sudden changes in direction and tight corners. A subtle example of this motion is when the horse leans over while grazing, without moving its feet. A more obvious example is when a racehorse leans into a turn. The horse is not curving its spinal

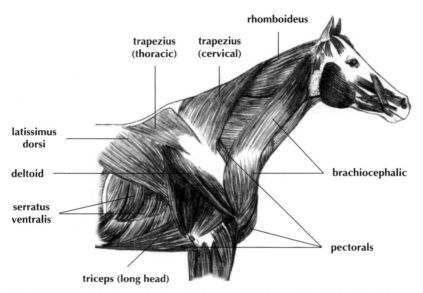

Fig. 6–50. Outside (lateral) view of the superficial muscles of the shoulder and upper arm.

column around the turn. It is leaning the inside legs under its body (adduction), and the outside legs away from its body (abduction).

Trapezius—This fan-shaped muscle has two parts: cervical and thoracic. The cervical part of the trapezius is discussed in Chapter 3, *Neck*. The thoracic part attaches along the supraspinous ligament from the first through the tenth thoracic vertebrae. It narrows as it travels to insert onto the scapular spine. The trapezius is instrumental in holding the scapula in place against the body. It draws the scapula upward and back.

Rhomboideus—Another fan-shaped muscle, the rhomboideus lies under the trapezius and originates in the same region along the spine. From the spine, the rhomboideus runs to the inner side of the upper edge of the scapula. It fixes the scapula to the strong nuchal ligament and to the tops of the first few thoracic vertebrae (withers). In motion, its function is to pull the upper part of the scapula upward and forward. It also aids in rotating the horse's barrel between the forelegs. When the foreleg is fixed in a standing position, the rhomboideus raises the neck.

Latissimus dorsi—This is a strong, wide, triangular flexor muscle. It is originates on the part of the spinal column that forms the back and

MUSCLES OF THE SHOULDER & UPPER ARM

Name	Origin	Insertion	Function
Trapezius	along spine from head to just behind withers	spine of scapula	lift scapula up and back
Rhomboideus	along spine from head to just below withers	inside surface of upper edge of scapula	lift scapula up and forward; rotates barrel
Latissimus dorsi	thoracic and lumbar vertebrae	teres tuberosity of humerus	pull foreleg up and back
Brachiocephalic	skull between and behind ears	deltoid tuberosity of humerus	extend and raise shoulder; extend elbow joint
Pectorals	sternum	inside of humerus and scapula	adduct foreleg
Serratus ventralis	top underside of scapula	cervical vertebrae & ribs to behind elbow	pair: raise barrel; single: swing scapula back & forth
Deltoid	spine of scapula	deltoid tuberosity of humerus	flex and abduct shoulder joint
Supraspinatus	supraspinous fossa of scapula	upper end of humerus	extend & support shoulder joint; advance foreleg
Infraspinatus	infraspinous fossa of scapula	upper end of humerus	flex & support shoulder joint; abduct upper arm

Fig. 6–51. Part 1.

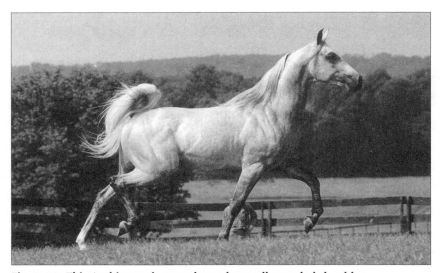

Fig. 6–52. This Arabian endurance horse has well-muscled shoulders.

loin by the lumbodorsal fascia (a wide band of tendinous tissue draped over the loins and back). The muscle narrows as it travels from this expansive beginning to run underneath the shoulder/girth area, ending at the teres tuberosity on the shaft of the humerus. The latissimus dorsi muscle works to pull the foreleg upward and backward (or the body forward if the foreleg is on the ground).

Brachiocephalic—This is a heavy, strong muscle that is responsible for most of the shoulder's motion. It extends from the horse's head to the upper arm. The brachiocephalic begins at the point where the skull meets the spine and ends by attaching near the deltoid tuberosity. The brachiocephalic covers the front of the point of the shoulder and works to pull the shoulder up and forward (extension). When the foreleg is fixed in a standing position, the brachiocephalic acts to extend the elbow joint.

Pectorals—The function of the pectoral muscles is to adduct the foreleg. They also advance the body when the leg is placed on the ground. The origins and insertions of these muscles are discussed in Chapter 5, *Chest*.

Serratus ventralis—This is the largest muscle in the shoulder girdle. The serratus ventralis fans outward and downward from its attachment at the top underside of the scapula, ending in a curved line along the cervical vertebrae (neck) and ribs to behind the elbow.

MUSCLES OF THE SHOULDER & UPPER ARM			
Name	**Origin**	**Insertion**	**Function**
Teres major	back edge of scapula	teres tuberosity of humerus	flex shoulder joint; adduct upper arm
Coracobrachialis	inside bottom of scapula	inside shaft of humerus	adduct forearm
Subscapularis	subscapular fossa	top inside of humerus	adduct foreleg
Triceps	lower back edge of scapula	olecranon	flex shoulder; extend elbow
Tensor fascia antebrachii	lower part of latissimus dorsi	olecranon	flex shoulder; extend elbow; tense forearm fascia
Biceps brachii	lower end of scapula	upper front of radius	extend shoulder; flex elbow

Fig. 6–53. Part 2.

Together the serratus ventralis muscles on each side form a sling to support the trunk between the forelegs. To accomplish this, it contains inelastic tendinous tissue that does not stretch, making the muscle very strong. When both sides contract they raise the barrel. Operating individually, they swing each scapula forward and backward, shifting the horse's weight to the leg on the corresponding side.

Other Shoulder and Upper Arm Muscles

Deltoid—This muscle originates at the scapular spine and inserts onto the deltoid tuberosity of the humerus. As the name implies, the deltoid muscle is somewhat triangular in shape. It is a strong muscle that serves to flex and abduct the shoulder joint.

Supraspinatus—This muscle originates on the supraspinous fossa of the scapula and runs to the upper end of the humerus. It extends the

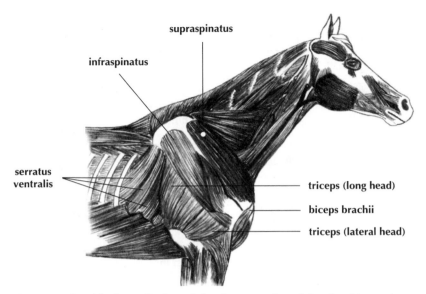

Fig. 6–54. Outside (lateral) view of the deep muscles of the shoulder and upper arm.

shoulder joint and advances the foreleg, but also functions as a ligament to strengthen and support the joint, preventing dislocation. This muscle can be felt just above the scapular spine.

Infraspinatus—The infraspinatus muscle originates on the infraspinous fossa of the scapula and inserts onto the upper end of the humerus. It flexes the shoulder joint. It also acts as a ligament of the shoulder and works to abduct the upper arm. This muscle can be felt just below the scapular spine.

Teres major—This deep muscle extends from the back edge of the scapula near the top, running across the outer surface of the shoulder joint. It inserts onto the inner surface of the humerus at the teres tuberosity. It flexes the shoulder joint and adducts the upper arm. A companion to this muscle is the small *teres minor*.

Coracobrachialis—The small coracobrachialis muscle originates on the inside of the scapula at the bottom, and inserts onto the inner side of the shaft of the humerus. This muscle adducts the forearm. Working in concert with the subscapularis and pectoral muscles, it also flexes the shoulder joint.

Subscapularis—This muscle originates on the subscapular fossa. It inserts on the top and inside of the humerus. Its function is to adduct

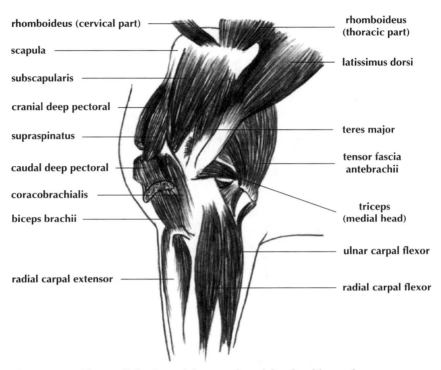

rhomboideus (cervical part)

rhomboideus (thoracic part)

scapula

latissimus dorsi

subscapularis

cranial deep pectoral

supraspinatus

teres major

tensor fascia antebrachii

caudal deep pectoral

coracobrachialis

triceps (medial head)

biceps brachii

ulnar carpal flexor

radial carpal extensor

radial carpal flexor

Fig. 6–55. Inside (medial) view of the muscles of the shoulder and upper arm. The rhomboideus has been reflected upward to reveal the structures beneath.

the leg and to prevent the leg from moving outward. It also supports the shoulder joint.

Triceps—The triceps muscle has three parts, or "heads." Of the three, the long head is the largest. It is considered a shoulder muscle because it originates on the lower back edge of the scapula and inserts onto the olecranon of the elbow. Its function is to flex the shoulder and extend the elbow. The two shorter heads of the triceps muscle function only to extend the elbow, and are more completely described in the Elbow section.

Tensor fascia antebrachii—This thin, broad muscle originates on the lower border of the latissimus dorsi muscle and inserts onto the olecranon of the elbow and deep fascia (connective tissue) of the forearm. Its action is very similar to the triceps, but it also puts tension on the fascia of the forearm.

Biceps brachii—This muscle contains inelastic tendinous tissue,

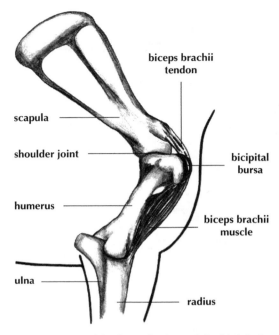

biceps brachii tendon

scapula

shoulder joint

humerus

ulna

bicipital bursa

biceps brachii muscle

radius

Fig. 6–56. Outside (lateral) view of the bicipital bursa at the front of the shoulder.

making it very strong. It originates on the lower end of the scapula and runs across the front of the shoulder joint to insert on the upper front surface of the radius (forearm bone). It extends the shoulder as it flexes the elbow, fixing both joints in a normal standing position.

Bursa of the Shoulder and Upper Arm

The major bursa (fluid-filled sac) that may occur in the shoulder area is the *bicipital bursa*. It is located at the front of the shoulder joint, between the top of the humerus and the biceps brachii tendon. It protects the bone and tendon from friction as the tendon slides over the joint.

Blood Vessels of the Shoulder and Upper Arm

The main artery supplying blood to the foreleg is the *axillary artery.* All major arteries in the shoulder and down the foreleg branch off this vessel. It begins at the shoulder joint, then curves down the upper arm as the *brachial artery.* (It is eventually reduced to the common digital artery supplying the pastern and foot.) Three branches run upward from the axillary to supply the shoulder muscles: the *suprascapular, subscapular,* and *thoracodorsal arteries.* As the brachial artery runs down the humerus, it has several branches as well.

The veins of the shoulder are companions to the arteries, and have the same names. They travel approximately the same paths to drain the area of blood. There is an additional vein in the upper arm region called the *cephalic vein.* It drains directly into the jugular vein rather than into the axillary vein.

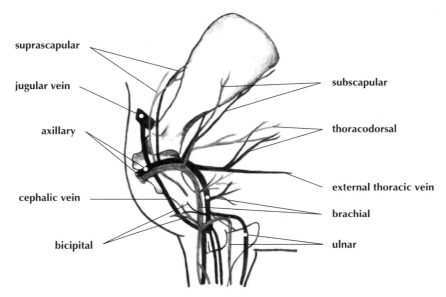

Fig. 6–57. Inside (medial) view of the major blood vessels of the shoulder and upper arm of the right leg.

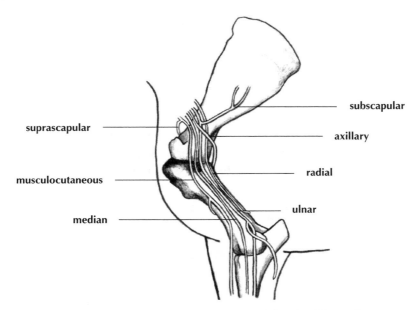

Fig. 6–58. Inside (medial) view of the major nerves of the shoulder and upper arm of the right leg.

Nerves of the Shoulder and Upper Arm

The *brachial plexus* is a set of nerves that supplies sensation and motion to the entire foreleg. One of its members is the *suprascapular nerve,* which runs across the front edge of the scapula. In this position, it is vulnerable to injury, resulting in "sweeney," where the supraspinatus and infraspinatus muscles atrophy (shrink). Other important nerves in the shoulder are the *subscapular, musculocutaneous,* and *axillary nerves.*

Elbow

In the horse, the *elbow* is the uppermost joint of the foreleg that is not within the shoulder girdle. In a normal standing position the elbow is slightly extended at about 150° (the angle between the humerus and the radius). The elbow's range of motion is 55° – 60°.

Bones

The elbow joint is formed by the junction of the lower end of the humerus and the upper ends of the *radius* and *ulna.* These bones have special shapes to make up the joint surface. To provide a larger supporting surface for the humerus, the upper end of the radius is slightly dished and enlarged. In its surface, the ulna has a *semilunar notch* at the point where the ulna projects past the radius. The dished end of the radius and the semilunar notch of the ulna meet to form a smooth half-circle. The condyles of the humerus fit neatly into this half-circle forming the elbow joint.

The ulna projects behind the elbow joint, forming the point of the elbow. At this location it is called the *olecranon.*

The following three terms are similar, but have distinct meanings:

1. Elbow—the general area on the outside of the horse.
2. Point of the elbow—the olecranon process of the ulna.
3. Elbow joint—the joint between the bones.

Elbow (Cubital) Joint

The elbow is a hinge joint, meaning its only actions are flexion and extension. Flexor muscles on the front of the joint and extensor muscles on the back provide power for these actions. As in all four-legged animals, the extensor muscles of this joint are stronger than the flexor muscles, since one of their purposes is to support the body weight, in addition to keeping the elbow joint extended while the horse is standing.

Ligaments

The elbow joint is held together by *collateral ligaments* on either side. There are also short ligaments between the radius and ulna.

Muscles

Extensor Muscles

The extensor muscles open the elbow joint by pulling the olecranon up, which draws the forearm back. The two extensor muscles of the elbow are the triceps and the *anconeus*. The triceps has three separate heads or origins. The long

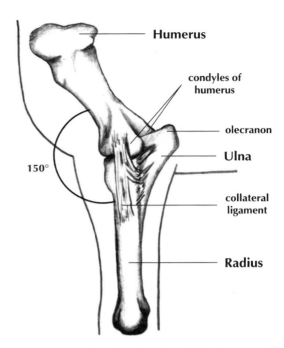

Fig. 6–59. Outside (lateral) view of the bones and ligaments of the elbow.

head acts on the shoulder and is described in the Shoulder section. The two shorter heads are called the lateral head *(see Figure 6–54)* and medial head *(see Figure 6–55)*. They originate on each side of the humerus. At their lower end, all three heads of the triceps insert onto the olecranon. The triceps is the longest extensor muscle of the elbow.

Underneath the triceps is the anconeus muscle. This short muscle covers and protects the back of the elbow joint. The anconeus begins on the lower end of the humerus and inserts onto the outside of the olecranon. It aids in extending the elbow.

Flexor Muscles

The flexor muscles of the elbow close the joint by pulling the radius forward. The biceps brachii muscle and the brachialis muscle are the flexors of the elbow joint. The two heads of the biceps originate on the lower end of the scapula and attach at the top of the radius, on the front and inside surface. The biceps is also considered a shoulder muscle. The brachialis muscle originates near the top of the humerus and attaches on the inside front of the elbow joint below

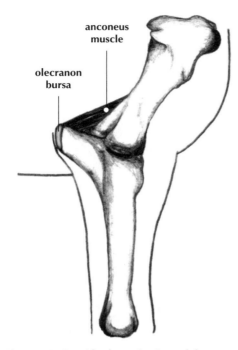

anconeus muscle

olecranon bursa

Fig. 6–60. Outside (lateral) view of the anconeus muscle and olecranon bursa.

the biceps. The essential action of both muscles is to flex the elbow.

Bursa of the Elbow

Some horses have a small bursa between the olecranon and the tendons of the triceps muscles. Inflammation of this *olecranon bursa* can result a capped elbow.

Forearm

The forearm is that part of the horse's foreleg between the elbow and the knee. The *chestnuts*—small masses of horn on the inside of the forearm just above the knee—are found in this area. The top layer of the chestnut can (and should) be easily trimmed away.

Bones

The *radius* and *ulna* are the two bones of the forearm. The radius is a large, well developed bone. At the top it is part of the elbow joint and at the bottom it is part of the carpal joint, or knee. The ulna is a small, short bone that is fused to the back of the radius. There is no movement between the radius and ulna. At their upper end they are bound together by ligaments *(see Figure 6–59)*. The ulna fuses with the radius about halfway down. Furthermore, the ligaments between the radius and ulna ossify (change into bone) as the horse matures. The olecranon of the ulna forms the point of the elbow. It prevents the forearm from rotating backward and outward. The function of the olecranon is that of a lever—it increases the power of the triceps muscles attaching to it.

The normal standing position of the radius is more or less vertical. The position of the radius is an important factor in the horse's foreleg conformation. If the radius is tilted forward, the horse is calf kneed. If the radius is tilted backward, the horse is buck kneed.

Muscles and Ligaments

Many of the strong muscles of the shoulder attach to the upper radius and ulna. They include the triceps, biceps, brachialis, tensor fascia antebrachii, and anconeus muscles, described in the Shoulder section.

Muscles activating the lower leg also originate at the upper ends of the radius and ulna, and pass over the forearm. The radial carpal extensor is the most prominent muscle on the front of the forearm. Also

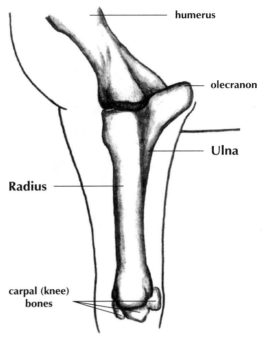

Fig. 6–61. Outside (lateral) view of the bones of the forearm.

along the forearm are the oblique carpal extensor, radial carpal flexor, ulnar carpal flexor, and lateral ulnar. Because these muscles primarily act on the knee, they are described in the Knee section.

The muscles described in this section activate the entire lower leg. Most become tendons just above the knee—in fact, the horse has no muscles below the top of the knee. The lower leg moves entirely via the actions of tendons and ligaments.

Common digital extensor—This muscle originates on the front of the lower humerus, and also on the top of the radius. Its tendon attaches at several places as it runs down the front of the leg, finally ending on the top of the coffin bone. It serves to extend the joints of the lower leg, including the knee and *digit* (fetlock, pastern, and coffin joints). As it passes over the knee it is surrounded and protected by a tendon sheath. At the fetlock it is joined by the two branches of the suspensory ligament, which emerge from behind the fetlock joint.

Lateral digital extensor—This muscle originates on the side of the lower humerus, near the origin of the common digital extensor. As its

139

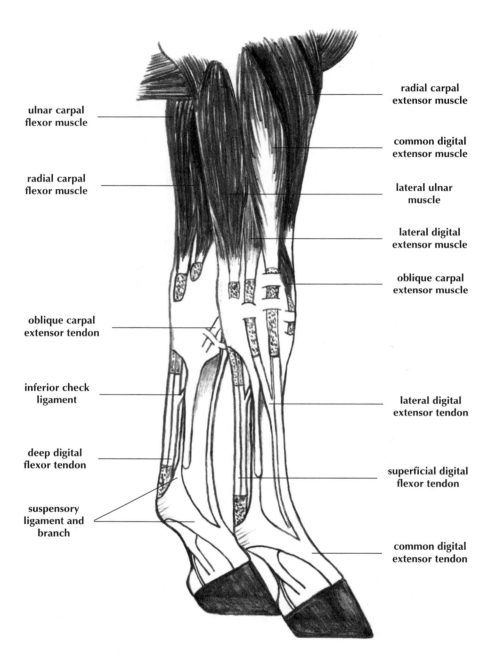

ulnar carpal
flexor muscle

radial carpal
flexor muscle

oblique carpal
extensor tendon

inferior check
ligament

deep digital
flexor tendon

suspensory
ligament and
branch

radial carpal
extensor muscle

common digital
extensor muscle

lateral ulnar
muscle

lateral digital
extensor muscle

oblique carpal
extensor muscle

lateral digital
extensor tendon

superficial digital
flexor tendon

common digital
extensor tendon

Fig. 6–62. Muscles, tendons, and ligaments of the foreleg.

MUSCLES OF THE FOREARM			
Name	**Origin**	**Insertion**	**Function**
Common digital extensor	front of lower humerus, side of upper radius	top of coffin bone	extend joints of lower foreleg
Lateral digital extensor	side of lower humerus & upper radius	front and top of long pastern bone	extend joints of lower foreleg
Superficial digital flexor	bottom of humerus	sides of pastern bones	flex joints of lower foreleg
Deep digital flexor	bottom of humerus, inside of olecranon, back of radius	underside of coffin bone	flex joints of lower foreleg

Fig. 6–63.

tendon passes over the knee it is surrounded and protected by a tendon sheath. A branch joins the common digital extensor to the lateral digital extensor, at the bottom edge of the knee. For most of its length it runs next to the common digital extensor tendon, then slips underneath it at the fetlock. Here there is a bursa between the tendon and the fetlock joint. The lateral digital extensor tendon inserts on the front and top of the long pastern bone.

Superficial digital flexor—The superficial digital flexor muscle runs closest to the outside of the leg, along the back. It originates at the bottom of the humerus. As its tendon passes over the knee it is surrounded and protected by a tendon sheath that it shares with the deep digital flexor tendon. It inserts on the sides of the pastern bones. The function of the superficial digital flexor is to flex the joints of the lower foreleg, including the knee, fetlock, and pastern joints. Closely associated is the *superior check ligament.* (A check ligament runs from bone to tendon, instead of from bone to bone like most ligaments. Its function is to "check," or limit the tendon's action, preventing overstretching.) It originates on the back surface of the radius and fuses with the superficial digital flexor tendon just above the knee.

Deep digital flexor—This muscle runs underneath the superficial digital flexor. It originates with that muscle at the bottom of the humerus. It also has other points of origin on the inside of the olecranon and on the back of the radius. It inserts on the underside of the coffin bone. The function of the deep digital flexor is to flex the joints of the lower foreleg, including the knee, fetlock, pastern, and coffin joints. Its check ligament, the *inferior check ligament,* originates just below the knee and joins the deep digital flexor tendon midway down the cannon.

Blood Vessels of the Forearm

The *median artery* and *transverse cubital artery* supply blood to the forearm. Likewise, there are several veins that carry blood away from the forearm, including the cephalic, the *medial cubital,* and two *median veins.*

Nerves of the Forearm

There are several nerves of the brachial plexus that supply the forearm with sensation and motion. The *radial nerve* travels down the back of the humerus and then slips around it to the outside of the leg. It supplies the extensor muscles on the front of the forearm. As it runs across the shaft of the humerus, it can be vulnerable to injury. The *median* and *ulnar nerves* supply the flexor muscles at the back of the leg.

Knee (Carpus)

Although *"knee"* is the common term for this joint, the knee (or carpus) of the horse corresponds anatomically to the human wrist. It is a hinge joint—capable of flexion and extension—with a wide range of motion.

Bones

This is a very complex joint composed of numerous small, cuboidal (cube-shaped) bones. Between the radius and the cannon bone there are two rows of small carpal bones. The upper row contains the *radial, intermediate,* and *ulnar carpal bones.* The lower row is made up of the *first, second, third,* and *fourth carpal bones,* although the first is sometimes missing. The larger *accessory carpal bone* projects backward from the inner side of the knee. The projection is visible from the outside. Because of its projecting position, the accessory carpal bone forms a lever for the attachments of some of the muscles that bend the knee.

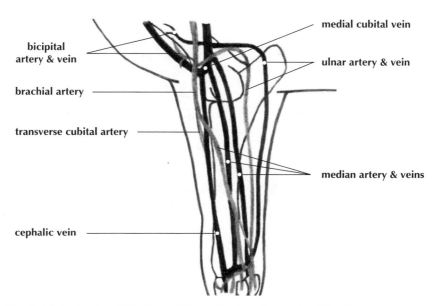

Fig. 6–64. Inside (medial) view of the major blood vessels of the forearm.

bicipital
artery & vein

brachial artery

transverse cubital artery

cephalic vein

medial cubital vein

ulnar artery & vein

median artery & veins

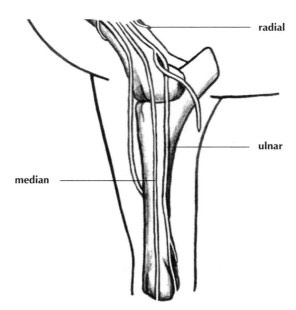

Fig. 6–65. Inside (medial) view of the major nerves of the forearm.

radial

ulnar

median

143

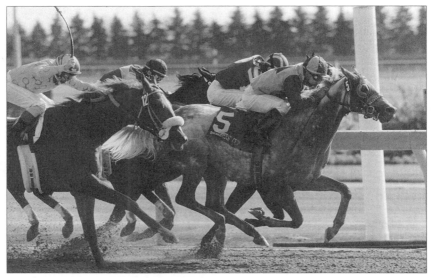
Fig. 6–66. The knee is capable of a wide range of motion.

Carpal Joints

The entire carpal joint actually contains three major joints. The *radiocarpal joint* is formed by the lower end of the radius and the upper surface of the top row of carpal bones. This joint permits hinge-like flexion and extension between the radius and carpal bones. The *intercarpal joint* lies between the two rows of carpal bones and allows some flexion and extension at this location. The third major joint, the *carpometacarpal joint*, is formed by the bottom of the lower row of carpal bones and the upper end of the cannon bone (third metacarpal bone). It has very little movement.

In addition, numerous small intracarpal joints are formed between each adjacent carpal bone. Although these joints have very limited movement, they absorb a great deal of concussion and are a vital part of the horse's shock-absorbing system.

All the joints of the knee are enclosed within a single, extensive joint capsule. The carpal joint capsule, much like a long sleeve, reaches from the radius to the cannon bone. Within the joint capsule, however, are three separate synovial sacs corresponding to each major joint. These sacs produce synovial fluid, which lubricates the joint surfaces.

Front View

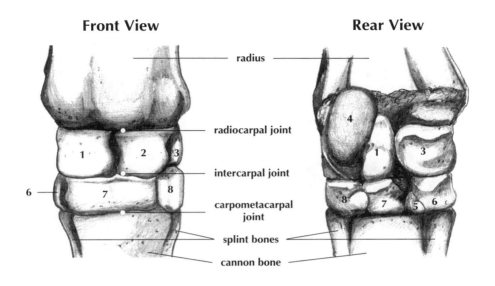

radius

radiocarpal joint

intercarpal joint

carpometacarpal joint

splint bones

cannon bone

Rear View

Inside View

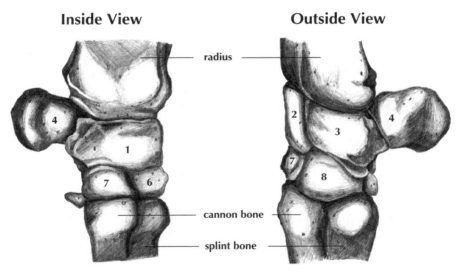

radius

cannon bone

splint bone

Outside View

Fig. 6–67. Four views of the bones and major joints of the knee:

1. radial carpal bone
2. intermediate carpal bone
3. ulnar carpal bone
4. accessory carpal bone

5. first carpal bone
6. second carpal bone
7. third carpal bone
8. fourth carpal bone

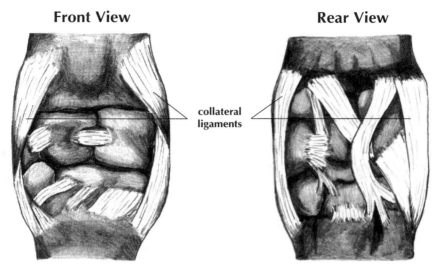

Front View   **Rear View**

collateral
ligaments

Fig. 6–68. Ligaments of the knee.

Ligaments of the Knee

There is a series of short, strong ligaments that bind the carpal bones, including the accessory carpal bone, together. There are also larger *collateral ligaments* on each side of the knee, running from the radius to the cannon bone. In addition, there is an annular ligament at the back of the knee. Annular ligaments are broad, ring-shaped, fibrous ligaments that support a joint.

Carpal Annular Ligament

The *carpal annular ligament* is a broad, strong support structure wrapped horizontally around the back of the knee, running from the accessory carpal bone to the carpal bones on the inside of the leg. It helps form the *carpal canal,* which encloses the superficial and deep digital flexor tendons and the radial carpal flexor tendon, as well as the blood vessels and nerves that supply the lower leg.

Muscles of the Knee

Because the knee is a hinge joint, there are extensor (straightening) muscles on the front and outside of the leg, and flexor (bending) muscles on the back. (**Note:** The terms "radial" and "ulnar" refer to the bone on the side of the forearm over which a muscle passes: either the radius or ulna.)

146

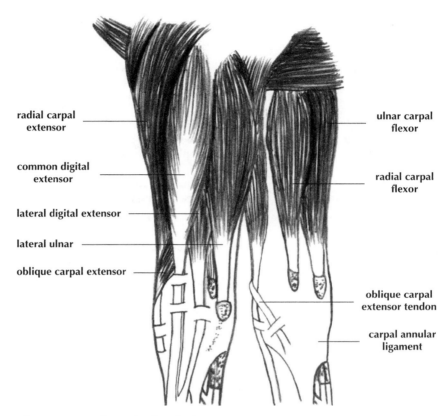

radial carpal
extensor

common digital
extensor

lateral digital extensor

lateral ulnar

oblique carpal extensor

ulnar carpal
flexor

radial carpal
flexor

oblique carpal
extensor tendon

carpal annular
ligament

Fig. 6–69. Muscles activating the knee.

Extensor Muscles

There are two major extensor muscles on the front of the foreleg that act on the knee. They function to extend the knee and to fix it in the normal standing position.

Radial carpal extensor—This is the most prominent muscle on the front of the forearm. It originates on the bottom of the humerus, runs along the outside of the upper elbow, and down the front of the foreleg. Just above the knee it becomes a tendon, surrounded and protected by a tendon sheath as it runs over the carpal bones. The tendon inserts on the upper front of the cannon bone.

Oblique carpal extensor—This muscle originates at the upper part of the radius, curls diagonally around the outside of the knee, and attaches to the top of the inside splint bone. As it runs over the knee it is surrounded and protected by a tendon sheath.

MUSCLES OF THE KNEE			
Name	**Origin**	**Insertion**	**Function**
Radial carpal extensor	bottom of humerus	upper front of cannon bone	extend and fix knee
Oblique carpal extensor	upper part of radius	top of inside splint bone	extend and fix knee
Radial carpal flexor	bottom of humerus	outside upper back of cannon bone	flex knee; extend elbow
Ulnar carpal flexor	bottom of humerus and olecranon	back of accessory carpal bone	flex knee; extend elbow
Lateral ulnar	bottom and back of humerus	top of accessory carpal bone and outside splint bone	flex knee; extend elbow

Fig. 6–70.

In addition, the common digital and lateral digital extensor tendons pass over the front and outside of the knee and help to extend it.

Flexor Muscles

There are three major flexor muscles on the back of the foreleg that act on the knee. They function to flex the knee and extend the elbow.

Radial carpal flexor—This muscle originates on the humerus just above the elbow joint. It inserts via a thin tendon on the outside of the upper back surface of the cannon bone. As it passes over the knee it is surrounded and protected by a tendon sheath.

Ulnar carpal flexor—This muscle has two origins, one on the humerus just above the elbow joint, and another on the olecranon. From these origins it runs down and attaches to the back of the accessory carpal bone.

Lateral ulnar—This muscle originates on the bottom and back of the humerus and inserts onto the tops of the accessory carpal bone and outside splint bone.

148

In addition, the superficial and deep digital flexor tendons pass over the back of the knee and help to flex it.

Cannon
Bones

The *cannon bone* forms part of the knee joint at its top and part of the fetlock joint at its bottom. Its normal position is vertical. On each back corner of the cannon bone is a splint bone. Together, these three bones of the foreleg

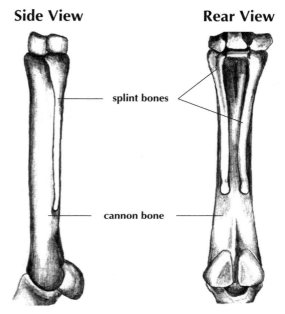

Side View　　**Rear View**

splint bones

cannon bone

Fig. 6–71. Bones of the cannon.

are known as the metacarpals. The cannon bone is the large metacarpal or third metacarpal.

Splint Bones

The *splint bones* in the foreleg are called the second and fourth, or medial and lateral metacarpal bones. The inside splint bone (medial metacarpal) is often slightly larger than the outside splint bone (lateral metacarpal). These bones are remnants, from when ancient horses had toes instead of hooves.

At the top, each splint bone is part of the carpal joint, or knee. At the bottom, the bone tapers down, ending on the side of the cannon bone about three inches above the fetlock. The triangular shape of a splint bone narrows from nearly an inch wide to as little as $1/16$ inch. At the small end there is a small bony knob that may be visible through the skin. The lower end does not have any direct support, but is in contact with the cannon bone and attached to it by the *interosseous ligament*. In horses over five years old this ligament usually ossifies (changes into bone), fusing the splint bone to the cannon bone. Splint bones have little useful value other than providing a

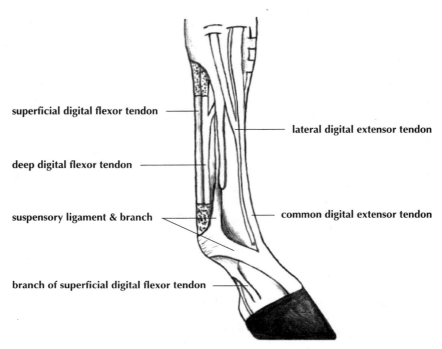

superficial digital flexor tendon

lateral digital extensor tendon

deep digital flexor tendon

suspensory ligament & branch

common digital extensor tendon

branch of superficial digital flexor tendon

Fig. 6–72. Outside (lateral) view of the tendons and ligaments of the cannon.

channel called the *metacarpal groove* for the flexor tendons and suspensory ligament, and also lending some support to the carpal bones.

Tendons and Ligaments of the Cannon

Passing down the front of the cannon bone are the flat, closely related tendons of the lateral digital extensor and the common digital extensor muscles. The superficial and deep digital flexor tendons run along the back of the cannon bone. The inferior check ligament is located between the suspensory ligament and the flexor tendons. The suspensory ligament of the fetlock runs next to the cannon bone underneath all these structures. Because its primary function is to support the fetlock, it is discussed in that section.

Blood Vessels of the Cannon

The lateral and medial *dorsal metacarpal arteries* supply the front of the cannon area with blood. The common digital, or *medial pal-*

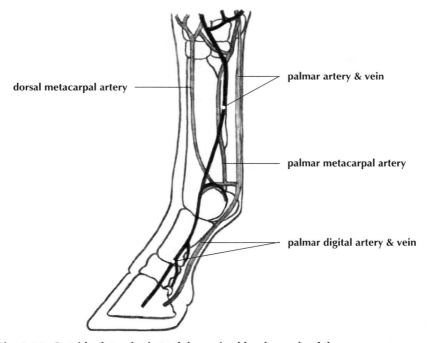

dorsal metacarpal artery

palmar artery & vein

palmar metacarpal artery

palmar digital artery & vein

Fig. 6–73. Outside (lateral) view of the major blood vessels of the cannon.

mar artery supplies the back of the cannon. This artery is the largest in the cannon area. Smaller, deeper arteries include the lateral and medial *palmar metacarpal arteries.* About three-fourths of the way down, the medial palmar artery divides into the lateral and medial *palmar digital arteries.*

The veins tend to follow the same general paths as the arteries and have similar names. The lateral and medial *palmar veins* drain the area of blood, returning it to the general circulation.

Nerves of the Cannon

Because there are no muscles below the knee, the nerves in the cannon area are sensory, not motor—they supply the area with sensation. The lateral and medial *palmar nerves* traverse either side of the back of the cannon, in a groove between the suspensory ligament and the flexor tendons. There is a communicating branch between them about mid-cannon.

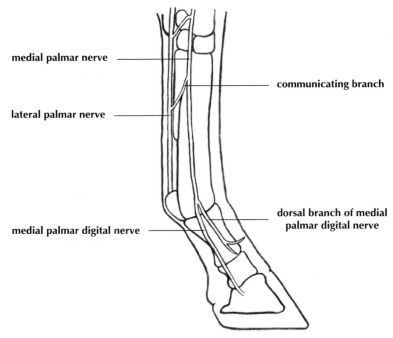

medial palmar nerve

communicating branch

lateral palmar nerve

medial palmar digital nerve

dorsal branch of medial palmar digital nerve

Fig. 6–74. Outside (lateral) view of the major nerves of the cannon.

Fetlock

The *fetlock joint,* always under tremendous stress, has two roles: shock absorption and locomotion. It is a hinge joint—capable of flexion and extension. Flexion is the position of the fetlock when the foot is being cleaned or shod. This is also called volar flexion. Extension is when all the joints of the lower leg are in a straight line, as when the horse extends the foreleg while galloping. In a normal standing position, the fetlock is partially hyperextended (also called partial dorsal flexion). This position allows the pastern to assume a slope equal to the angle of a well-shaped hoof. If, when the horse is galloping, the back of the fetlock hits the ground, it is called extreme hyperextension or overdorsiflexion.

Horses have an *ergot* under the bottom curve of the fetlock. It is a horny structure similar to the chestnut, usually hidden by hair. If it is so large that it gets in the way, it should be trimmed.

Bones

The fetlock is the joint formed by the bottom of the cannon bone and the top of the *long pastern bone*. This bone's normal standing position is slightly tilted at a 47° – 54° angle with the ground. Located at the back of the fetlock joint are the paired, roughly pyramid-shaped bones called *sesamoid bones.* These bones act as a pulley, increasing the leverage of the tendons that pass over them.

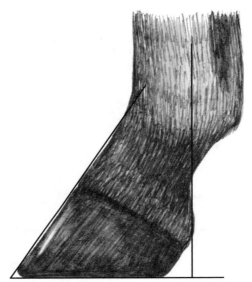

Fig. 6–75. The fetlock is partially hyperextended (bent backward).

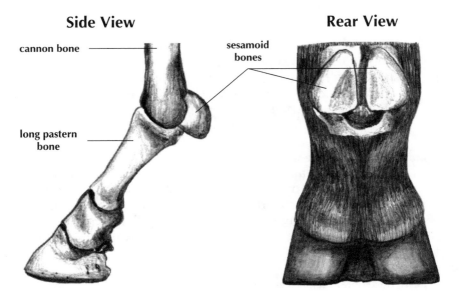

Side View

cannon bone

long pastern bone

Rear View

sesamoid bones

Fig. 6–76. The bones of the fetlock.

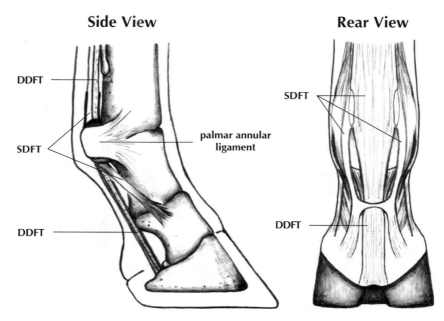

Side View

DDFT

SDFT

DDFT

palmar annular
ligament

Rear View

SDFT

DDFT

Fig. 6–77. The SDFT and DDFT at the back of the fetlock. On the rear view, the palmar annular ligament has been removed to show the branches of the sdft.

Tendons and Ligaments of the Fetlock

The tendons and ligaments of the fetlock hold it together, support its shock-absorbing movements, and enhance its locomotor function. The *collateral ligaments* of the fetlock joint and of the sesamoids hold the bones of the joint together. They and other structures are discussed here from superficial to deep.

Palmar Annular Ligament

The *palmar annular ligament* of the fetlock wraps horizontally around the back of the fetlock. This is a broad, strong support structure. It encloses the superficial and deep digital flexor tendons in their sheath, the sesamoidean ligaments, binding these structures close to the sesamoid bones. It attaches onto the outsides of the sesamoid bones.

Superficial Digital Flexor Tendon

The superficial digital flexor tendon (SDFT) runs down the back of the leg. It is surrounded and protected by a tendon sheath beginning about two inches above the sesamoid bones. It shares this sheath with the deep digital flexor tendon. As the SDFT branches just below the fetlock, it leaves the sheath and forms a loop through which the deep digital flexor tendon glides. Each branch inserts on either side of the lower long pastern bone and upper *short pastern bone.*

Deep Digital Flexor Tendon

The deep digital flexor tendon (DDFT) lies underneath the superficial flexor. After the SDFT leaves the common tendon sheath, it forms a loop through which the DDFT continues in the sheath down the back of the pastern. The tendon sheath ends just above the navicular bone in the foot. The DDFT then inserts on the underside of the coffin bone in the foot.

Suspensory Ligament

The *suspensory ligament* lies in the metacarpal groove created by the cannon and splint bones. It is a wide, thick band that originates on the upper back surface of the cannon bone and on the lower row of carpal bones.

At the lower quarter of the cannon it divides into two branches. Each branch passes to the outside face of the corresponding sesamoid bone, to which a large segment of the ligament attaches, nearly encasing the bone. The rest of the ligament passes downward and forward to the front surface of the long pastern bone where it merges with the common digital extensor tendon. There is a bursa (fluid-filled sac) between the suspensory's extensor branch and the upper end of the long pastern bone.

The suspensory ligament is more elastic than other ligaments. This is because it contains tendinous tissue. In young horses, it even has a small

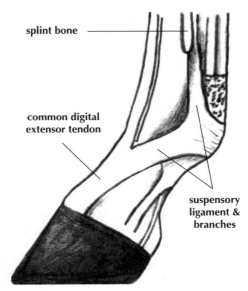

Fig. 6–78. Outside (lateral) view of the suspensory ligament supporting the fetlock.

155

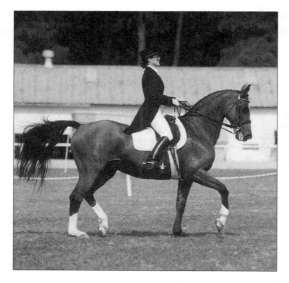

Fig. 6–79. Overdorsiflexion of the right rear fetlock joint—the fetlock nearly touches the ground.

amount of muscle tissue in its deep part (which is why it is also known as the interosseous muscle). Its main function is to support the fetlock, guarding against extreme hyperextension (or overdorsiflexion) of the joint. The two branches that join the common digital extensor tendon limit extreme flexion of the pastern joint.

Collateral Ligaments of the Fetlock

The *collateral ligaments* of the fetlock joint are short ligaments running from the bottom of the cannon bone to the top of the long pastern bone. They stabilize the fetlock joint.

Sesamoidean Ligaments

There are many small ligaments which fix the sesamoid bones in place at the back of the fetlock and pastern. They include the intersesamoidean ligament, the distal sesamoidean ligaments, the collateral sesamoidean ligaments, and the short sesamoidean ligaments.

Intersesamoidean ligament —The intersesamoidean ligament fills the space between the two sesamoid bones. It forms a groove for the flexor tendons to slide across.

Distal sesamoidean ligaments —There are three pairs of distal sesamoidean ligaments. The *straight sesamoidean ligament* attaches above to the bases of the sesamoid bones and the intersesamoidean ligament, and below to the short pastern bone. It stabilizes the pas

156

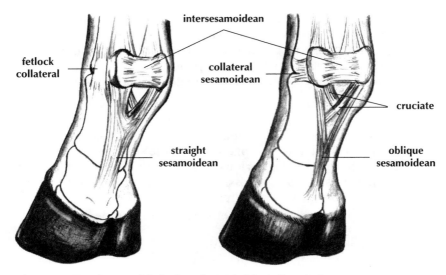

Fig. 6–80. Two layers of fetlock and sesamoidean ligaments.

tern joint. The *oblique sesamoidean ligament* attaches above to the base of the sesamoid bones and the intersesamoidean ligament, and below to the long pastern bone. The *cruciate ligaments* arise from the base of the sesamoids, cross each other, and insert on the opposite upper end of the back side of the long pastern bone.

Collateral sesamoidean ligaments—The collateral sesamoidean ligaments run horizontally from the outside of each sesamoid bone to the outside of the lower cannon bone and upper long pastern bone.

Short sesamoidean ligaments—The short sesamoidean ligaments extend from the front surface of the sesamoid bones directly to the back of the long pastern bone.

Suspensory Apparatus

The *suspensory apparatus* is a vital shock absorber for the leg. It is also one of the main supporting structures of the horse's fetlock, which is under heavy strain, even in the normal standing position. Under normal circumstances, the suspensory apparatus prevents the back of the fetlock from hitting the ground. The structures of suspensory apparatus begin at the knee and consist of:
- suspensory ligament
- superficial and deep flexor tendons and their check ligaments
- sesamoidean ligaments

The sesamoid bones are considered to be ossified parts of the suspensory apparatus. Weight is received and transmitted to the long pastern bone directly via the suspensory apparatus functioning through the sesamoid bones like a pulley.

The suspensory apparatus is an integral part of the stay apparatus.

Stay Apparatus

The stay apparatus is a system of muscles, tendons, and ligaments in the horse's leg. It works together with the suspensory apparatus to allow the horse to "lock" its lower leg joints with no muscular effort. This mechanism makes it possible for the horse to sleep while standing. The structures involved are:

- biceps brachii tendons (both origin and insertion)
- lacertus fibrosis tendon
- radial carpal extensor tendon
- common digital extensor tendon
- serratus ventralis muscle (thoracic portion)
- triceps muscle (long head)
- SDFT and superior check ligament
- DDFT and inferior check ligament
- suspensory ligament and its branches
- distal sesamoidean ligaments

Except for the *lacertus fibrosis tendon*, all of these structures are described earlier in this chapter. The lacertus fibrosis is a long tendinous band through the biceps brachii and the fascia (connective tissue) of the forearm. It ends by merging with the radial carpal extensor tendon. Its function is to assist the stay apparatus by stabilizing the knee, keeping it from buckling forward.

These structures work together to hold the legs in a normal standing position. For example, the serratus ventralis muscle supports the horse's body weight, which would normally flex the shoulder. But the biceps brachii tendons and the triceps muscle prevent this action by extending it. The SDFT and DDFT help by fixing the elbow joint. Of course, the bones from the elbow to the fetlock are situated in a more-or-less straight line, so it takes very little effort (by the lacertus fibrosis) to stabilize them. The fetlock joint, however, is under the constant heavy strain created by the horse's body weight. The suspensory apparatus, as part of the stay apparatus, holds it securely in the normal standing position.

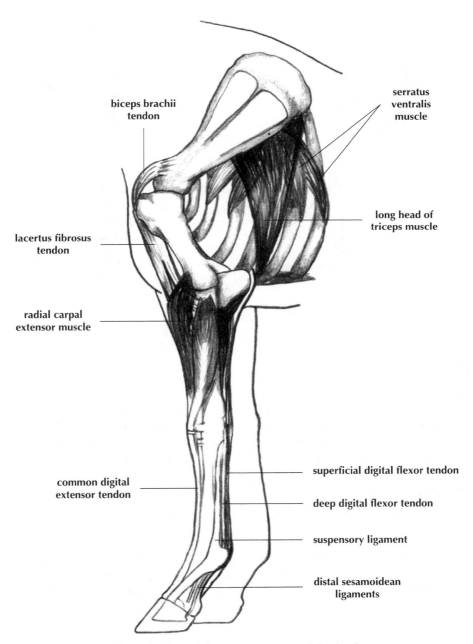

Fig. 6–81. Outside (lateral) view of the stay apparatus of the foreleg.

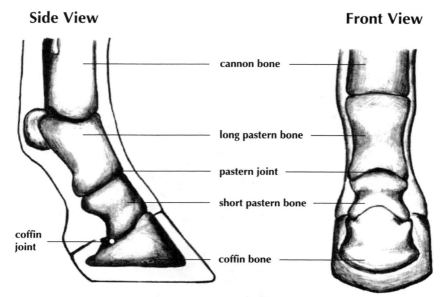

Side View

Front View

cannon bone

long pastern bone

pastern joint

short pastern bone

coffin joint

coffin bone

Fig. 6–82. Bones of the pastern.

Pastern

Bones

The pastern is the area between the fetlock and the coronet. The underlying bones are the long and short pastern bones (first and second phalanges). These bones are both slightly tilted in their normal standing position, at a 47° – 54° angle with the ground.

Pastern Joint

The *pastern joint* between the long and short pastern bones is capable of limited flexion and extension. This motion contributes to the flexion of the whole leg in motion, and extension while the bottom of the hoof is planted on the ground. The joint can also slightly flex from side to side, and even rotate a little when manipulated by hand. The lower end of the short pastern bone forms the coffin joint with the coffin bone in the foot.

Front View

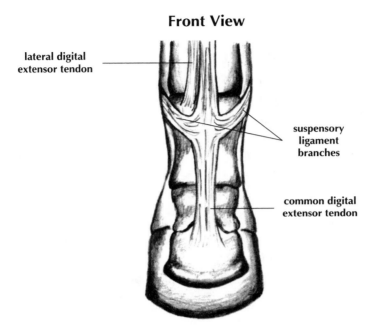

lateral digital
extensor tendon

suspensory
ligament
branches

common digital
extensor tendon

Fig. 6–83. Front view of the tendons and ligaments of the pastern.

Tendons and Ligaments

The common digital extensor tendon continues down the front of the pastern, flattening and widening as it goes. It inserts on the top of the coffin bone. The deep digital flexor tendon continues down the back of the pastern, over a tough plate of fibrocartilage before inserting on the underside of the coffin bone.

The pastern joint is stabilized by three sets of paired ligaments running from the long pastern bone to the short pastern bone. The *collateral ligaments* are located at the sides of the pastern. The other two pairs are *palmar ligaments*, located at the back of the pastern. Aiding these ligaments is the straight sesamoidean ligament, described in the Fetlock section.

The *proximal digital annular ligament* is made of upper and lower bands, forming a structure that resembles a butterfly bandage. Its four corners attach to the four back corners of the long pastern bone.

The *ligament of the ergot* runs from the back and bottom of the fetlock to insert on the palmar annular ligament. The ergot is actually an extension of the ligament. The ligament is vestigial, which means it has no modern function. It is a leftover from when horses had toes.

Side View

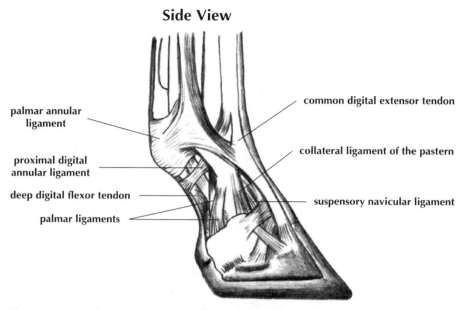

palmar annular ligament

proximal digital annular ligament

deep digital flexor tendon

palmar ligaments

common digital extensor tendon

collateral ligament of the pastern

suspensory navicular ligament

Fig. 6–84. Outside (lateral) view of the tendons and ligaments of the pastern. The bottom of the proximal digital annular ligament has been removed to reveal the structures beneath.

Rear View

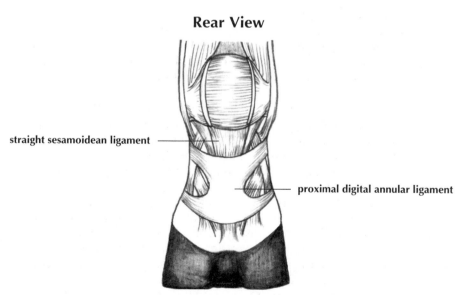

straight sesamoidean ligament

proximal digital annular ligament

Fig. 6–85. Rear (caudal) view of the tendons and ligaments of the pastern.

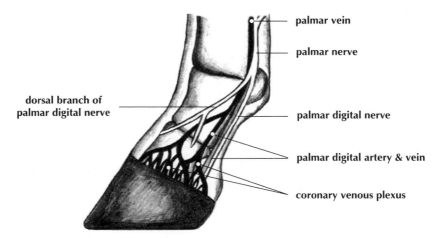

palmar vein

palmar nerve

dorsal branch of
palmar digital nerve

palmar digital nerve

palmar digital artery & vein

coronary venous plexus

Fig. 6–86. Outside (lateral) view of the major blood vessels and nerves of the pastern.

Blood Vessels of the Pastern

The common digital, or medial palmar artery supplies the pastern and foot with blood. Above the fetlock it divides into lateral and medial palmar digital arteries. These branches pass over each side of the fetlock and continue down the pastern and eventually supply the foot. Likewise, the lateral and medial palmar digital veins drain blood from the foot, sending it back up the leg.

Nerves of the Pastern

The lateral and medial *palmar digital nerves* run down the back of the pastern, on either side of the DDFT. They supply the pastern and foot with sensation. Each also has a dorsal branch that supplies the front of the pastern. 🐎

7

BODY

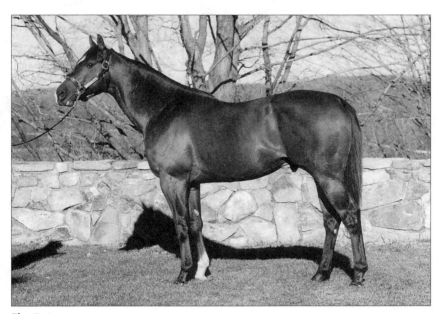

Fig. 7–1.

The body of the horse can be viewed in two parts: the back and the barrel. The back refers to the topline region between the end of the withers and the point of the croup. The barrel includes the chest cavity (or thorax) and the abdomen.

CONFORMATION OF THE BODY
Back

The *back* extends from the withers to the loins and supports much of the horse's weight. It also acts as a "suspension bridge" for the ribs, muscles, and other structures. Because it must support this weight—and often that of a rider—it is best if the horse has a relatively short, straight, wide back. Collection is also easier to accomplish for a horse with a shorter back. But overall, the best length of the back is one that produces good balance in the individual horse.

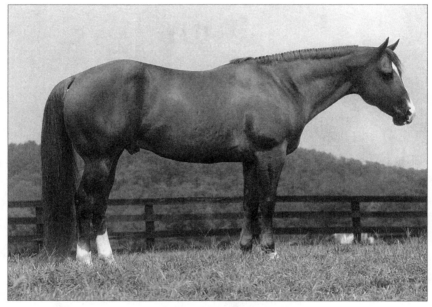

Fig. 7–2. This horse has a good, short, strong back.

The length of the back is determined by the length of each vertebra in the spinal column, rather than the number of vertebrae. Some breed enthusiasts contend that their horses' backs are shorter because the spinal columns have fewer vertebrae. Actually, research shows that the number of vertebrae varies more among individuals than among breeds. The backs of Arabian or Morgan horses may appear shorter than those of other breeds (which is a good trait), and they may differ more frequently than other breeds. But they generally have the same number of vertebrae.

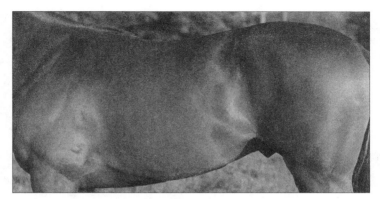

Fig. 7–3. A Thoroughbred's back.

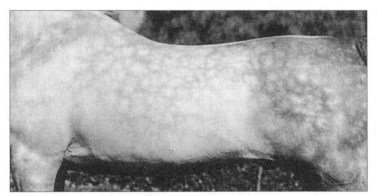

Fig. 7–4. An Arabian's back.

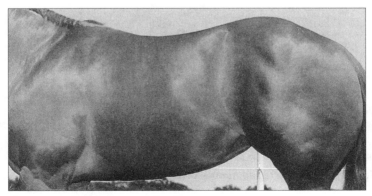

Fig. 7–5. A Quarter Horse's back.

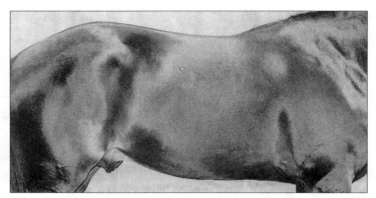

Fig. 7–6. A Standardbred's back.

Loin

The *loin* is a muscular portion of the horse's back that extends from the last rib to the *point of the croup*. The point of the croup should be about even with the peak of the withers or lower (see Chapter 4, *Withers,* for an illustration).

The loin is called the coupling because it supports the lumbar vertebrae, and transfers power from the hindlegs forward (impulsion). It performs these functions most effectively when it is short and well developed. A good rule of thumb is to have no more than about three

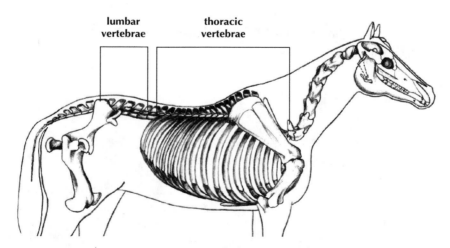

Fig. 7–7. The thoracic and lumbar vertebrae make up the back and loin.

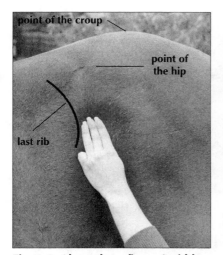

Fig. 7–8. About three fingers' width between the last rib and the point of the hip.

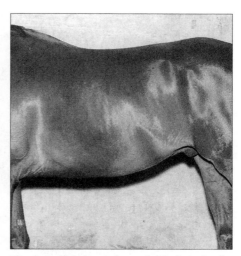

Fig. 7–9. This horse has a fairly long back, which is likely to tire and sag under stress.

fingers' width between the last rib and the point of the hip. A horse that is "well coupled" or "short coupled" in the loin has enough muscling to tense its spinal column to raise and propel the forehand. These muscles should be strong and supple.

Conformational Faults of the Back

Long Back and Long Loin

A long back is often accompanied by a long loin. A horse's back is considered long if it measures more than about one-third of the topline. A long loin creates a weak back and limits impulsion from the hindquarters. A horse's loin is considered long if it is more than about a hand's width across.

The back and loins work in concert to allow a horse to collect or "gather" itself: the back muscles straighten and stiffen the spinal column, and the loin muscles contract to pull the hindquarters forward. Unnecessary length in this area limits the horse's ability to collect quickly and powerfully. A longer back may give a more comfortable ride, but it is prone to tire and sag under stress, which can lead to muscle or ligament injury. It also prevents the horse from executing lateral (sideways) movements easily.

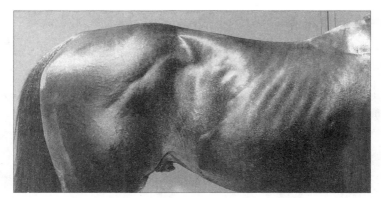

Fig. 7–10. A long loin limits impulsion from the hindquarters.

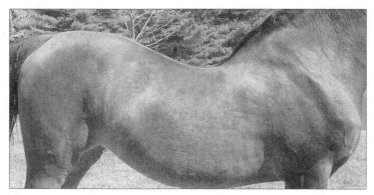

Fig. 7–11. A "sway back" does not provide adequate support.

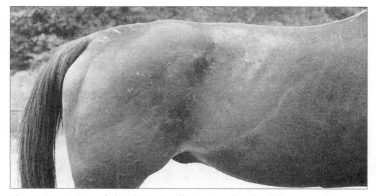

Fig. 7–12. A "roach back" is inefficient and inflexible.

Short Back

A short back is one that measures less than one-third of the total body length. Bending and flexing through the barrel is more difficult for a short-backed horse. This lack of flexibility also contributes to a choppy stride and limits the horse's foreleg scope. A horse with a short back is also more prone to interfere. However, a short back is generally not considered as serious a fault as a long back, and in fact can enable the horse to change direction with speed and agility.

Sway Back

A horse is *sway backed* when there is an exaggerated dip between the withers and loin. Sway backs are often the result of an overly long back and loin. The unnecessary length stresses the back ligaments, which weaken and sag. Sway back may also be caused by aging, pregnancy, and nutritional deficiencies, particularly lack of calcium.

Roach Back

The opposite of a sway back, a *roach back* has a concave arch along the topline, especially in the loin. Because this horse's spinal column is already curved up, its upward range of motion is limited. This motion is necessary to elevate the back and engage the hindquarters during collection. Also, the horse is usually less flexible laterally.

Barrel

The *barrel* on a well-conformed horse is deep and wide to accommodate the heart and expanding lungs. Traditionally, the *heartgirth*, defined as the distance around the horse just behind the forelegs, should be greater than the horse's height. In racehorses, a huge barrel is a sign of a sprinter, but a stayer's body is longer instead of heavier.

A spacious rib cage protects the heart, lungs, and other internal organs within it. Many of the muscles associated with the neck and legs attach to the ribs. The shape of the rib cage partly determines the limitations of the barrel. The ribs should be well arched and project backward instead of down. There should also be large spaces between the ribs to allow room for lung expansion. Together, these two traits create a long, deep underline and heartgirth (for power); and a short, straight back and loin (for strength). Such a horse has *"well-sprung ribs"* or is *"well ribbed up."*

Fig. 7–13. The shape of the rib cage influences the conformation of the barrel.

short loin

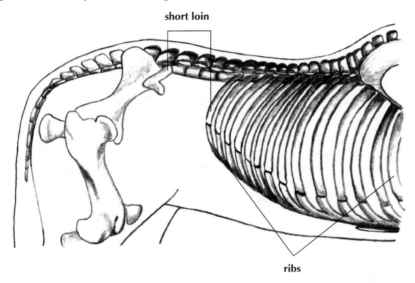

ribs

Well-sprung ribs. The ribs are rounded and project backward, creating a rounded barrel and a short loin.

long loin

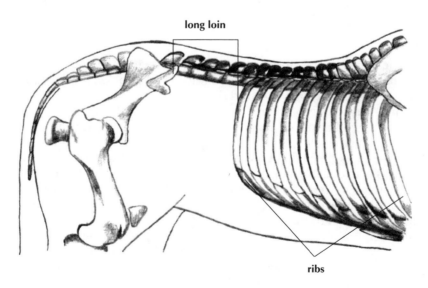

ribs

Not well-sprung ribs. The ribs are flat and project straight down, creating a slab-sided horse with a long loin.

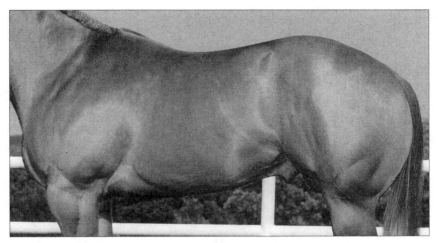

Fig. 7–14. A deep chest cavity.

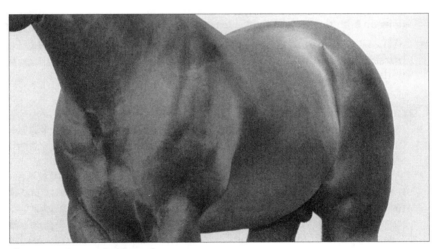

Fig. 7–15. A rounded barrel.

Viewed from the side, the deepest point of the barrel should be the heartgirth, which is a straight line from the back of the withers to the girth area. The underline, or abdominal area, should rise cleanly to the groin. The underline should slope gradually, not sharply up toward the flank.

Viewed from the front, the barrel should be plainly visible on either side of the horse. It should also be symmetrical.

Flank

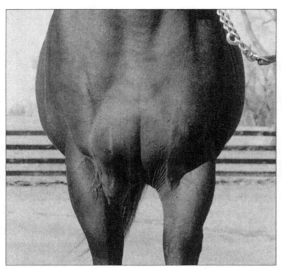

The *flank* of the horse is on the lower body between the ribs and hip. It should give the horse's middle a balanced appearance. On a hardworking horse with good muscle tone in its abdomen, the flanks may be cut up high. Racehorses are especially known for this characteristic.

Flank movements indicate a horse's wind capacity and breathing rate. The horse's respiration should be slow and regular (12 – 18 per minute) without panting or jerkiness.

Fig. 7–16. The barrel should have the same proportions on both the left and right sides of the horse.

Conformational Faults of the Barrel

A *"slab-sided"* horse has short, flat, straight, or upright ribs. The horse has little room for development of heart and lung capacity, which limits its performance potential.

High flanks should be discriminated against in a horse that does not have good muscle tone—or one with a weak loin. A horse that is excessively "tucked up" like a greyhound has little strength for fast turns or maneuvers. Such a horse is referred to as *"hound-gutted"* or *"wasp-waisted."* Further, the horse should not have too much of a "waist" between the belly and the flank.

On the other hand, if the barrel is too wide, the horse must swing the hindquarters around the barrel during normal movement, resulting in wasted motion. A *"hay belly,"* where the abdomen drops below the chest line, may indicate lack of fitness of the abdominal muscles.

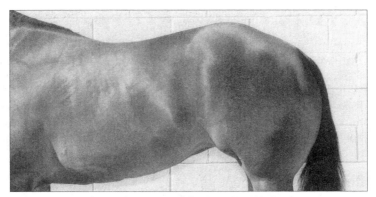

Fig. 7–17. A horse with a normal flank and body depth.

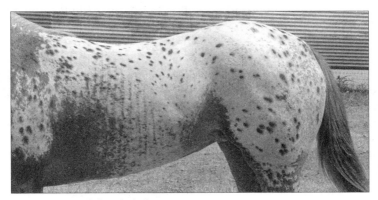

Fig. 7–18. A "slab-sided" horse.

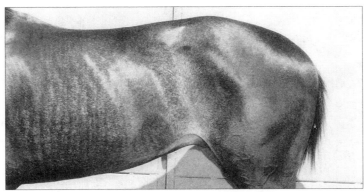

Fig. 7–19. A "hound-gutted" or "wasp-waisted" horse.

ANATOMY OF THE BODY

The anatomy of the back, *thorax,* and *abdomen* is extremely complex due to the presence of the internal organs—the respiratory, circulatory, digestive, and reproductive systems are completely or partially enclosed by the barrel. To simplify their discussion, we will address the internal body systems separately in Chapter 14, *Body Systems.* The following section describes the structures that give the barrel shape, allow movement, and support the internal organs.

Bones

The back and barrel are supported and moved by a complex system of bones, cartilage, muscles, and ligaments. The bones involved are the thoracic and lumbar vertebrae, the ribs, and the sternum (breastbone).

Vertebrae

The *vertebrae* of the *spinal column* protect the spinal cord and provide attachment sites for muscles. This section of the spinal column is strong and relatively rigid, as compared to cats, for example. It does not flex very far in any direction. The vertebrae are joined by *intervertebral discs.* These discs are cartilaginous (made of cartilage) pads that absorb shock as well as create a joint. If the intervertebral

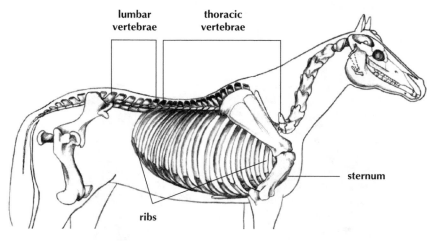

Fig. 7–20. Outside (lateral) view of the bones of the back and barrel.

discs are fairly thick, the spinal column will be more flexible. As the horse ages, the discs often become calcified and hardened, especially in performance horses. This is why the horse's back stiffens with age.

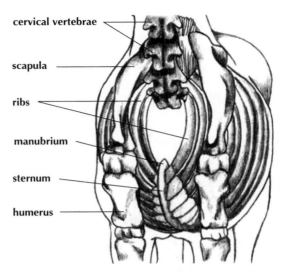

Labels on figure:
cervical vertebrae
scapula
ribs
manubrium
sternum
humerus

Fig. 7–21. Front (cranial) view of the bones of the barrel.

Thoracic

Starting at the base of the horse's skull and moving toward the tail, the *thoracic vertebrae* are the second "set" of vertebrae in the spinal column. They immediately follow the cervical vertebrae (the first "set" in the neck), and extend to the middle of the back. There are usually 18 thoracic vertebrae. Horses have been known to have 19, and 17 is not uncommon. The first 6 or 7 thoracic vertebrae are located behind the scapula (shoulder blade).

The thoracic vertebrae are composed of a *body* (a round mass of bone), an *arch* that forms the foramen through which the spinal cord travels, and several *spinous processes*. The spinous processes (projections) provide attachment and support for other bones, muscles, ligaments, and nerves. The names of the spinous processes are:

- *dorsal spinous process* above
- *ventral process* (or ventral crest) below
- *transverse process* (or lateral process), one on each side
- *articular process*, one on each end (cranial/caudal)

The thoracic vertebrae have tall dorsal spinous processes. The first 10 or so thoracic vertebrae are the tallest and form the outline of the withers. The height of the dorsal spinous processes determines whether a horse is high withered, low withered, roach backed, or sway backed. Moving toward the tail, the dorsal spinous processes become shorter. Conversely, the transverse processes become longer, extending further out on each side. Occasionally the transverse processes of the last two thoracic vertebrae are fused together.

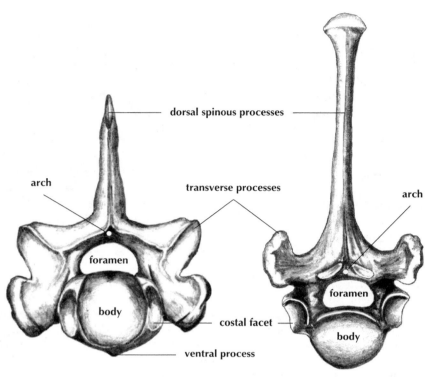

dorsal spinous processes

arch

transverse processes

arch

foramen

foramen

body

costal facet

body

ventral process

Fig. 7–22. Left: Rear (caudal) view of the 1st thoracic vertebra. Right: Front (cranial) view of the 7th thoracic vertebra.

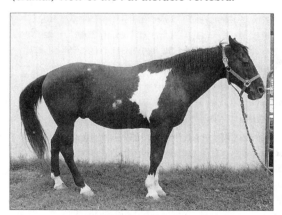

Fig. 7–23. The low withers and roach back on this horse are determined by the height of the dorsal spinous processes.

The thoracic vertebrae are unique because they form joints with the ribs. Each thoracic vertebra (except the last one) has four joint surfaces called *costal facets* on its body. Each costal facet forms half a "socket." A facet on the adjoining vertebra forms the other half of the socket. The rib forms a joint with this socket and with similarly placed facets on the transverse processes of the vertebra. *(See Figures 7–25 and 7–26.)*

Lumbar Vertebrae

Following the thoracic vertebrae are the *lumbar vertebrae,* the third "set" of vertebrae in the spinal column. There are usually six lumbar vertebrae, extending from mid-back to the point of the croup. Some horses have been known to have five, especially those with 19 thoracic vertebrae. The lumbar vertebrae have the same basic construction as the thoracic vertebrae. However, the transverse processes are longer, sometimes 4 inches long, at the third or fourth lumbar vertebrae. The lumbar vertebrae are also distinguished from thoracic vertebrae in that they do not form joints with the ribs. This part of the spinal column is even less flexible than the thoracic part.

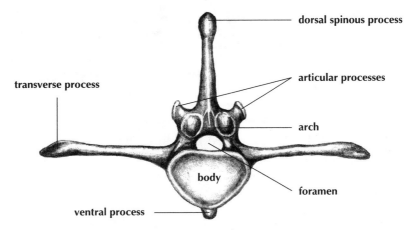

Fig. 7–24. Rear (caudal) view of a lumbar vertebra.

Ribs

The *ribs* form the skeleton of the thoracic walls on each side of the horse. These flexible, curved bones are arranged in 18 opposing pairs, although there are sometimes 19 pairs. (The number of ribs depends on the number of thoracic vertebrae, because the ribs are attached to these vertebrae.) The ribs protect the vital organs, and also serve as attachment sites for muscles. For example, the first nine ribs are attachment sites for the serratus ventralis muscle activating the shoulder. The intercostal spaces—the gaps between the ribs—are also well muscled.

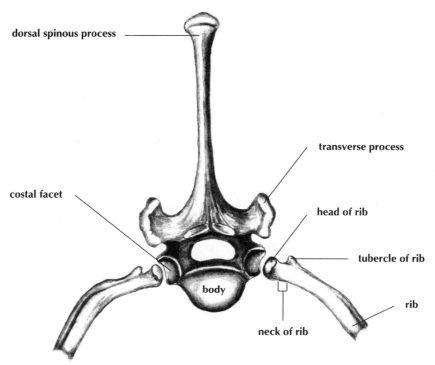

dorsal spinous process

transverse process

costal facet

head of rib

tubercle of rib

body

rib

neck of rib

Fig. 7–25. Front (cranial) view of the joints between the ribs and a thoracic vertebra.

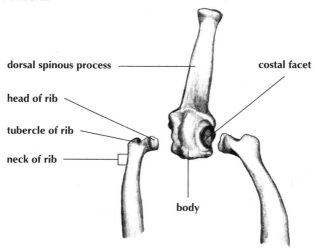

dorsal spinous process

costal facet

head of rib

tubercle of rib

neck of rib

body

Fig. 7–26. The same connection with a different vertebra at a different angle.

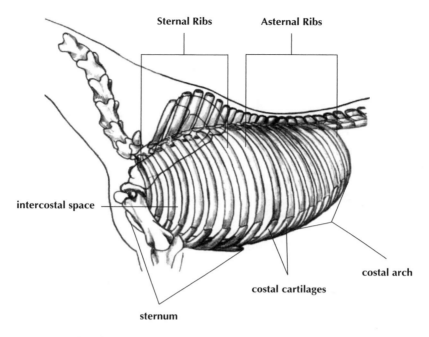

Sternal Ribs   Asternal Ribs

intercostal space

costal arch

costal cartilages

sternum

Fig. 7–27. The ribs form the walls of the thorax.

The first rib is the shortest and is directed slightly forward and down. The second rib is vertical and the remaining ribs are (ideally) sloped backward and down.

Although they vary in length and curvature, each rib consists of a curved shaft and two ends, or extremities. The top of the rib (vertebral extremity) has a *head, neck,* and *tubercle* by which it attaches to the spinal column. The head of the rib is a smooth, rounded surface connected to the shaft by a narrow neck. The head forms a joint between two costal facets of the thoracic vertebrae. The tubercle is a small, knobby extension, slightly back from the neck of the rib, that forms a joint with the transverse process of the adjacent thoracic vertebrae. The bottom of the rib (sternal extremity) is extended by a cartilage, called the *costal cartilage.*

Sternal Ribs

The first eight pairs of ribs are called the *sternal* or *"true" ribs.* They called "true" because they are joined directly to the sternum by the costal cartilages.

Asternal Ribs

Asternal, or *"false" ribs* are not joined directly to the sternum. There are usually 10 of these ribs, but 11 or 9 are not unusual. At the sternal extremity of each rib, the costal cartilages angle forward and fuse together, forming one common connection called the *costal arch.* The last one or two pairs of asternal ribs are called *"floating ribs"* because their sternal extremities are often not attached to those of adjacent ribs.

Sternum

The *sternum,* or breastbone, forms the floor of the thorax. This bone is composed of eight joined segments called *sternebrae.* The sternebrae fuse as the horse ages. It is canoe-shaped, with the "stern" of the canoe in the chest region and the "bow" in the thorax. The rearmost tip of the sternum is called the *xiphoid cartilage.* It is located at about the girth area on the dorsal midline on the underside of the thorax. It serves as an attachment point for the diaphragm muscle.

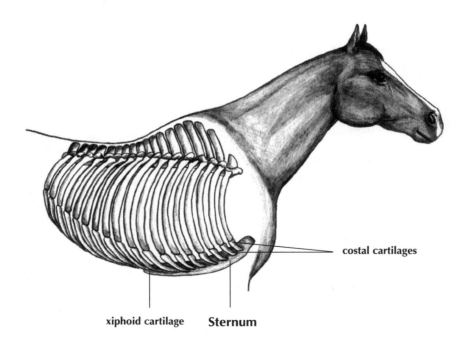

costal cartilages

xiphoid cartilage   **Sternum**

Fig. 7–28. The sternum forms the floor of the thorax.

Fascia and Ligaments of the Body

Fascia is the body's connective tissue. A large sheet of very strong, tendinous fascia is draped over the horse's back and loins. It is called the *lumbodorsal fascia* (or sometimes the thoracolumbar fascia). It aids the abdominal muscles in supporting the heavy weight of the internal organs. Several of the abdominal muscles originate or insert on the lumbodorsal fascia.

The *supraspinous ligament* in the back is a continuation of the nuchal ligament in the neck. It serves much the same purpose: to support the vertebrae and assist the back and abdominal muscles.

Small supporting ligaments surround the vertebrae: between the dorsal spinous processes, below the bodies, and under the transverse processes.

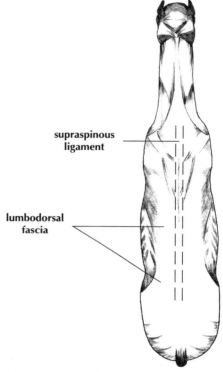

supraspinous ligament

lumbodorsal fascia

Fig. 7–29. Top (dorsal) view of the fascia. The dotted line shows the position of the supraspinous ligament beneath the lumbodorsal fascia.

Muscles of the Body
Back Muscles

The back muscles support and move the vertebrae. They flex and extend the spinal column, both vertically and laterally (side-to-side). The major muscles of the back are listed below.

Longissimus dorsi—The longissimus dorsi is the longest and largest muscle in the horse's body. It runs from the sacrum (point of the croup) to the neck, connecting to each thoracic and lumbar vertebra. The vertebrae are connected from transverse process to dorsal spinous process, from transverse process to transverse process, and

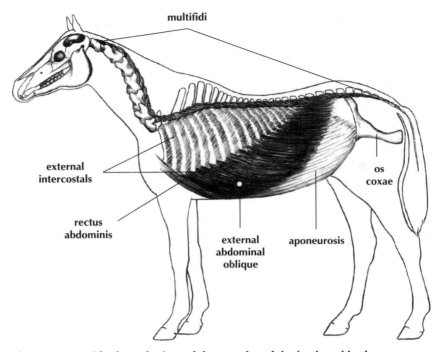

Fig. 7–30. Outside (lateral) view of the muscles of the back and body.

from dorsal spinous process to dorsal spinous process. The longissimus dorsi has half of its mass on each side of the spinal column and is the most powerful extensor of the back and loins when both sides act together. It holds the spinal column rigid, allowing the horse to pick up its forehand. Each half may also act independently, flexing the spinal column laterally. The muscle also assists in respiration and extending the horse's neck.

Multifidi—This complex set of muscles runs from the articular processes of each vertebra to the dorsal spinous process of the previous vertebra. In this way, the mutifidi weave the vertebrae together. When both sides contract at once, they extend, or straighten, the spinal column. When only one side contracts, it flexes, or bends, the spinal column laterally.

Psoas, major and minor—These muscles are primarily hip flexors, but they also help the longissimus dorsi to hold the spinal column rigid, preventing it from flexing vertically. They are discussed and illustrated in Chapter 8, *Hindlegs.*

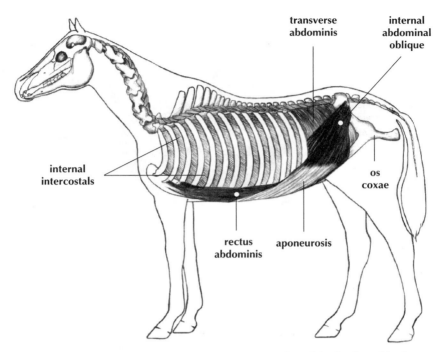

transverse
abdominis

internal
abdominal
oblique

internal
intercostals

os
coxae

rectus
abdominis

aponeurosis

Fig. 7–31. Outside (lateral) view of the deeper muscles of the back and body: the external abdominal oblique muscle from Figure 7–30 has been removed.

Latissimus dorsi—Primarily a shoulder flexor, this muscle also supports the thorax and draws the thorax forward when the leg is fixed. It is discussed and illustrated in Chapter 6, *Forelegs.*

Abdominal Muscles

The abdominal muscles are strong, extensive muscles that form most of the abdominal wall. They are arranged in layers, but each muscle runs in a different direction. This provides effective support of the internal organs, including the digestive and reproductive systems (especially of the mare during pregnancy). The abdominal muscles compress the abdomen, aiding in defecation, urination, exhalation, coughing, and birthing. They also arch the back and flex the trunk laterally by acting on one side only. Following is a list of the four abdominal muscles on each side of the body.

External abdominal oblique—This muscle is the most superficial. It originates on the outside of the ribs and the lumbodorsal fascia. The

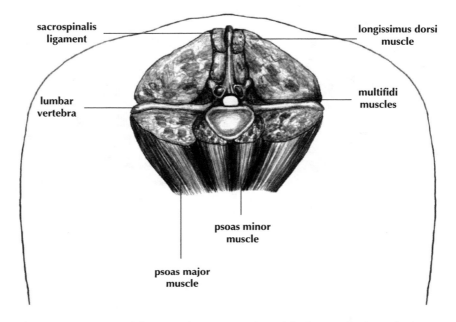

Fig. 7–32. Front (cranial) view of a cross-section of the horse's body at the loin.

muscle then becomes a broad, flat tendon called an aponeurosis, which inserts at the dorsal midline. Here it meets the opposite tendon.

Internal abdominal oblique—Just under the external abdominal oblique, the internal abdominal oblique originates from a deeper portion of the lumbodorsal fascia, the *inguinal ligament*, and the ilium (one of three bones that form the pelvis). It inserts in the same manner as the external abdominal oblique, becoming a broad tendon and meeting the opposite tendon at the dorsal midline.

Rectus abdominis—This hammock-shaped muscle runs along the floor of the abdomen. It originates on the sternum and the first few ribs. Eventually it becomes the *prepubic tendon*, which inserts on the pubis (another of three pairs of fused bones that form the pelvis).

Transverse abdominis—This is the deepest of the abdominal muscles. It originates at the deepest fascia of the back and inserts at the dorsal midline.

MUSCLES OF THE BACK

Name	Origin	Insertion	Function
Longissimus dorsi	each vertebra from sacrum to neck	each vertebra from sacrum to neck	pair: extend spine; single: flex spine laterally; support vertebrae; aid respiration
Multifidi	each vertebra from sacrum to neck	each vertebra from sacrum to neck	pair: extend spine; single: flex spine laterally
Psoas, major & minor	last few thoracic vertebrae; lumbar vertebrae	lesser trochanter of femur; lower front of os coxae	help to hold spine horizontal
Latissimus dorsi	thoracic and lumbar vertebrae	teres tuberosity of humerus	support & draw thorax forward

Fig. 7–33.

MUSCLES OF THE ABDOMEN

Name	Origin	Insertion	Function
External abdominal oblique	outside of ribs	dorsal midline	• support internal organs
Internal abdominal oblique	lumbodorsal fascia, inguinal ligament, and ilium	dorsal midline	• aid defecation, urination, exhalation, coughing, and birthing
Rectus abdominis	sternum and first few ribs	pubis	• pair: arch back
Transverse abdominis	lumbodorsal fascia	dorsal midline	• single: flex barrel laterally

Fig. 7–34.

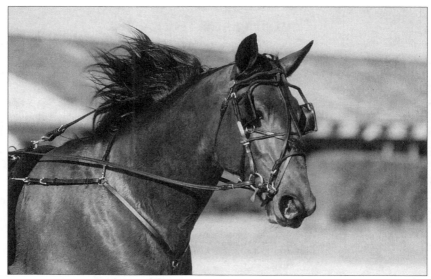

Fig. 7–35. The diaphragm muscle is of critical importance, allowing intake of air into the lungs.

Respiratory Muscles

The muscles of respiration are attached to the thoracic vertebrae, the ribs and their cartilages, and the sternum. They expand the thorax for inhalation, and contract the thorax for exhalation. The most important of these are the external intercostal muscles, internal intercostal muscles, and the diaphragm.

External intercostals—The external intercostal muscles extend downward and backward from each rib to the next rib in back. The action of these muscles increases the size of the thorax by rotating the ribs upward and forward.

Internal intercostals—The internal intercostal muscles are the next layer beneath the external intercostals. These muscles extend from each rib downward and forward to the previous rib. They rotate the ribs backward, decreasing the size of the thorax.

Diaphragm—This unpaired, dome-shaped muscle is the principle muscle of inhalation, and is therefore of critical importance. It lies behind the lungs, effectively separating the thorax and abdomen. It originates on the costal cartilages of the last true rib and the false ribs, and also on the lumbar vertebrae and xiphoid cartilage. It inserts via a common tendon, much as the abdominal muscles do.

MUSCLES OF RESPIRATION

Name	Origin	Insertion	Function
External intercostals	each rib	next rib backward	rotate ribs up and forward to increase size of thorax
Internal intercostals	each rib	previous rib forward	rotate ribs down and forward to decrease size of thorax
Diaphragm	costal cartilages of last true ribs and false ribs; lumbar vertebrae; xiphoid cartilage	a central tendon	principle muscle for inhalation

Fig. 7–36.

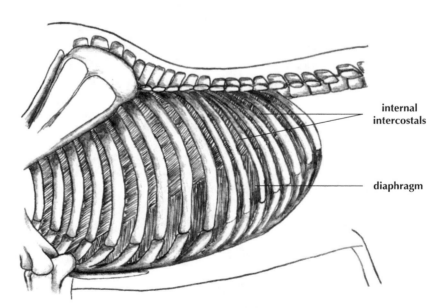

internal intercostals

diaphragm

Fig. 7–37. Outside (lateral) view of the deep respiratory muscles. The rear half of the internal intercostals have been removed, revealing the diaphragm beneath the ribs.

Nerves

All along the spinal column, pairs of spinal nerves emerge from between the vertebrae. Each pair in the thorax and loin is named for the vertebra in front of it. For example, the second thoracic spinal nerve emerges from between the second and third thoracic vertebrae. There are 18 pairs of *thoracic spinal nerves*. Their branches supply the longissimus dorsi and the multifidi muscles.

The *intercostal nerves* are also branches of the thoracic nerves. They run with a corresponding artery and vein down the rear border of each rib. The last thoracic nerve gives rise to the *costoabdominal nerve*. This nerve is just like the intercostal nerves, but it runs behind the last rib and so has a different name. The intercostal and costoabdominal nerves supply the abdominal and respiratory muscles.

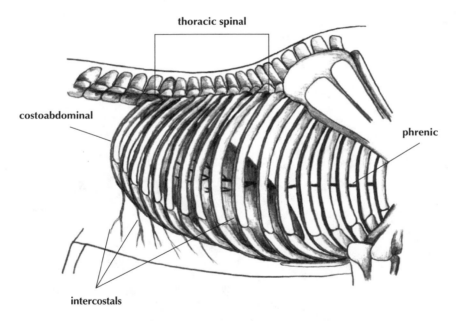

Fig. 7–38. Outside (lateral) view of the major nerves of the body.

There are six pairs of *lumbar spinal nerves*. Some of them supply the abdominal muscles, and many contribute to the *lumbar plexus* nerve group of the hindleg. (See Chapter 14, *Body Systems,* for an illustration.)

The *phrenic nerve* begins as the sixth and seventh cervical nerves. It supplies the diaphragm muscle, causing it to contract.

8

HINDLEGS

A horse's hindlegs should be straight, strong, and well muscled to aid in the forward propulsion of the body. The hindlegs supply much more power toward locomotion than the forelegs. Their connection to the spinal column is direct, giving them a solid base for propulsion, and the muscles are larger and stronger in the hindlegs than in the forelegs.

Because the hindlegs drive extremely hard to push a horse forward, the column of bones in the hindleg, from the hindquarters to the foot, is a system designed to spread concussion evenly. Any conformational defect in the hindlegs causes excess stress due to uneven distribution of concussion.

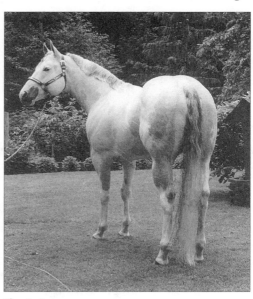

Fig. 8–1.

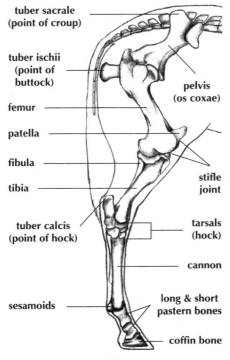

tuber sacrale
(point of croup)

tuber ischii
(point of
buttock)

femur

patella

fibula

tibia

tuber calcis
(point of hock)

sesamoids

pelvis
(os coxae)

stifle
joint

tarsals
(hock)

cannon

long & short
pastern bones

coffin bone

Fig. 8–2. The column of bones is designed to spread pressure evenly.

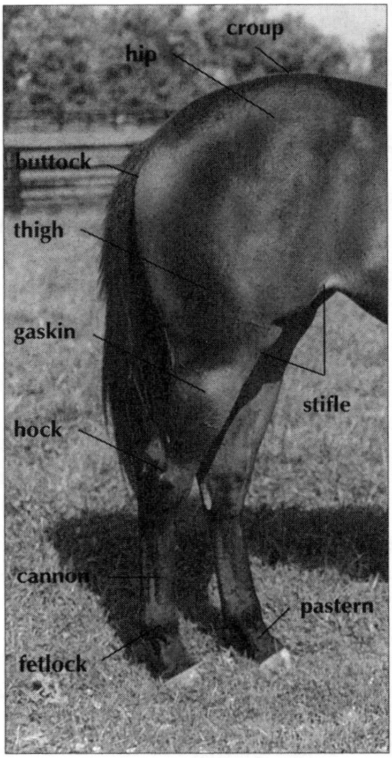

hip
croup
buttock
thigh
gaskin
hock
stifle
cannon
pastern
fetlock

Fig. 8–3. Parts of the hindleg.

CONFORMATION OF THE HINDLEG
From the Side

Viewed from the side, the angles of the stifle and hock should appear neither too straight nor too angled. On a horse standing with the cannons vertical, a line dropped straight down from the *point of the buttock* should touch the *point of the hock* and the back of the cannon on its way to the ground.

The terms *"straight behind"* or *"post-legged"* indicate excessively straight legs when viewed from the side. In this case there is very little angle between the thigh and gaskin. The hock and pastern are also straight, and the imaginary line will fall through the cannon instead of behind it. A horse with this defect is easily injured by heavy work, and is prone to arthritis, bone spavin, and upward fixation of the patella.

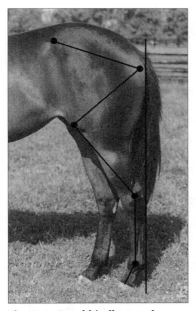

Fig. 8–4. Good hindleg conformation viewed from the side.

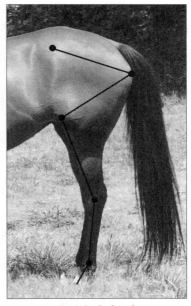

Fig. 8–5. Straight behind.

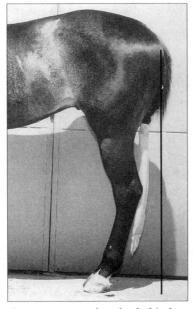

Fig. 8–6. Camped under behind.

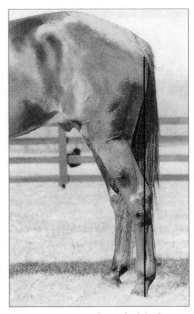

Fig. 8–7. Camped out behind.

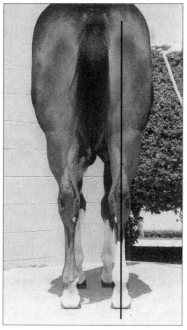

Fig. 8–8. Good hindleg conformation from the rear.

"Camped under behind" describes a leg that is placed too far forward when viewed from the side. In this case, a straight line from the point of the buttock falls too far behind the cannon. This fault is also called "standing under."

A leg that is placed too far back when viewed from the side is called *"camped out behind."* The imaginary line falls through the middle of the cannon. This fault is often accompanied by upright pasterns.

From the Rear

Viewed from the rear, the leg should be straight with no deviation of the hock. An imaginary line dropped from the point of the buttock to the ground should bisect the hock, cannon, fetlock, and pastern. Two conformational faults of the

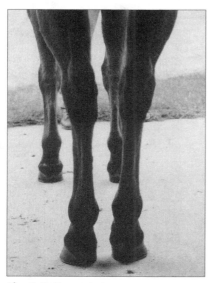

Fig. 8–9. Base narrow.

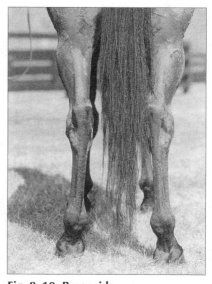

Fig. 8–10. Base wide.

hindleg that can be seen from the rear are *base narrow* and *base wide*. A base narrow horse is narrower between the feet than between the hindlegs at the gaskin. A base wide horse has a wider distance between the feet than between the hindlegs at the gaskin.

Hindquarters

The *hindquarters* consist of the upper part of the hindleg: the croup, pelvis (hip to buttock), and thigh. The hindquarters are shaped by layers of large, powerful muscles. The longer the bones, the longer and more powerful are the muscles that attach to them. To an extent, the type of muscling varies among breeds. Working Quarter Horses are known for their bulky hindquarter muscles. Arabian endurance horses have smooth, flat muscling.

From behind, the hindquarters should look "square," with the croup rounded and both sides symmetrical. The notable exception to this is the Quarter Horse, in which a pear shape is more desirable. Quarter Horses, draft horses, and overweight horses are sometimes *"double-rumped,"* meaning that a groove is visible down the center. At the other extreme, narrow hindquarters lack power and cause the hindlegs to be too close together.

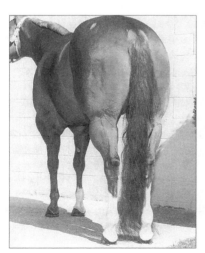

Fig. 8–11. Quarter Horses have bulky hindquarter muscles.

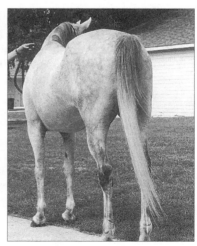

Fig. 8–12. Arabian horses have smooth, flat muscling.

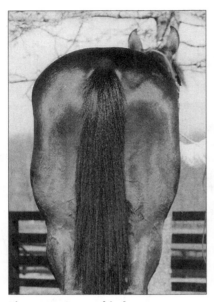

Fig. 8–13. Square hindquarters.

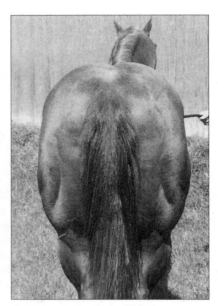

Fig. 8–14. Pear-shaped hindquarters.

Croup

The *croup* is the area along the horse's topline from the loin to the base of the tail *(see Figure 8–3)*. Seen from the side, the *point of the hip* should be in line with or just in front of the *point of the croup*. The point of the hip is a bony prominence that marks the front of the pelvis: the tuber coxae *(see Figure 8–2)*. The croup should be fairly long, as measured from the point of the hip to the point of the buttock. The point of the buttock marks the back of the pelvis: the tuber ischii. Ample length between the two points gives the muscles over the croup more power and leverage.

Ideally, the croup should be about the same height or lower than the withers. However, different breeds and types do vary a little. Draft horses and Shetland ponies are sometimes higher at the croup than at the withers. This may be acceptable for the work they do, but it is not necessarily desirable. It is best if the withers are slightly higher than the croup, because this conformation shifts the center of gravity forward and allows the hindlegs to work under the body. It also helps to fit a saddle better.

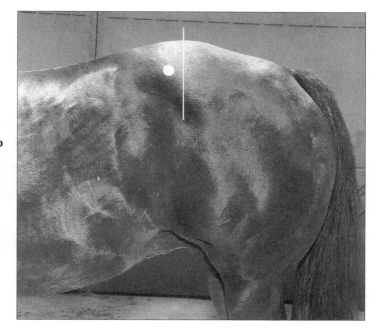

Fig. 8–15. The point of the hip should be just in front of the point of the croup.

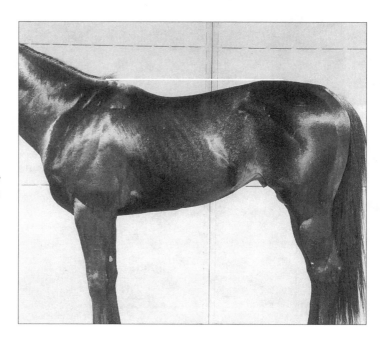

Fig. 8–16. The point of the croup should be about the same height or lower than the peak of the withers.

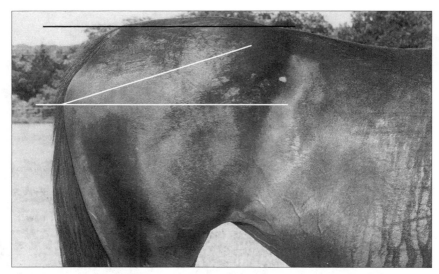

Fig. 8–17. A high tail carriage can make the croup appear more level than it is.

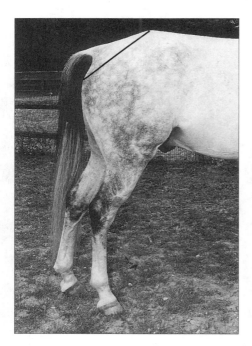

Fig. 8–18. If the croup is severely angled, and the point of the buttock is too low, the horse is called "goose-rumped."

Flat Croup

The angle of the croup is the slope from the point of the hip to the point of the buttock relative to the ground. A flat croup allows a horse to develop a long, ground-covering stride. Arabians often have flat, level croups, which is one reason why endurance competitors often prefer this breed. For the same reason, the current preference of Warmblood breeders, especially in horses used for dressage, is a lower and flatter croup.

Sometimes the angle of the croup can be deceptive. A high tail carriage can make the croup appear more level than it is. Sway-backed horses develop a more level croup over time.

Steep Croup

If the croup is severely angled, and the point of the buttock is too low, the horse is called *"goose-rumped."* A steep croup is usually short, which reduces the range of motion necessary to generate speed. A short croup also provides fewer points for muscle attachment, which further reduces speed and efficiency. However, a fairly steep croup allows a horse to get its hindlegs "under itself." This is an advantage for activities such as barrel racing, reining, and cutting. Tennessee Walking Horses tend to have steep croups, which enables them to perform their specific gaits efficiently. Draft horses that have this conformational trait gain leverage for pulling heavy objects.

Hunter's Bump

If, when seen from the side, the point of the croup is sharp, it is sometimes called *"hunter's bumps"* or "jumper's bumps." This is an injury caused by sacro-iliac subluxation, which is the tearing of the ligaments at the sacro-iliac joint. This allows the sacrum of the spinal column to displace from the ilium of the pelvis. A weak loin and long back are often contributing factors, as they reduce the horse's ability to properly gather

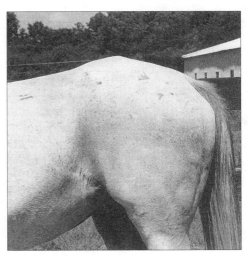

Fig. 8–19. Hunter's bump.

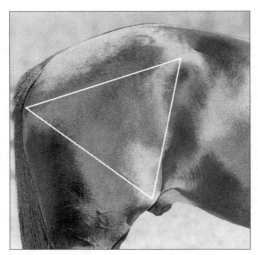

and collect itself (see Chapter 7, *Body*). Either side of the pelvis may be affected. Seen from behind, it is obvious that one side of the croup is higher than the other. The feature is more prominent if there is also muscle atrophy over the croup.

Fig. 8–20. If the croup and thigh are fairly long, the hindquarters have a triangular shape.

Thigh

The *thigh* area lies between the hip and the stifle. The thigh should be long and more-or-less perpendicular to the ground, creating deep hindquarters when viewed from the side.

Viewed from the rear, the inside of the thigh and outside of the stifle should be well developed and wide. Again, very well-developed muscles here and in the buttocks are standard for the Quarter Horse.

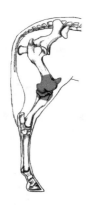

Stifle

The *stifle* should be about the same height as the elbow. It should also be in a well-forward position, giving a rectangular shape to the thigh from a side view. A stifle that is too far back indicates a short thigh and from the side has a V-shape instead of rectangular. Full muscling that arches smoothly over the stifle denotes strength and contributes to the rectangular shape when viewed from the side or rear. In fact, viewed from the rear, the stifle should be the widest part of the hindquarters.

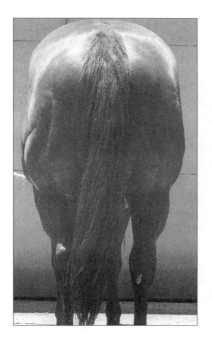

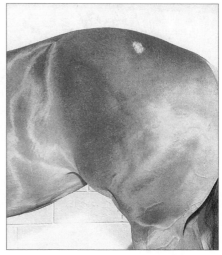

Fig. 8–21. Left: A correct stifle viewed from the rear. The stifle should be the widest part of the hindquarters. Above: A correct stifle viewed from the side.

Gaskin

The *gaskin*, or second thigh, lies between the stifle and the hock. It should be a little shorter than the thigh, but still long. A long gaskin provides greater distance between the hock and the hip. The correspondingly longer muscles exert more pull, lengthen the stride, and increase hindleg swing action. Sprinters need a slightly longer gaskin than other athletes might.

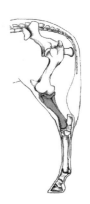

The gaskin plays an integral part in a horse's "driving force" and should be well muscled. Although the muscling varies by breed, the muscles should be well developed on both the inside and outside of the leg, because they give the horse power to run, jump, and pull.

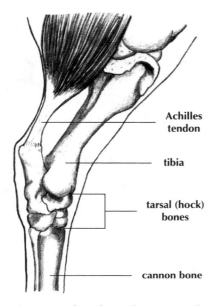

Achilles
tendon

tibia

tarsal (hock)
bones

cannon bone

Fig. 8–22. The tuber calcis (point of the hock) and the Achilles tendon.

From a side view, the width of the gaskin depends on the point of the hock and the Achilles tendon. This is because the Achilles tendon forms the back line of the lower gaskin and attaches to the point of the hock. The farther back these structures are, the wider the gaskin and the better the leverage.

From a rear view, the inside of the gaskin may be curved slightly inward in some horses, like the Arabian, or may be almost vertical, as in the Quarter Horse. The outside of the tibia (the major bone of the gaskin) is heavily muscled, while the inside is directly under the skin. Since the muscles can be seen so clearly in the gaskin, they indicate the horse's overall condition.

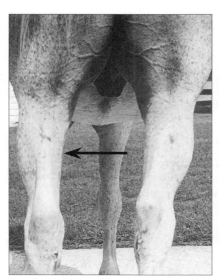

Fig. 8–23. The inside of an Arabian gaskin may be curved slightly inward.

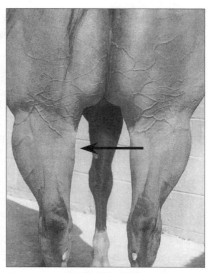

Fig. 8–24. The inside of a Quarter Horse gaskin may be almost vertical.

Hock

A good *hock* is of ample size to bear the horse's weight. But it should be in proportion with the structure of the horse's entire body—neither too fine nor too coarse.

From the side, the hock should be wide: as wide and strong as the gaskin. Ideally, the point of the hock is long, so that the lever it forms has increased length and power. The hock should be clean cut, with no roundness or "meatiness." The joint should have a neat look with thin, supple skin covering it so that the bones stand out clearly.

Correct placement of the hock is essential for power and shock absorption. When viewed from the rear, the leg should be straight with no deviation of the hock joint. Since a horse must collect and balance itself, the hocks suffer the least interference when they move in parallel planes with the cannons and fetlocks.

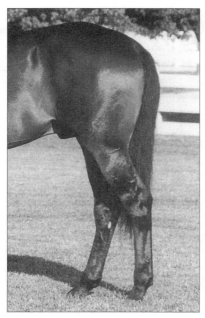

Fig. 8–25. Good hock conformation in proportion with the entire body.

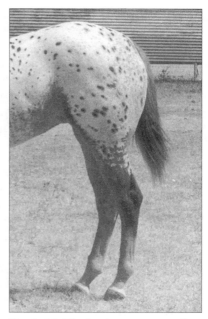

Fig. 8–26. The hocks are too small for the body.

Angulation of the Hock

When viewed from the side, the hock should appear neither too straight nor too angled. Angulation can be estimated by dropping an imaginary line from the point of the buttock to the ground. On a horse standing with the cannons vertical, the line should touch the point of the hock and run down the back of the cannon on its way to the ground.

The angle of the hock affects the power and length of the stride to a certain extent. A relatively straight hock, accompanied by a long, straight gaskin and short cannon, gives a running horse its lengthy stride. Together, these features allow full extension of the hindlegs and, consequently, full use of the power in the hindquarters.

On the other hand, a stock horse usually works better with more angulation in the hock. This conformation, combined with a short cannon, enables the horse to execute pivots, sliding stops, and roll-backs more easily because it can "get its hocks under it." Tennessee Walking Horses and Paso horses often have even more angulation in the hocks. Breeders believe these horses can cover ground more comfortably than horses with straighter legs.

Conformational Faults of the Hock

Viewed From the Side

The point of the hock should be about halfway between the stifle and the ground. Some people prefer *"low-set"* hocks (actually short cannons) because the horse has more power for pushing and quick turns. If too extreme, however, low-set hocks result in sickle hocks and reduced stride length. Others prefer *"high"* hocks. With this conformation, the cannon bone is lengthened, and the tibia is shortened. If extreme, this causes the horse to be camped under behind and increases concussion on the hindlegs.

Sickle hocks and *straight hocks* are deviations in the angle of the hock as seen from the side. A horse with sickle hocks appears to be camped under from the hock down—the cannon slopes forward. This is due to excessive angulation of the hock. Sickle hocks place increased strain on the back of the hock, predisposing the horse to curbs, bone spavin, and bog spavin. Generally, horses with this characteristic are not as fast as horses with straighter legs. The importance given to this characteristic depends on the horse's activity or breed, as mentioned in the previous section.

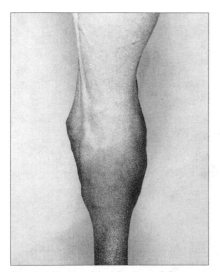

Fig. 8–27. Good hock viewed from the front.

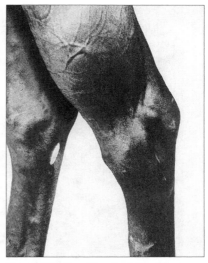

Fig. 8–28. Good hock viewed from the side.

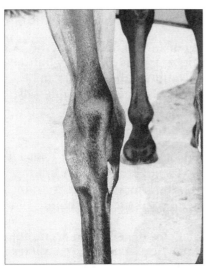

Fig. 8–29. Good hock viewed from the rear.

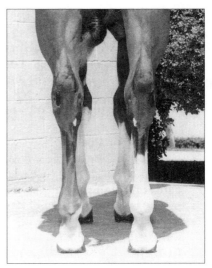

Fig. 8–30. Correctly set hock viewed from the rear.

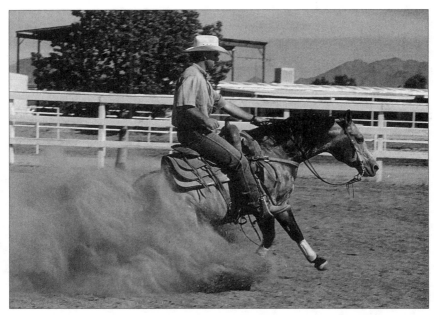

Fig. 8–31. A more angulated hock allows a reining horse to work with its hocks under its body.

An overly straight hock increases the tension on the front of the joint capsule of the hock. The "too straight" leg may be easily injured by hard work. Bog spavin and upward fixation of the patella can be attributed to a straight hock, but like sickle hocks, some people will attribute more importance to this conformation than others.

Viewed From the Rear

"Cow hocks" and *"bow legs"* are both deviations of the hock, viewed from the rear. In the case of cow hocks, the hocks are set closer together than the fetlocks. If extreme, this conformation causes strain on the insides of the hocks and stifles, and predisposes to bone spavin.

As with sickle hocks, the importance of cow hocks varies according to the horse's use and/or breed. Cow hocks are a common characteristic of draft horses. In dressage horses, mild cow hocks allow a longer stride, which is called over-reaching. A toed-out stance usually accompanies cow hocks.

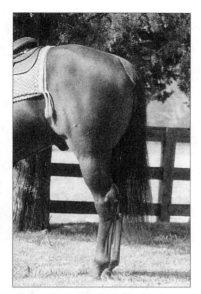

Fig. 8–32. "Low-set" hocks.

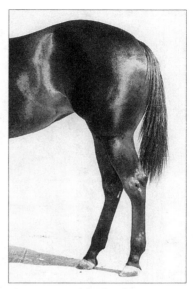

Fig. 8–33. "High" hocks.

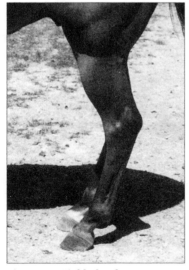

Fig. 8–34. Sickle hocks.

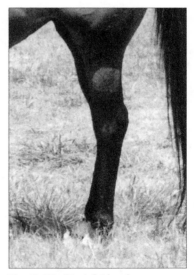

Fig. 8–35. Straight hocks.

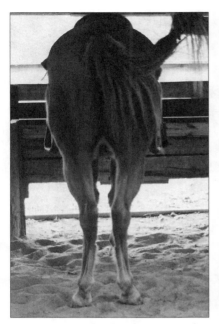

Fig. 8–36. Cow hocks: the points of the hocks turn inward.

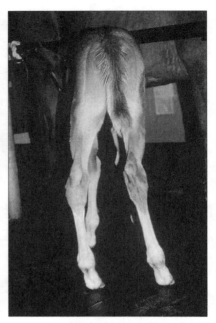

Fig. 8–37. This foal is bow-legged on the left and cow-hocked on the right.

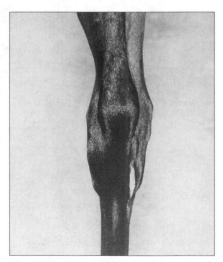

Fig. 8–38. Narrow, thin hocks are weak and unable to adequately dissipate concussion.

With bow legs (also called bandy legs or bow hocks), the hocks are set farther apart than the fetlocks. This frequently causes interference between the hind feet. Quarter Horses sometimes have this fault. Bow-legged horses are often toed-in.

Another type of poor hock conformation is a narrow, thin hock. This type of hock is weak and unable to adequately dissipate concussion. If the horse also has long, thin hindquarters and gaskins, it is called "cat-hammed." In the opposite situation, "beefy hocks," the hocks are too thick and meaty.

Cannon, Fetlock, and Pastern

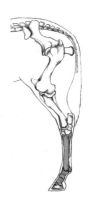

Conformation of the lower hindleg is similar to that of the lower foreleg. The *cannon* area between the hock and the fetlock should be short, although it is usually longer and wider than in the foreleg. Like the forelegs, the flexor tendons at the back of the cannon should be sharply defined.

The hind *fetlock* should be well set back and sturdy because it joins with the *pastern* to provide a springy gait. To compensate for a longer and wider cannon, normal hind pasterns should be slightly more upright and shorter than the front pasterns, sloping at an angle of 49° – 56°.

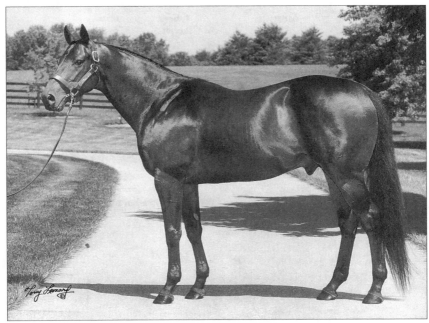

Fig. 8–39. Proper hindleg angulation is essential for adequate shock absorption.

ANATOMY OF THE HINDLEG
Hindquarters

The hindquarters area includes the croup, pelvis, and thigh. The croup is the area between the loin and the dock of the tail. The pelvis is the area between the croup and the hip joint. The thigh is located between the hip joint and the stifle.

Bones of the Hindquarters

The underlying bones of the hindquarters include the sacrum, os coxae, and femur. These bones form the structural basis for the entire hindquarters area.

Sacrum

Located in the croup area, the sacrum forms the roof of the pelvic cavity. This roughly triangular bone is made of the five sacral vertebrae, which are fused together.

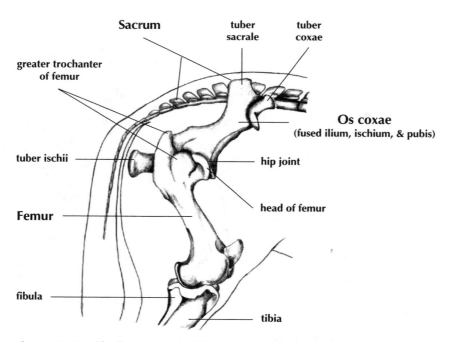

Fig. 8–40. Outside (lateral) view of the bones of the hindquarters.

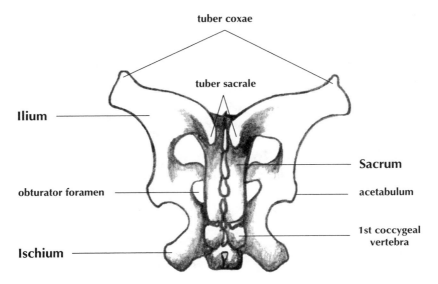

tuber coxae

tuber sacrale

Ilium

Sacrum

obturator foramen

acetabulum

1st coccygeal
vertebra

Ischium

Fig. 8–41. Top (dorsal) view of the bones of the hindquarters.

Os Coxae

The major bone of the pelvis is the *os coxae*, or hip bone. It is relatively immobile. Together with the pelvic ligaments, it forms the walls of the pelvic cavity, which contains the internal organs, and in mares forms the birth canal. The os coxae also provides many points of attachment for the large hindquarter muscles.

The os coxae is made of three pairs of bones (with left and right halves) that are all fused together in the mature horse. The largest of the three bones is the *ilium*. Each half of the ilium is roughly triangular, giving the appearance of a *wing* on either side. The floor of the pelvis is formed by the *ischium* and *pubis*. The ischium is a roughly square bone with the sides curved inward. Where the two halves of the ischium join is a ridge called the *spine of the ischium*. The pubis is the smallest of the three bones.

The prominences at the tops of the wings of the ilium are called the *tuber sacrale*. Together, the two tuber sacrale form the point of the croup. The prominence that forms the point of the hip is called the *tuber coxae*. The prominence that forms the point of the buttock is called the *tuber ischii*.

The ilium, ischium, and pubis on each side of the pelvis meet at a cup-shaped "socket" called the *acetabulum*. This is where the femur inserts to form the hip joint.

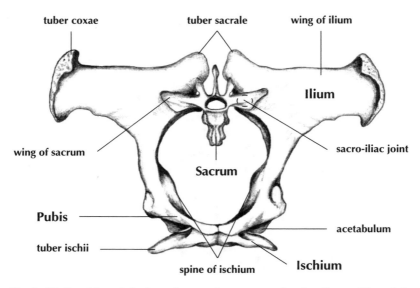

Fig. 8–42. Front (cranial) view of a mare's os coxae, showing the position of the sacrum between the wings of the ilium.

Femur

The *femur* is the underlying bone in the horse's thigh. It is the largest and strongest of the long bones. The *head of the femur* is ball-shaped, inserting into the acetabulum to form the hip joint.

The shaft of the femur has several prominences for muscle attachment. The largest is the *greater trochanter*, which rises above the femoral head on the outside of the bone. It can be felt beside the joint, beneath the layers of muscle. (The hip joint is several inches behind, and a couple of inches lower than the point of the hip.) A smaller prominence, the *lesser trochanter,* is located on the inside (medial) surface, near the top of the femur. The *third trochanter* is an even smaller rise on the inside surface, about one-third of the way down the bone.

The lower end of the femur joins with the tibia and patella to form the stifle joint.

Joints of the Hindquarters

Sacro-Iliac Joint

In the hindleg, the connection between the spinal column and rest of the leg is direct, at the *sacro-iliac joint.* This is in contrast to the foreleg, where the connection is purely muscular. As a consequence of the bony connection, propulsive forces are transmitted directly to the spinal column—but so is concussion.

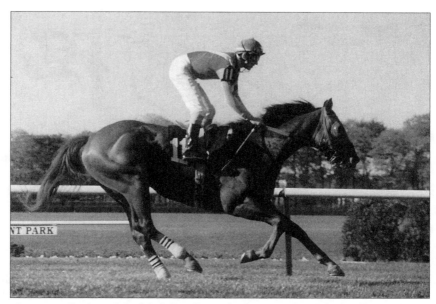

Fig. 8–43. Flexion of the hip joint allows the horse to draw the hindleg well underneath the body.

The sacrum lies centered below the ilial wings. Each wing of the sacrum forms a joint with the corresponding wing of the ilium. The joints are broad, flat, and virtually immobile.

Hip Joint

The *hip joint* between the os coxae and the femur has a normal standing angle of about 115°. To varying degrees, it is capable the following types of movement:

- flexion—the femur moves forward
- extension—the femur moves backward
- abduction—the femur moves away from the horse's midline
- adduction—the femur moves toward the horse's midline
- rotation—the femur twists left and right
- circumduction—the femur moves around the joint in a circle

Ligaments of the Hindquarters

Sacro-iliac Ligaments

Supporting the sacro-iliac joints and forming what is called the "pelvic girdle" are the *dorsal* and *lateral sacro-iliac ligaments*. The

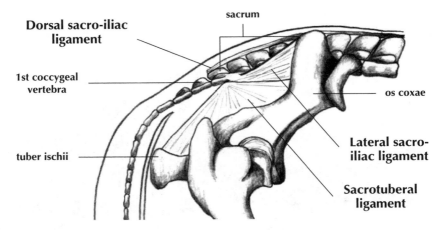

Fig. 8–44. Outside (lateral) view of the sacro-iliac and pelvic ligaments.

dorsal sacro-iliac ligament is a cord that runs from the tuber sacrale to the dorsal spinous processes of the sacrum. Continuous to it is the lateral sacro-iliac ligament. This broad, triangular ligament attaches the wing of the ilium to the sacrum and tail fascia (connective tissue). Surrounding and reinforcing the joint from underneath is the *ventral sacro-iliac ligament.*

Pelvic Ligaments

On each side of the pelvis is a *sacrotuberal ligament.* This structure is a broad sheet of fibrous connective tissue. It runs from the sacrum and first two coccygeal vertebrae to the spine of the ischium and tuber ischii. It completes the outside wall of the pelvic cavity.

Hip Joint Ligaments

The strong ligaments of the hip joint anchor the femoral head within the acetabulum. The *accessory ligament* of the hip joint is unique to equids. It connects the prepubic tendon (a tendon of the rectus abdominis muscle, described in Chapter 7, *Body*), to the femoral head, limiting hip abduction. This is why a horse cannot effectively "cow kick," where it kicks out to the side. The *transverse ligament* encircles the acetabulum, binding down the accessory ligament.

Within the hip joint is the *round ligament:* a short, but very strong band. It limits hip adduction by securing the top of the femoral head to the inside of the acetabulum. It is also called the ligament of the femoral head.

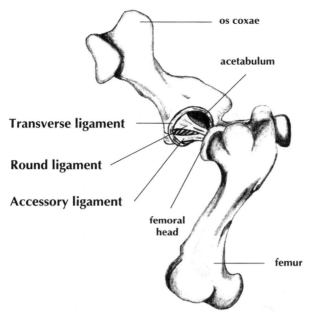

Fig. 8–45. Hip joint ligaments.

Fascia of the Hindquarters

The deep fascia is a thin, fibrous, strong connective tissue covering much of the muscle mass. It serves as a point of attachment for many hindquarter muscles. Draped over the croup is the *gluteal fascia.* Just behind the gluteal fascia, and continuous with it, is the *tail fascia* around the base of the horse's tail. The *fascia lata* (also continuous with the gluteal fascia),

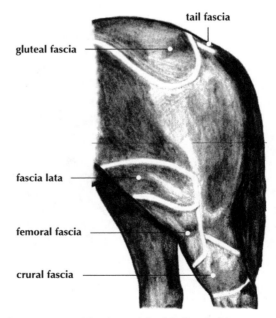

Fig. 8–46. Outside view of the hindleg fascia.

covers the stifle area, attaching to the patella and its ligaments. Below the fascia lata is the *femoral fascia* over the quadriceps muscle, and below that is the *crural fascia*. The superficial muscles of the entire hindquarters region are connected to these sheets of tissue.

Muscles of the Hindquarters

Many of the large hindquarter muscles have broad and/or multiple origins and narrower insertions. This arrangement gives the strong muscles the leverage necessary to propel the horse forward.

Some of these muscles also attach to nearby soft tissues: ligaments or deep fascia. For example, the biceps femoris partially inserts on the sacro-iliac ligaments and the crural fascia.

Extensor Muscles

Extending the hip joint pulls the horse's femur, and the entire hindleg, backward. Therefore, the extensor muscles of the hip figure strongly in kicking, rearing, and forward motion. They are mostly located behind the thigh.

Middle gluteal—Often called the gluteus medius, this is the largest muscle in the horse and forms the mass of the upper hindquarters. It has a broad origin along the top of the pelvis, including the tuber

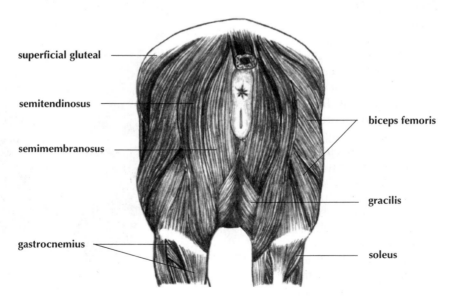

Fig. 8–47. Rear (caudal) view of the hindquarter muscles.

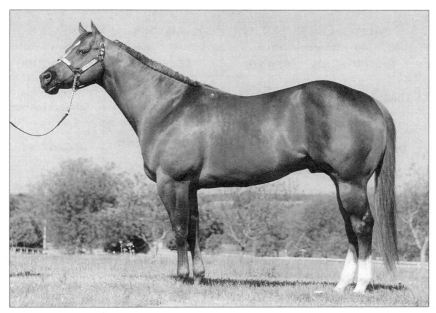

Fig. 8–48. The mass of the upper hindquarters is formed by the middle gluteal.

sacrale, wing of the ilium, tuber coxae, and gluteal fascia. It inserts on the greater trochanter of the femur. This powerful muscle extends the hip joint, and also helps to abduct the hindleg.

Deep gluteal—This muscle originates on the spine of the ischium, traveling over the upper hip to insert on the greater trochanter of the femur. It pulls the top of the femur upward and inward, which abducts the hindleg. This muscle is also called the gluteus profundus.

Biceps femoris—This muscle is large and complex, originating along the croup (sacrum, coccygeal vertebrae, and surrounding soft tissues) and also on the lower pelvis (the spine of the ischium and tuber ischii). It passes behind the femur before inserting on the back of the femur, outside of the patella, front of the tibia, and nearby soft tissues. Another tendon continues down the back of the gaskin to the point of the hock. The biceps femoris extends and abducts the hip joint, and helps extend the hock, as part of the reciprocal apparatus (described in the Hock section). It also affects the stifle: one part extends it and another part flexes it. The biceps femoris is one of the three "hamstring" muscles. The groove between it and the semitendinosus muscle is visible on most horses, curving down the hindquarters.

MUSCLES OF THE HINDQUARTERS—EXTENSORS

Name	Origin	Insertion	Function
Middle gluteal	upper pelvis	greater trochanter of femur	extend hip; abduct hindleg
Deep gluteal	spine of the ischium	greater trochanter of femur	abduct hindleg
Biceps femoris	upper pelvis; ischium	back of femur; outside of patella; front of tibia; point of hock	extend and abduct hip; extend and flex stifle; extend hock
Semitendinosus	upper pelvis; ischium	inside stifle; front of tibia; point of hock	extend hip & hock; flex stifle; rotate hindleg
Semimembranosus	upper pelvis; ischium	bottom inside of femur	extend hip; adduct hindleg
Adductor	underside of os coxae	bottom inside of femur; top of tibia	extend hip; adduct hindleg; rotate hindleg
Gracilis	prepubic tendon; pubis; accessory ligament	inside top of tibia; medial patellar ligament	adduct hindleg; stabilize hip
Internal/External obturators	underside of os coxae	trochanteric fossa of femur	adduct and rotate thigh
Quadratus femoris	underside of ischium	lesser trochanter of femur	extend hip; adduct thigh

Fig. 8–49.

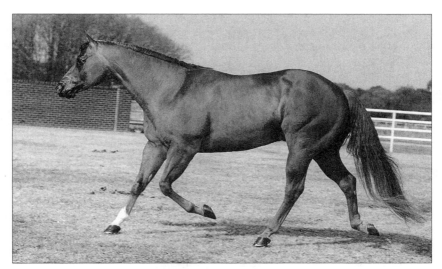

Fig. 8–50. The groove between the biceps femoris and the semitendinosus muscles is clearly visible.

Semitendinosus—This muscle runs behind the biceps femoris, forming the bulge of the buttock. It originates on the top of the croup (the sacrum, coccygeal vertebrae, and surrounding soft tissues) and also on the lower pelvis (the tuber ischii). It inserts on the inside of the stifle and also the front of the tibia near the top. Another tendon continues down the gaskin to insert on the point of the hock. Its function is to extend the hip and hock joints and to flex the stifle. It also rotates the leg to the inside. The semitendinosus is another of the clearly defined "hamstring" muscles. It is easily seen in conditioned athletes.

Semimembranosus—The third "hamstring" muscle, the semimembranosus lies a little in front of the semitendinosus, under the biceps femoris. It originates on the top of the rump (the sacrum, coccygeal vertebrae, and surrounding soft tissues) and also on the lower pelvis (the tuber ischii). It then passes behind the femur to insert on the bottom inside of that bone. The semimembranosus aids in hip extension and adducts the leg.

Adductor—This is the largest muscle on the inside of the horse's thigh. It runs from the underside of the pelvis to the bottom of the femur, on the inside back surface. It also inserts on the top of the tibia. It extends the hip joint, adducts the leg, and rotates the thigh to the inside.

219

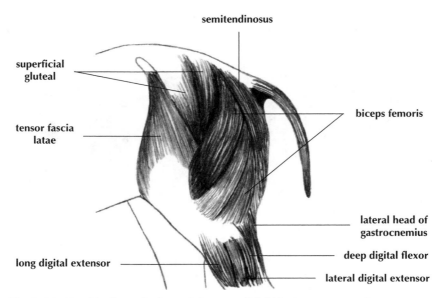

superficial gluteal

semitendinosus

biceps femoris

tensor fascia latae

lateral head of gastrocnemius

deep digital flexor

long digital extensor

lateral digital extensor

Fig. 8–51. Outside (lateral) view of the superficial hindquarter muscles.

Gracilis—This broad muscle covers the inside of the thigh. It originates on the prepubic tendon (see Chapter 7, *Body*), the pubis, and the accessory ligament. It inserts at the top of the tibia, on the inside surface. It also inserts on nearby fascia and the medial patellar ligament of the stifle. This muscle adducts the hindleg and stabilizes the hip joint by acting against the powerful abductor muscles on the outside of the thigh.

External/Internal obturators—These muscles originate on the underside of the pelvis near the obturator foramen. They insert on the trochanteric fossa of the femur, located at the base of the greater trochanter. The external obturator lies outside the pelvis; the internal obturator lies inside the pelvis. They adduct and rotate the thigh.

Quadratus femoris—This muscle originates on the underside of the ischium and inserts near the lesser trochanter of the femur. It extends the hip joint and adducts the thigh.

Flexor Muscles of the Hindquarters

Flexing the hip joint pulls the horse's femur, and the entire hindleg, forward. The flexor muscles of the hip are mostly located in the front of the thigh.

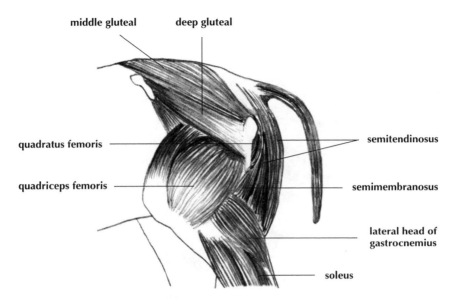

middle gluteal

deep gluteal

quadratus femoris

quadriceps femoris

semitendinosus

semimembranosus

lateral head of gastrocnemius

soleus

Fig. 8–52. Outside (lateral) view of the deep hindquarter muscles.

Tensor fascia latae—This is the hindleg muscle that is furthest forward. It originates on the tuber coxae, fanning out to insert on the fascia latae, which attaches to the patella. It tenses the fascia, flexing the hip joint and extending the stifle. It also abducts the hindleg.

Superficial gluteal—This muscle begins on the tuber coxae, outside (lateral) border of the ilium, and gluteal fascia. It inserts on the third trochanter of the femur. It functions to flex and abduct the hip. This muscle is also called the gluteus superficialis.

Psoas major and Iliacus—These two muscles are often considered as a single muscle called the iliopsoas. The psoas major originates on the lumbar vertebrae. The iliacus originates on the underside of the wing of the ilium. Both muscles insert on the lesser trochanter of the femur. Together they flex the hip joint and rotate the thigh outward.

Psoas minor—This small muscle originates on the last few thoracic vertebrae and the first few lumbar vertebrae. It inserts on the lower front of the os coxae. It flexes the pelvis, swiveling the hip forward into the loin.

Sartorius—This thin muscle originates on the tuber coxae and surrounding soft tissues. It then runs diagonally across the thigh, and inserts on the tibia and medial patellar ligament of the stifle with the

Inside View

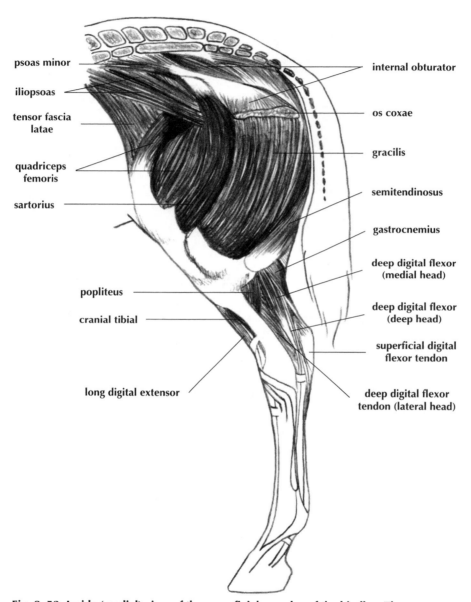

psoas minor

iliopsoas

tensor fascia latae

quadriceps femoris

sartorius

popliteus

cranial tibial

long digital extensor

internal obturator

os coxae

gracilis

semitendinosus

gastrocnemius

deep digital flexor (medial head)

deep digital flexor (deep head)

superficial digital flexor tendon

deep digital flexor tendon (lateral head)

Fig. 8–53. Inside (medial) view of the superficial muscles of the hindleg. The vertebrae and os coxae are shown in cross–section.

Inside View

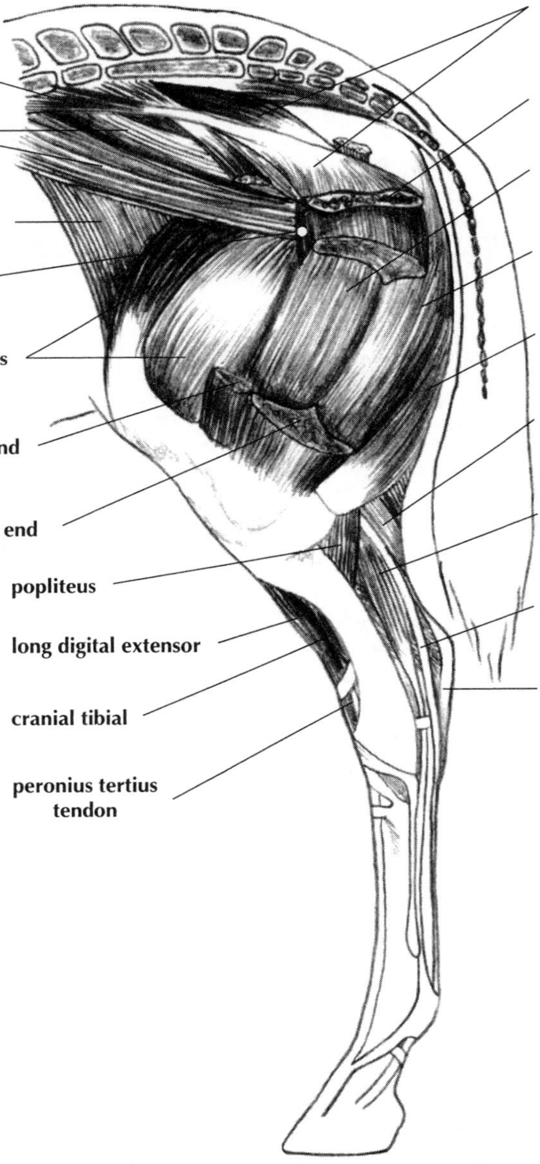

psoas minor

iliopsoas

tensor fascia latae

pectineus

quadriceps femoris

sartorius—cut end

gracilis—cut end

popliteus

long digital extensor

cranial tibial

peronius tertius
tendon

internal obturator

os coxae

adductor

semimembranosus

semitendinosus

gastrocnemius

deep digital flexor
(medial head)

deep digital flexor
(deep head)

superficial digital
flexor tendon

Fig. 8–54. Inside (medial) view of the deep muscles of the hindleg. The gracilis and sartorius have been removed to reveal the muscles underneath. The vertebrae and os coxae are shown in cross–section.

MUSCLES OF THE HINDQUARTERS—FLEXORS			
Name	Origin	Insertion	Function
Tensor fascia latae	tuber coxae	fascia latae	flex hip; extend stifle; abduct hindleg
Superficial gluteal	tuber coxae; outside of ilium; gluteal fascia	third trochanter of femur	flex and abduct hip
Psoas major	lumbar vertebrae	lesser trochanter of femur	flex hip; rotate thigh
Iliacus	underside of wing of ilium	lesser trochanter of femur	flex hip; rotate thigh
Psoas minor	last few thoracic vertebrae; first few lumbar vertebrae	lower front of os coxae	flex pelvis, swiveling hip forward
Sartorius	tuber coxae	tibia and medial patellar ligament	flex hip; adduct hindleg; rotate thigh
Pectineus	front of pubis	inside surface of femur	flex hip; adduct hindleg
Quadriceps femoris	lower pelvis; shaft of femur	patella	flex hip; extend stifle

Fig. 8–55.

tendon of the gracilis. The sartorius flexes the hip joint, adducts the leg, and rotates the thigh.

Pectineus—This is a small cylindrical muscle that is under the gracilis. It originates on the front of the pubis, and inserts on the inside surface of the femur. It flexes the hip joint and adducts the leg.

Quadriceps femoris— This muscle group flexes the hip joint, but its primary function is to extend the stifle. It is discussed in more detail in the Stifle section.

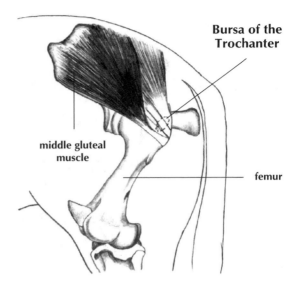

Bursa of the Hindquarters

The *bursa of the trochanter* lies between the tendon of the middle gluteal muscle and the greater trochanter of the femur. It protects both structures from pressure and friction.

Fig. 8–56. Outside (lateral) view of the bursa between the tendon of the middle gluteal muscle and the greater trochanter.

Blood Vessels of the Hindquarters

The main artery supplying blood to the hindleg is the *external iliac artery*. All other arteries in the hip, thigh, and down the hindleg branch off this vessel. It begins in front of the hip joint. Then the *medial circumflex femoral artery* branches off the external iliac artery, and travels across the femur toward the back of the hindleg.

The external iliac artery becomes the *femoral artery* as it passes over the front of the femur. Midway down the femur, the *saphenous artery* branches off the femoral artery and travels down the back of the thigh.

There is an opening on each side of the floor of the pelvis called the obturator foramen. The *obturator artery* passes through this opening before merging with the medial circumflex femoral artery.

The veins in the hindquarters are companions to the arteries, and have the same names. They travel approximately the same paths to drain the area of blood, sending it back toward the heart.

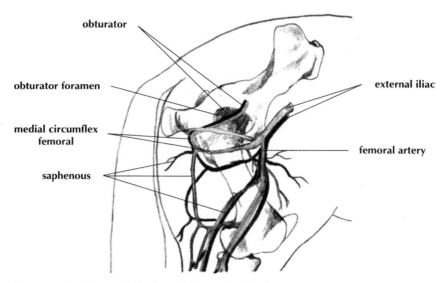

Fig. 8–57. Inside (medial) view of the major blood vessels of the hindquarters.

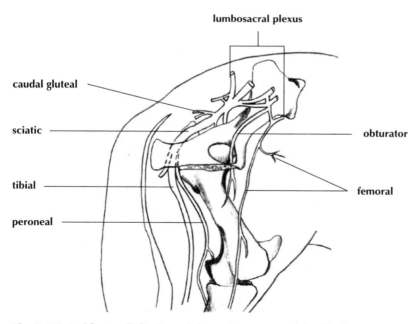

Fig. 8–58. Inside (medial) view of the major nerves of the hindquarters.

Nerves of the Hindquarters

The *lumbosacral plexus* supplies sensation and motion to the entire hindleg. It is a set of nerves formed by the fourth, fifth, and sixth *lumbar spinal nerves,* and the first and second *sacral spinal nerves.*

One of its nerves is the *obturator nerve,* which runs from the top of the pelvis and through the obturator foramen, supplying the muscles on the inside of the thigh. Compression of this nerve during foaling can cause temporary "foaling" paralysis. The *femoral nerve* supplies the muscles at the front of the thigh. Below the hip joint, the *sciatic (ischiatic) nerve*—the largest nerve in the horse's body—branches into the *tibial nerve* and *peroneal nerve.* These nerves supply the muscles at the back of the thigh. Other important nerves in this area include the *cranial* and *caudal gluteal nerves,* which supply the gluteals and several other muscles.

Tail Area

The underlying bones of the horse's tail are the *coccygeal vertebrae.* There are approximately 18 of these bones, becoming smaller as they progress down the tail. The final coccygeal vertebra is pointed.

The muscles of the tail begin in the croup area. Long tendons run on either side of the coccygeal vertebrae. The tail muscles are paired

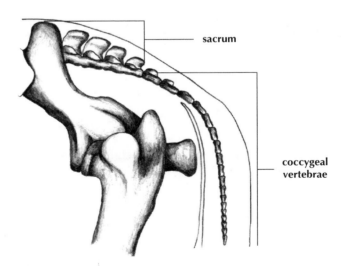

sacrum

coccygeal
vertebrae

Fig. 8–59. Outside (lateral) view of the bones of the tail.

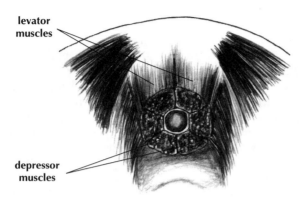

levator muscles

depressor muscles

Fig. 8–60. Rear (caudal) view of the tail muscles.

and lie in layers around the vertebrae. This arrangement allows the horse to move its tail in any direction. The muscles are broadly divided into two categories: *levator (extensor)* and *depressor (flexor)*. When both the left and right sides contract together, the levator muscles pull the tail up, and the depressor muscles pull the tail down. When one side contracts independently, the muscle moves the tail to that side.

Stifle

The stifle is the forward part of the hindleg just below where it joins the flank. In a normal standing position, it is slightly extended: the angle at the back of the leg should be about 150°. The stifle joint is a hinge joint in the horse, corresponding to the human knee. It is the largest joint in the horse's body. When the strong muscles of the hindleg extend the stifle joint, they propel the horse forward.

Bones

There are three bones making up the stifle joint: the *femur, tibia,* and *patella.* At the lower end of the femur are two round projections that look like knuckles. They are called the *lateral* and *medial condyles.* The medial condyle is a little larger than the lateral.

At the upper end of the tibia is a narrow ridge called the *tibial spine,* which fits neatly between the femoral condyles. It stabilizes the stifle.

There are two thick, C-shaped cartilages called *menisci* (singular = meniscus) that separate the femur and tibia. They help to keep the joint in position and absorb shock.

A thin bone called the *fibula* is attached to the outside of the tibia. It narrows as it travels down the tibia, ending about halfway down without forming a joint.

At the front of the stifle is a small bone called the *patella* (kneecap). It rides on the *trochlear groove,* which is a track-like structure be-

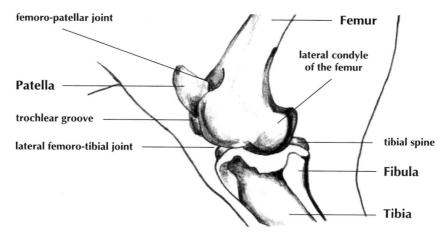

femoro-patellar joint

Femur

lateral condyle
of the femur

Patella

trochlear groove

lateral femoro-tibial joint

tibial spine

Fibula

Tibia

Fig. 8–61. Outside (lateral) view of the bones and joints of the stifle.

tween the femoral condyles. The patella helps to reduce friction and transmits extension power from the femur to the tibia.

Joints

Although collectively referred to as the "stifle joint," the three bones in the stifle create two separate joint spaces. They are the *femoro-tibial joint* and the *femoro-patellar joint*. The femoro-tibial joint connects the femur and tibia. It is divided into two halves (lateral and medial) by the tibial spine. The femoro-patellar joint is the largest articulation in the stifle, connecting the femur and patella. Each of these joints has its own joint capsule. The linings of the joint capsules produce synovial fluid, which lubricates the joint surfaces.

Ligaments

The stifle joint is held together by many ligaments. The femur is connected to the tibia by the *lateral* and *medial cruciate ligaments* crisscrossing each other within the joint. The femur is connected to the patella by the *collateral ligaments* and the *femoro-patellar ligaments* on either side, and by the quadriceps femoris muscle. The patella is connected to the tibia by the *medial, middle,* and *lateral patellar ligaments*. The patellar ligaments are under constant tension from the quadriceps femoris muscle, unless the horse is lying down. The menisci also have small ligaments anchoring them to the femur and tibia.

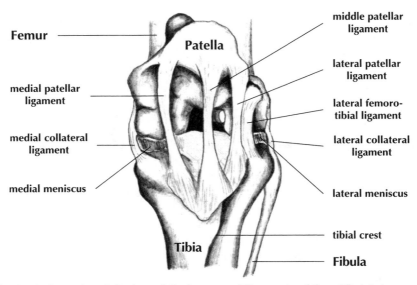

Fig. 8–62. Front (cranial) view of the bones and ligaments of the stifle joint.

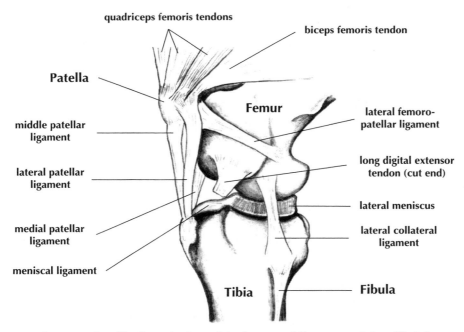

Fig. 8–63. Outside (lateral) view of the bones and ligaments of the stifle joint.

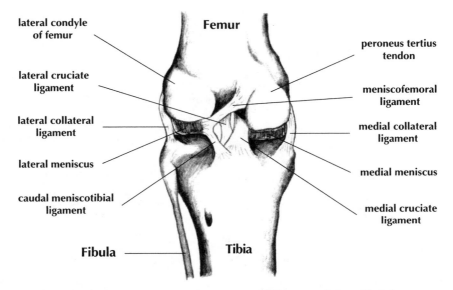

lateral condyle of femur

Femur

peroneus tertius tendon

lateral cruciate ligament

meniscofemoral ligament

lateral collateral ligament

medial collateral ligament

lateral meniscus

medial meniscus

caudal meniscotibial ligament

medial cruciate ligament

Fibula

Tibia

Fig. 8–64. Rear (caudal) view of the bones and ligaments of the stifle joint.

Muscles of the Stifle

The stifle is surrounded, except in front, by heavy muscles. The efficiency of the joint depends on these muscles.

The stifle joint and hock joint always move in unison, extending together and flexing together. Stifle flexion and hock extension cannot happen simultaneously. This "reciprocal apparatus" is discussed in more detail in the Hock section.

Extensor Muscles

The major extensor of the stifle is the *quadriceps femoris muscle (see Figure 8–52).* This large, fan-shaped muscle group has four different parts, or "heads":

- *rectus femoris muscle*
- *lateral vastus muscle*
- *intermediate vastus muscle*
- *medial vastus muscle*

They originate on the lower pelvis and along the shaft of the femur, covering the front and sides of the thigh. All four heads insert on the patella. They pull on the patella, affecting the patellar ligaments and

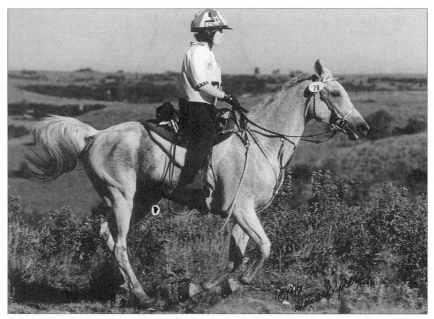

Fig. 8–65. The quadriceps femoris muscle extends this endurance horse's stifle.

thus moving the tibia. The quadriceps femoris also helps to flex the hip joint.

Flexor Muscles of the Stifle

Flexion of the stifle is the result of many muscles acting at a distance with multiple actions. The hamstring muscles are integral. They include the biceps femoris, semitendinosus, and semimembranosus muscles, discussed in the Hindquarters section as hip extensors *(see Figures 8–51 and 8–52).*

Helping to flex the stifle are the extensor muscles of the hock and lower hindleg. They include the *gastrocnemius* (discussed in the Hock section) and the *superficial digital flexor muscle* (discussed in the Gaskin section).

The *popliteus* muscle also flexes the stifle. It is located behind the stifle on the inside of the hindleg. It originates on the lateral condyle of the femur and inserts on the inside of the tibia. The popliteus primarily flexes the stifle, but also slightly rotates the leg inward. *(See Figure 8–67.)*

Gaskin
Bones

The gaskin is the area of the hindleg between the stifle and the hock. The *tibia* and *fibula* are the underlying bones of the gaskin. The tibia is the larger bone situated on the inside of the leg, while the fibula is much smaller and is located on the outside of the leg.

The wide top end of the tibia forms the stifle joint with the femur and patella. The

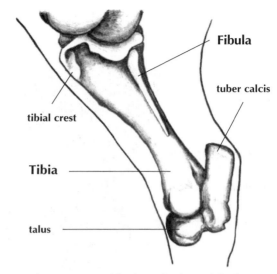

Fig. 8–66. Outside (lateral) view of the bones of the gaskin.

shaft of the tibia is slender and triangular. On the shaft a few inches below the top is a broad, vertical ridge called the *tibial crest* (also called the tibial tuberosity). The patellar ligaments and biceps femoris muscle attach here. The lower end of the tibia forms the hock joint with the tarsal bones.

The small *fibula* has a head and shaft, but no enlargement at the lower end. It fuses with the tibia about halfway down that bone.

Muscles

Several hindquarter muscles insert near the top of the tibia. They include the biceps femoris, semitendinosus, gracilis, and popliteus muscles, described in the Hindquarters and Stifle sections.

Muscles and tendons activating the hock originate near the top of the tibia, and pass over the gaskin. They include the gastrocnemius, soleus, cranial tibial, and peroneus tertius tendon. They are described in the Hock section.

The muscles described in the current section activate the entire lower hindleg, including the *digit*, composed of the fetlock, pastern, and coffin joints. They become tendons just above the hock. The lower leg moves entirely via tendons and ligaments.

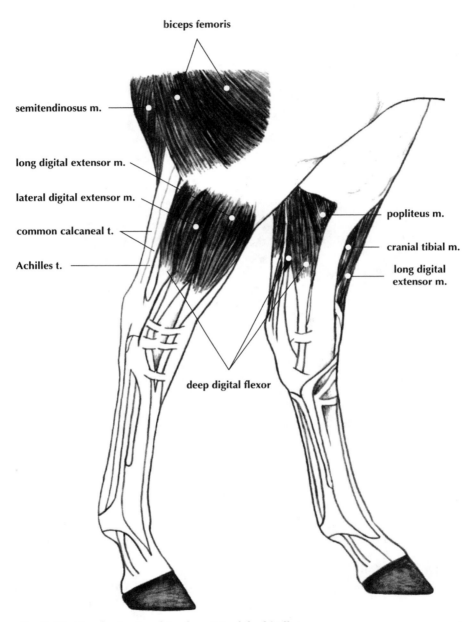

biceps femoris

semitendinosus m.

long digital extensor m.

lateral digital extensor m.

common calcaneal t.

Achilles t.

popliteus m.

cranial tibial m.

long digital extensor m.

deep digital flexor

Fig. 8–67. Muscles (m.) and tendons (t.) of the hindleg.

234

MUSCLES OF THE GASKIN			
Name	**Origin**	**Insertion**	**Function**
Long digital extensor	front of lower femur	top of coffin bone	extend digit; flex hock
Lateral digital extensor	side of tibia and fibula; collateral ligament of stifle	long digital extensor tendon	extend digit; flex hock
Superficial digital flexor	back of lower femur	point of hock; side of pastern bones	flex stifle, fetlock, and pastern joints; extend hock
Deep digital flexor	back of tibia/fibula	underside of coffin bone	flex digit; extend hock

Fig. 8–68.

Long digital extensor—This muscle originates on the front of the lower femur. Its tendon attaches at several places as it runs down the front of the leg, eventually ending on the top of the coffin bone. As it passes over the hock it is surrounded and protected by a tendon sheath. It is joined by the lateral digital extensor tendon near the top of the cannon. The long digital extensor flexes the hock, and extends the digit.

Lateral digital extensor—This muscle originates on the side of the tibia, fibula, and the lateral collateral ligament of the stifle. As its tendon passes over the hock it is surrounded and protected by a tendon sheath. It joins the long digital extensor tendon near the top of the cannon, assisting it in flexing the hock and extending the digit.

Superficial digital flexor—This round, tendinous muscle originates on the back side of the lower femur and travels down the back of the gaskin. Its tendon attaches to the point of the hock before continuing down the back of the cannon. It extends the hock and also helps to flex the stifle and fetlock joints. (**Note:** There is no superior check ligament in the hindleg as there is in the foreleg.)

Deep digital flexor—In the hindleg, this muscle group has three heads, all of which originate on the back of the tibia and fibula. The lateral digital flexor is the deepest and largest head. It also has the broadest origin, wrapping around the back and sides of the tibial shaft for over half that bone's length. The medial digital flexor muscle is the second head, and the caudal tibial muscle is the third and most superficial head of this muscle group. Together they extend the hock joint and flex the fetlock, pastern, and coffin joints.

Tendons of the Gaskin

The *common calcaneal tendon* is actually made of the tendons of many muscles, including the superficial digital flexor, biceps femoris, semitendinosus, and the Achilles or calcaneal tendon. The *Achilles tendon* is made up of the combined tendons of the gastrocnemius and soleus muscles. It forms the back of the lower gaskin, seen from the side.

The *peroneus tertius tendon* travels from the front of the femur to the tarsal (hock) bones. Just before it inserts, it divides into two heads: lateral and medial. This structure connects the stifle and hock so that they move together. When the stifle is flexed, the peroneus tertius automatically flexes the hock. (It also prevents the hock from overextending.) This tendon is also known as the fibularis tertius.

Blood Vessels of the Gaskin

The femoral artery runs down the front of the thigh. At about the stifle it becomes the *popliteal artery.* Just below the stifle, this artery branches into the *cranial* and *caudal tibial artery.* The cranial tibial artery travels down the front of the gaskin. The caudal tibial artery travels down the back of the gaskin, close to the tibia.

At about the level of the stifle, a branch called the *caudal femoral artery* leaves the main femoral artery. It travels toward the back of the gaskin, and is more superficial than the femoral artery. The caudal femoral artery is eventually rejoined by the saphenous artery from the hindquarters region. Together they become the *recurrent tibial artery* a few inches above the hock.

The veins in the gaskin are very similar to the arteries. One exception, however, is the *saphenous vein.* It has a long medial branch and a short lateral branch. The medial saphenous vein again divides into cranial and caudal branches. The cranial branch runs along the inside toward the front of the gaskin. The caudal branch runs down the back of the gaskin.

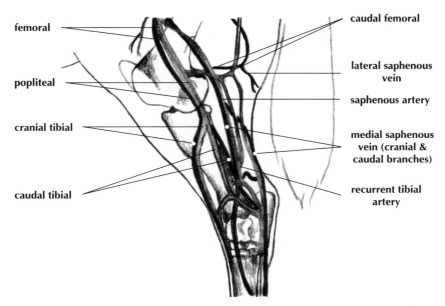

femoral

caudal femoral

popliteal

lateral saphenous vein

saphenous artery

cranial tibial

medial saphenous vein (cranial & caudal branches)

caudal tibial

recurrent tibial artery

Fig. 8–69. Inside (medial) view of the major blood vessels of the gaskin.

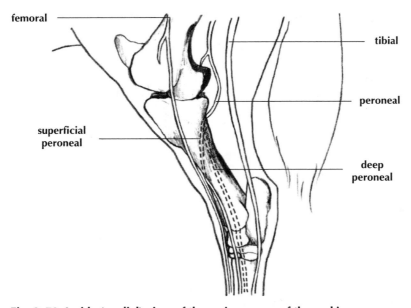

femoral

tibial

peroneal

superficial peroneal

deep peroneal

Fig. 8–70. Inside (medial) view of the major nerves of the gaskin.

Nerves of the Gaskin

The femoral nerve continues from the thigh, across the inside surface of the stifle, and down the gaskin. It supplies the quadriceps femoris muscle. At the back of the leg, just below the stifle, the *peroneal nerve* divides into superficial and deep branches. The *superficial peroneal nerve* travels down the inside front of the gaskin, supplying the lateral digital extensor muscle. The *deep peroneal nerve* travels down the outside, closer to the tibia, supplying the long and lateral digital extensor muscles. The tibial nerve also travels down the back of the gaskin. It supplies the popliteus, gastrocnemius, soleus, and the superficial and deep digital flexor muscles.

Hock (Tarsus)

The hock is the joint between the tibia and the cannon bone in the equine hindleg. The hock joint is anatomically equivalent to the human ankle.

Bones

The hock is a complex joint composed of many bones arranged in rows. The *talus* is the large bone between the tibia and the top row of tarsal bones. Behind the talus is another large bone called the *calcaneus*. Part of the calcaneus projects upward and backward to form the point of the hock. The projection is called the *tuber calcis*, and it acts as a lever for the tendons running over it, which extend and support the hock.

The remaining *tarsal bones* are smaller, and are arranged between the talus and cannon bone. In the front of the joint are the *central tarsal bone* and *third tarsal bone*. At the back of the joint are the *first* and *second tarsal bones*: these two are fused together. The *fourth tarsal bone* is vaguely L-shaped, and curves from the outside around to the back.

Joints

The hock is a hinge joint—capable of flexion and extension—with a wide range of motion. It is partially flexed at 150° in the normal standing position, which helps it to absorb concussion. It is helpful to keep in mind that flexing the hock brings the horse's hind foot *forward*. This motion is in contrast to flexing the knee, which brings the horse's forefoot *backward*.

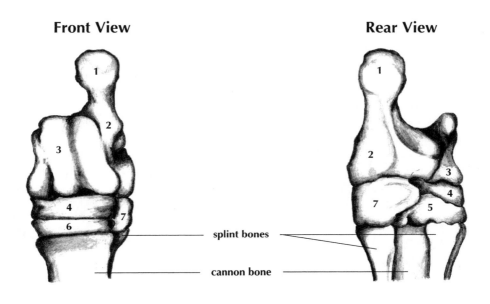

Front View

Rear View

splint bones

cannon bone

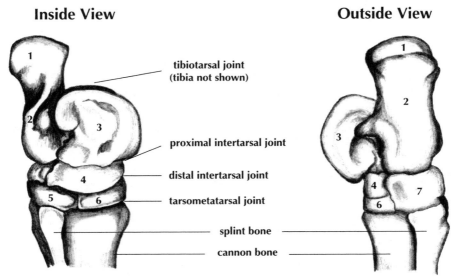

Inside View

Outside View

tibiotarsal joint
(tibia not shown)

proximal intertarsal joint

distal intertarsal joint

tarsometatarsal joint

splint bone

cannon bone

Fig. 8–71. Four views of the bones and major joints of the hock:

1. tuber calcis
2. calcaneus
3. talus
4. central tarsal bone
5. 1st and 2nd tarsal bones—fused
6. 3rd tarsal bone
7. 4th tarsal bone

The tarsal bones form one major joint, three minor horizontal joints, and several vertical joints (between each bone is a joint). The vertical joints are immobile. The major joint is the *tibiotarsal*, between the tibia and the talus. This is the joint that is most mobile, and allows the hock to flex. The three minor horizontal joints, from top to bottom are:

- *proximal intertarsal joint*
- *distal intertarsal joint*
- *tarsometatarsal joint*

Each has its own joint capsule, but there is frequently communication between them. The linings of the joint capsules produce synovial fluid, which lubricates the joint surfaces.

Ligaments of the Hock

The tarsal bones are bound together by short, strong ligaments. The *short collateral ligaments* on either side of the hock connect the tibia to the tarsal bones. The *long collateral ligaments* on either side of the hock connect the tibia to the cannon bone. Both sets prevent the hock joint from extending completely.

Across the front of the hock is the fan-shaped *dorsal tarsal ligament*. Traveling vertically along the back of the hock is the *plantar tarsal ligament*, which attaches the tuber calcis to the cannon bone. This is the structure involved in a "curb."

There are also three *annular ligaments* in the hock: the proximal, middle, and distal. Annular ligaments are broad, strong support structures that wrap horizontally over a joint. They strengthen and protect the hock joint, and bind down the tendons running under them.

Muscles and Tendons of the Hock

Extensor Muscles

The extensor muscles of the hock are located on the back of the hindleg, and attach to the tuber calcis.

Gastrocnemius—The large "gastroc" muscle originates on the back of the lower femur, forming the rear curve of the gaskin. It becomes a tendon about halfway down the gaskin before inserting onto the tuber calcis. It extends the hock and helps to flex the stifle (although these two actions cannot occur simultaneously). It is part of the Achilles tendon.

Soleus—This narrow muscle originates on the top of the fibula. It runs along the outside of the gastrocnemius muscle and is closely

Front View

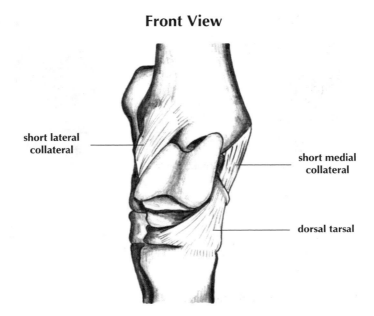

short lateral collateral

short medial collateral

dorsal tarsal

Inside View   ## Outside View

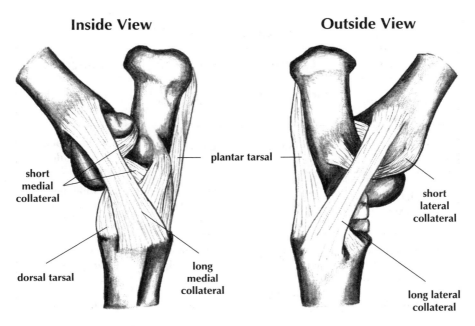

plantar tarsal

short medial collateral

short lateral collateral

dorsal tarsal

long medial collateral

long lateral collateral

Fig. 8–72. Ligaments of the hock.

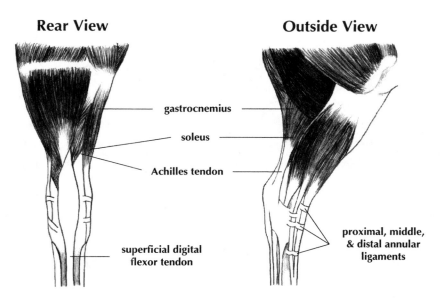

Rear View

Outside View

gastrocnemius

soleus

Achilles tendon

superficial digital
flexor tendon

proximal, middle,
& distal annular
ligaments

Fig. 8–73. Muscles activating the hock.

MUSCLES OF THE HOCK			
Name	**Origin**	**Insertion**	**Function**
Gastrocnemius	back of lower femur	tuber calcis	extend hock; flex stifle
Soleus	top of fibula	tuber calcis	extend hock; flex stifle
Superficial digital flexor	back of lower femur	point of hock; side of pastern bones	flex stifle, fetlock, and pastern joints; extend hock
Peroneus tertius tendon	front of femur	tarsal bones; top of cannon bone	prevents hock overextension
Cranial tibial	top outside of tibia	tarsal bones	flex hock

Fig. 8–74.

associated with it. In fact, its tendon joins that of the gastroc before inserting onto the tuber calcis. Its function is to assist the gastroc.

Superficial digital flexor—This very tendinous muscle originates on the back of the lower femur. Its tendon attaches to the tuber calcis, then continues down the leg before inserting on the short pastern bone and coffin bone. These attachments allow it to extend the hock joint and flex the fetlock joint.

In addition, the deep digital flexor tendons pass over the inside and back of the hock and help to ex-

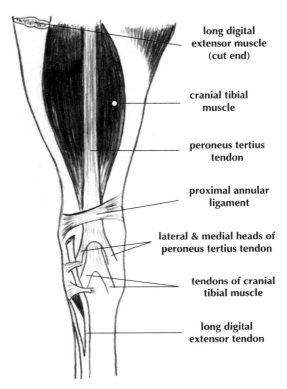

long digital extensor muscle (cut end)

cranial tibial muscle

peroneus tertius tendon

proximal annular ligament

lateral & medial heads of peroneus tertius tendon

tendons of cranial tibial muscle

long digital extensor tendon

Fig. 8–75. Front (cranial) view of the gaskin and hock, showing the peroneus tertius tendon.

tend and stabilize it. As they do, they are surrounded and protected by tendon sheaths. Strain and subsequent fluid accumulation within one of these sheaths causes the swelling known as "thoroughpin."

Flexor Muscles

The flexor muscles are located on the front of the leg, and attach to the tarsal bones.

Peroneus tertius tendon—Also called the fibularis tertius, this thin tendon runs from the front of the femur to the tarsal bones, traveling under the long digital extensor muscle. Just before it inserts, it divides into two heads: lateral and medial. The two heads attach to both the tarsal bones and the top of the cannon bone. This structure prevents the hock from overextending. Its vital contribution to the reciprocal apparatus is discussed in the next section.

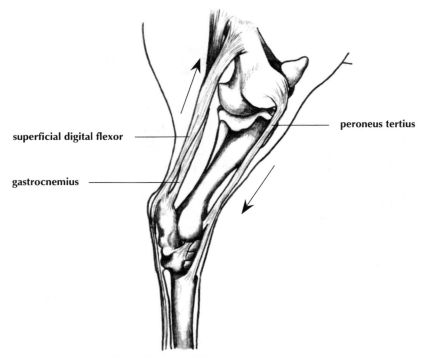

superficial digital flexor

gastrocnemius

peroneus tertius

Fig. 8–76. Outside (lateral) view of the reciprocal apparatus.

Cranial tibial—This muscle originates near the top and outside of the tibia. Its tendon passes between the two heads of the peroneus tertius tendon before it, too, divides into two heads. The medial head of the cranial tibial tendon is also known as the cunean tendon. The medial and lateral heads insert onto different tarsal bones. The cranial tibial muscle flexes the hock.

In addition, the long and lateral digital extensor tendons pass over the front and outside of the hock and help to flex it.

Reciprocal Apparatus

The hock has reciprocal action with the stifle, meaning that the stifle joint cannot flex without also flexing the hock joint. The structures on the back of the leg responsible for this reciprocal movement are the superficial digital flexor muscle and gastrocnemius muscle. The structure on the front of the leg is the peroneus tertius tendon. Together they are termed the *reciprocal apparatus.*

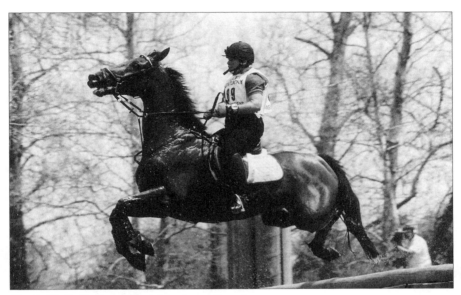

Fig. 8–77. Both the stifle and hock are flexed.

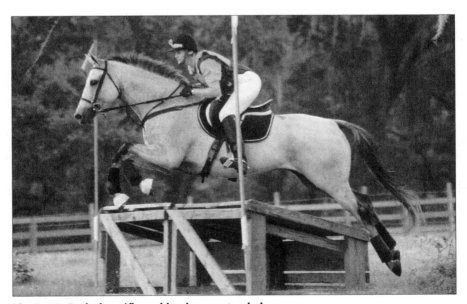

Fig. 8–78. Both the stifle and hock are extended.

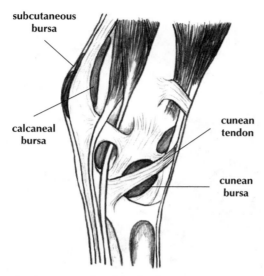

subcutaneous bursa

calcaneal bursa

cunean tendon

cunean bursa

Fig. 8–79. Bursae of the hock.

Bursae of the Hock

There are several places where bursae (plural of "bursa") may occur in the hock. The *cunean bursa* lies between the cunean tendon (the medial head of the cranial tibial tendon) and the tarsal bones. It protects both the tendon and the bones from pressure and friction.

There may be two bursae over the vulnerable tuber calcis. The *calcaneal bursa* is located on the side, and *subcutaneous bursa* is located at the very tip. This is the structure involved in a "capped hock."

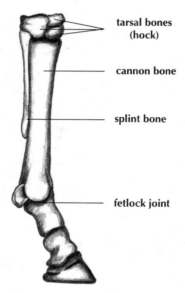

tarsal bones (hock)

cannon bone

splint bone

fetlock joint

Fig. 8–80. Bones of the cannon.

Cannon

The anatomy of the hind cannon is very similar to the fore cannon. The information in this section is an overview of the corresponding section in Chapter 6, *Forelegs*. Details unique to the hindleg, however, are mentioned throughout the section.

Bones

The *cannon bone* forms part of the hock joint at its top end and part of the fetlock joint at its lower end. The two *splint bones* form a joint with the lower row of *tarsal bones*. Together, these three bones of the hindleg are known as the *metatarsals*. The hind cannon bone is the large or third

Front View

Outside View

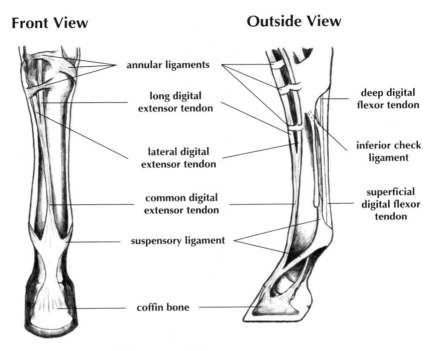

annular ligaments

long digital extensor tendon

lateral digital extensor tendon

common digital extensor tendon

suspensory ligament

coffin bone

deep digital flexor tendon

inferior check ligament

superficial digital flexor tendon

Fig. 8–81. Tendons and ligaments of the cannon.

metatarsal. It is a little longer than in the foreleg. Likewise, the splint bones are longer and slightly larger. In the hindleg, the splint bones are also called the second and fourth metatarsal bones.

Tendons and Ligaments

About one-third of the way down the cannon, the lateral digital extensor tendon merges with the long digital extensor tendon. Together they become the *common digital extensor tendon,* traveling down the front of the cannon. The superficial and deep digital flexor tendons run along the back of the cannon. The *inferior check ligament* is located between the suspensory ligament and the flexor tendons, but it is smaller than the corresponding check ligament in the foreleg. In fact, some horses do not have an inferior check ligament in the hindleg.

The *suspensory ligament* of the fetlock runs next to the cannon bone underneath the flexor tendons. It functions to support the fetlock.

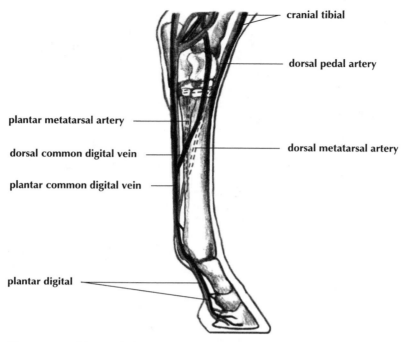

cranial tibial

dorsal pedal artery

plantar metatarsal artery

dorsal common digital vein

dorsal metatarsal artery

plantar common digital vein

plantar digital

Fig. 8–82. Inside (medial) view of the major blood vessels of the cannon.

Blood Vessels of the Cannon

At about the level of the hock, the cranial tibial artery becomes the *dorsal pedal artery*. Below the hock, it becomes the large *dorsal metatarsal artery*. This artery passes between the metatarsal bones, moving from the front of the hindleg to the back before continuing down the outside of the cannon. It then becomes the *distal perforating branch*.

Traversing the back of the leg are the lateral and medial *plantar arteries* and the deeper *plantar metatarsal* arteries. The distal perforating branch is joined by the two plantar arteries and the two plantar metatarsal arteries. Together they form the *distal plantar arch*. About three-fourths of the way down the cannon, it divides into the lateral and medial *plantar digital arteries* supplying the foot.

The veins follow the same general paths as the arteries and have similar names—the lateral and medial plantar veins drain the cannon area of blood, sending it back toward the heart.

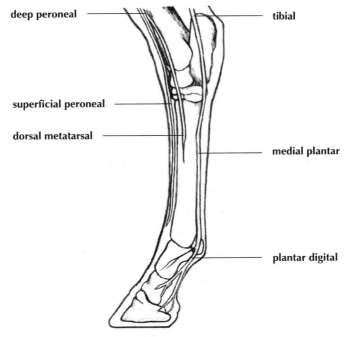

deep peroneal

tibial

superficial peroneal

dorsal metatarsal

medial plantar

plantar digital

Fig. 8–83. Inside (medial) view of the major nerves of the cannon.

Nerves of the Cannon

At the front of the leg, the *superficial peroneal nerve* continues down the cannon, ending about mid-cannon. At the hock, the *deep peroneal nerve* divides into lateral and medial branches. These branches become the lateral and medial *dorsal metatarsal nerves*.

Below the point of the hock, the *tibial nerve* divides into the lateral and medial *plantar nerves*. These nerves traverse either side of the back of the cannon, in a groove between the suspensory ligament and the flexor tendons.

Fetlock & Pastern

Like the cannon area, the anatomy of the hind fetlock and pastern is similar to that of the foreleg. One notable difference is the slope of the hind pastern: it has a normal standing position of 49° – 56°.

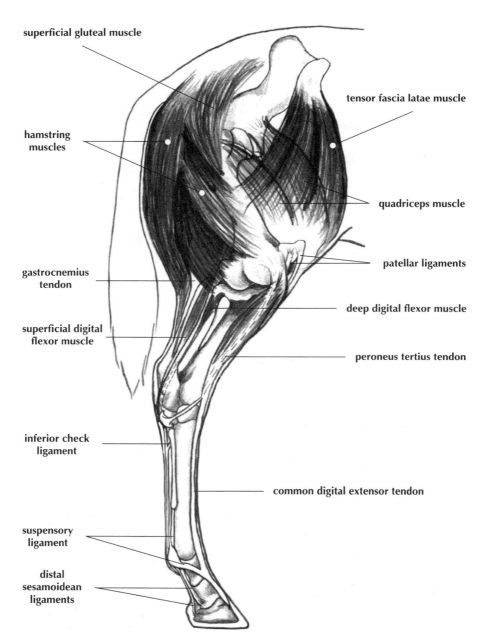

superficial gluteal muscle

tensor fascia latae muscle

hamstring
muscles

quadriceps muscle

patellar ligaments

gastrocnemius
tendon

deep digital flexor muscle

superficial digital
flexor muscle

peroneus tertius tendon

inferior check
ligament

common digital extensor tendon

suspensory
ligament

distal
sesamoidean
ligaments

Fig. 8–84. Stay apparatus of the hindleg and associated structures.

250

As in the foreleg, the hind fetlock joint is under the constant heavy strain of the horse's body weight. The *suspensory apparatus,* as part of the stay apparatus, holds the fetlock securely in the normal standing position.

The reader is referred to the corresponding sections in Chapter 6, *Forelegs.* The word "plantar" for the hindleg structures can be substituted for the word "palmar" for the foreleg structures to arrive at their proper names.

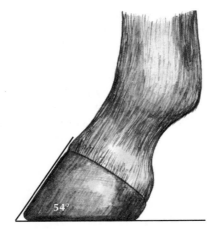

Fig. 8–85. The slope of the hind pastern is normally 49° – 56°.

Stay Apparatus

The *stay apparatus* is a system of muscles, tendons, and ligaments that allows the horse to "lock" its lower leg joints with little muscular effort. This mechanism, aided by the reciprocal apparatus, makes it possible for the horse to sleep while standing. The structures involved are:

- gluteal muscles
- tensor fascia latae muscle
- hamstring muscles
- quadriceps muscles
- patellar ligaments
- peroneus tertius tendon
- gastrocnemius muscle and tendon
- common digital extensor tendon
- superficial digital flexor tendon
- deep digital flexor tendon and inferior check ligament
- suspensory ligament and its branches
- distal sesamoidean ligaments

All of these structures are detailed earlier in this chapter or in Chapter 6, *Forelegs.*

The structures work together to hold the leg in a normal standing position. The hip is held in extension by the gluteal muscles and the hamstring muscles. The horse's body weight would logically tend to flex the stifle, but the peroneus tertius tendon prevents this action. In

251

turn, the gastrocnemius muscle stabilizes the hock, preventing the peroneus tertius from flexing the hock too much. The superficial digital flexor also extends the hock, assisting the gastrocnemius.

The horse's stifle has an additional locking mechanism. The patella can hook itself over the inner trochlear ridge of the femur. This eases the load on the quadriceps muscles considerably. Unlocking the patella requires the combined efforts of the quadriceps, biceps femoris, and tensor fascia latae muscles.

9

FEET

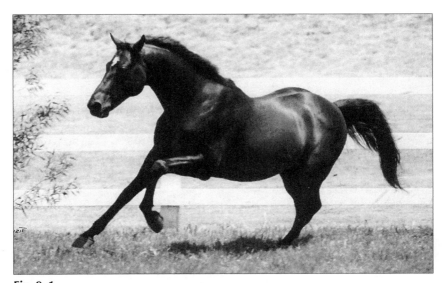

Fig. 9–1.

The feet bear all of the horse's weight, and often that of a rider. Every time the foot hits the ground, concussive forces pass through the foot up into the leg. The foot is designed to absorb much of this impact, preventing injury to the leg structures. Poor conformation causes uneven or ineffective distribution of concussive

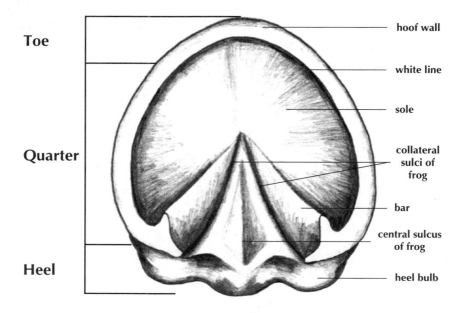

Toe

Quarter

Heel

hoof wall

white line

sole

collateral
sulci of
frog

bar

central sulcus
of frog

heel bulb

Fig. 9–2. The horse's foot is divided into three areas: toe, quarter, and heel.

forces, making the horse vulnerable to injury. Therefore, good foot conformation is essential to soundness.

The feet are indexes to the health and soundness of the whole horse. Therefore, most people consider the feet first when selecting a horse. If the feet are unsatisfactory, they waste no time examining the rest of the horse.

CONFORMATION OF THE FOOT
Influence of Leg Conformation

Conformation of the foot is influenced by the structure of the entire leg. To function correctly, proper alignment of the foot in relation to the leg is important. The foot should be placed squarely on the leg. From the front (or rear), a vertical line dropped straight down from the point of the shoulder (or buttock) should bisect the foot. From the side, a vertical line dropped through the center of the cannon should reach the ground just behind the heel bulbs. (These concepts are illustrated in Chapter 6, *Forelegs*, and Chapter 8, *Hindlegs*.)

Parts of the Foot

The external parts of the horse's foot include the hoof wall, bars, sole, and frog. The hoof wall is the horny outer covering of the foot. The bars, sole, and frog are located on the bottom of the foot.

Hoof Wall

The *hoof wall* can be divided into three areas: *toe, quarter,* and *heel.* The toe should be round and the heels broad. The wall is thickest at the toe and thinnest at the heels, allowing them to be flexible. The hoof wall should not be too dry and brittle, but should contain

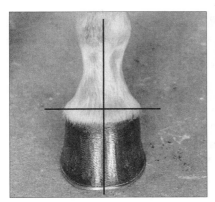

A. Front View.

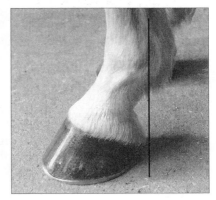

B. Side View.

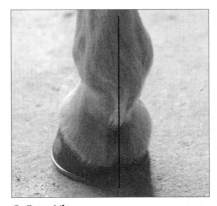

C. Rear View.

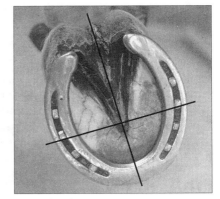

D. Bottom View.

Fig. 9–3. A well-conformed foot is symmetrical from all angles.

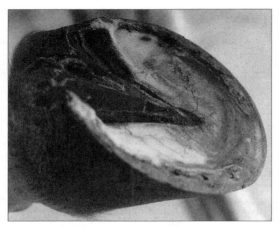

Fig. 9–4. Healthy frog, sole, and bars.

enough moisture to allow the heels to expand as the foot bears weight. There should be no major cracks or blemishes.

The bottom of the hoof should show even wear. The horn grows about ¼ – ½ inch per month. Hoof wall growth is normally faster in the summer and slower in the winter.

Bars

The *bars* of the hoof are formed by the wall as it turns inward and forward at the heels. The bars run on each side of the frog and converge toward one another, helping to preserve the width of the heel and prevent excessive expansion or contraction of the heel. This part of the wall and bar is commonly called the "buttress" of the hoof.

Frog

The *frog* divides the bottom of the foot into two equal halves, with the point of the frog aimed directly at the center of the toe. The frog should be large, well developed, and resilient.

Sole

The *sole* should be concave enough to prevent it from touching the shoe or the ground. It is closest to the ground surface just behind the toe. The sole prevents undue shock to vulnerable structures inside the foot and permits most of the horse's weight to be borne by the wall, and lesser amounts by the bars and frog. The sole of the hind foot is normally more concave than the forefoot.

Foot Size

The size of the horse's foot should be in proportion to the size of its body. A generous foot with good sole concavity is ideal. Sizable feet provide a solid base of support and good shock absorption. In addition, such feet indicate ample bone structure.

The two forefeet should be of similar size and shape, and the two hind feet should be of similar size and shape. It is normal for there to be *small* differences between the forefeet or hind feet.

While the two forefeet should match, and the two hind feet should match, there are distinct

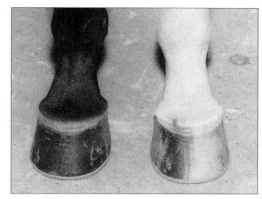

Fig. 9–5. Although these feet are different colors, they are equal in size and quality.

differences between the forefeet and the hind feet. The hind feet are narrower, and have toes that are more pointed. The hind feet are also more upright (have steeper hoof wall angles) than the forefeet.

Hoof Color

Tradition holds that a white or unpigmented hoof is drier or of poorer quality than a dark or pigmented hoof. Science has been unable to support this. White hooves appear to be of poorer quality because minor imperfections are more conspicuous on a white hoof than on a dark hoof, where the same blemish would go unnoticed. Good conformation, proper foot care, and an appropriate diet result in healthy, well-formed hooves, regardless of their color.

The Balanced Foot

A balanced foot is one that allows concussive forces to be distributed evenly. It is symmetrical when viewed from the front or back, and when picked up to view the bottom. The farrier balances the foot when the horse is trimmed. If an unshod hoof wears evenly on all sides and remains level between trimmings, it is an indication of even concussion, good conformation, and soundness. (Because a shoe interferes with the natural wearing of the hoof wall, it is impossible to make the same judgment on a shod foot.)

An unbalanced foot is most often the result of improper trimming or shoeing. It may also be due to poor foot or total leg conformation.

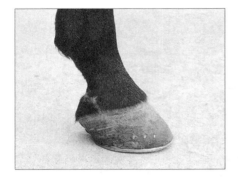 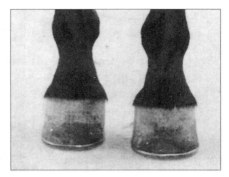

Forefeet

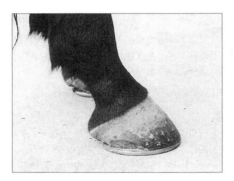 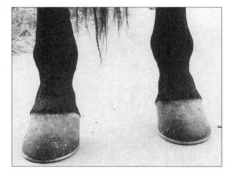

Hindfeet

Fig. 9–6. The angle of the hoof wall should equal that of the pastern. The hind feet are normally narrower and longer, with steeper angles, than the forefeet.

From the Front

The height and slope of the hoof wall should be the same on both sides. In this ideal situation, the coronet runs straight across the front of the foot, then slopes evenly down toward each heel.

From the Back

Viewed from the back, the two heel bulbs should be even in height. An easy way to examine heel height is to pick up the foot by cupping the front of the fetlock and allowing the pastern and foot to hang naturally. This position permits a good view of the heels.

From the Bottom

The bottom of the foot should also be symmetrical. A line drawn through the central sulcus of the frog to the center of the toe should divide the foot evenly *(see Figure 9–3)*. The heels, bars, and collateral sulci of the frog should be in the same position on each side.

Hoof Wall Angulation

The angle of the hoof wall should match that of the pastern, creating a straight, continuous line from the fetlock to the toe. For most horses, the angle of the forefeet is 47° – 54°. The hind hoof wall angles are steeper: most horses have angles of 49° – 56° in the hind feet. However, it is more important for the hoof wall and pastern angles to match each other than to conform to an "ideal" number.

Conformational Faults of the Foot

Too Large/Too Small

If the horse's feet are too big and wide (*mushroom-* or *puddle-footed*), the walls cannot provide enough support for the horse's weight. Good sole concavity is lost, resulting in a flat foot that is prone to dropped soles and sole bruises. These horses often have porous horn, which is difficult to keep properly moisturized.

Overly small or narrow feet create even greater problems. These feet do not expand during weight-bearing, and are therefore poor shock absorbers. Small or narrow feet also have less area over which to diffuse concussive forces. With excess concussion, the hoof wall becomes dry and brittle. Over time, the horse my be at risk for navicular syndrome, ringbone, and sole bruises.

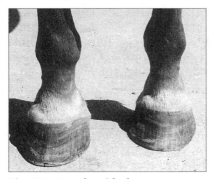

Fig. 9–7. Overly wide feet.

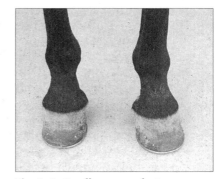

Fig. 9–8. Small, narrow feet.

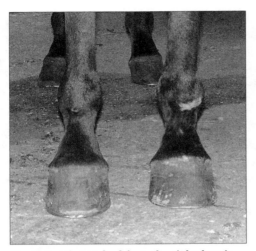

Fig. 9–9. Mismatched feet: the right foot is smaller than the left foot.

Both overly large and overly small feet are heritable characteristics. Small feet especially should be selected against because they create more serious foot problems.

Mismatched Feet

With *mismatched feet,* one forefoot (or less often, one hind foot) is different from the other in size, shape, and hoof wall angle. Mismatched feet are often caused by chronic foot pain. The horse bears less weight on the painful foot, reducing heel expansion. Therefore the frog does not expand and circulation in the foot is reduced. As the frog atrophies (shrinks), the heel grows taller, and the painful foot gradually becomes more narrow and upright.

Meanwhile, the opposite foot bears proportionally more of the horse's weight. It spreads and becomes flatter, which can also cause painful problems.

Toed-In/Toed-Out

Toed-in means that the horse's toes point in, toward each other (also called "pigeon-toed"). *Toed-out* means that the horse's toes point outward, away from each other (also called "splay-footed"). However, it is possible for only one foot to be affected.

Toeing-in and toeing-out are often caused by abnormal conformation higher up in the leg. However, these problems are most obvious in the feet. Toeing in and toeing out may cause the horse to move poorly, and to interfere while in motion (discussed later).

Trainers place different emphasis on these problems, depending on the severity of the fault and the level of the horse's activity. For example, Standardbred trainers may find a toed-in stance to be more acceptable on a pacer than on a trotter, because the risk of interference is less. But many people will accept slightly turned-out toes if the horse's cannons are parallel to each other. According to the

Fig. 9–10. Toed-in.

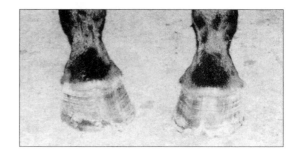

Fig. 9–11. Toed-out.

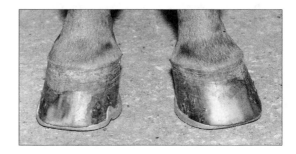

Hackney Judging Standards, "A slight toeing-out is not objectionable." Arabians and Trakehners are also sometimes toed-out in the hind feet, usually only from the fetlock down.

Uneven Coronet

An uneven coronet indicates that the foot was not balanced properly. It is therefore subject to uneven stress. The taller side of the wall hits the ground first, and pushes the coronet on that side upward. The shorter side then impacts the ground forcefully, which can cause bruising and lameness. With proper trimming, the coronet will realign itself.

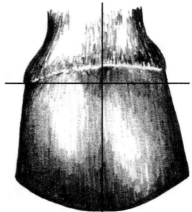

Fig. 9–12. Uneven coronet.

Club Foot

A *club foot* has developed when the hoof wall angle is nearly vertical, at 60° or more. It may occur in one or both forefeet. The heel is very high and the hoof becomes box-shaped. This condition is most often caused by contracture of the deep digital flexor tendon. Shortening of this tendon raises the heel. The hoof wall at the heel does not wear as fast as the toe, and becomes longer. Over time, the hoof wall at the heel grows down to the ground.

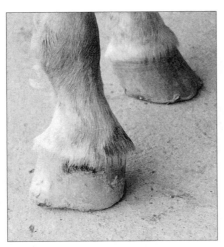

Fig. 9–13. Severe club foot.

Horses with a steep club foot are prone to toe bruising and laminitis because of the excess weight born by the toe. Tension on the tendon hyperflexes the knee (bends it forward), which can eventually cause problems there as well. If the condition is caught early and properly managed, the horse's performance does not usually suffer.

Hoof Rings

Rings on the surface of the hoof wall may be caused by a number of situations. Some are normal; others indicate illness or serious disease. However, all of these situations have a common underlying cause—changes in the rate of hoof wall growth. Rings may occur with:

- dietary changes, such as the addition of grain or lush pasture
- growth spurts, which often occur in spring
- high fever, causing "fever rings"
- inflammation (including laminitis), causing "founder rings"
- improper trimming or shoeing

Hoof Cracks

Hoof wall cracks may be called *toe cracks, quarter cracks,* or *heel cracks,* depending on their location. They vary in length and depth, and therefore in seriousness. Hoof wall cracks can be caused by abnormal foot conformation or trauma to the coronet. They can also be caused by improper shoeing, abnormal hoof moisture, or poor diet. Hoof cracks should be examined by a veterinarian or farrier—they

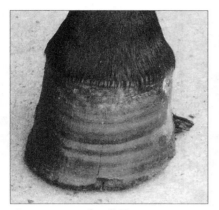

Fig. 9–14. Hoof wall rings.

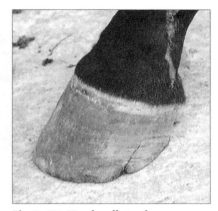

Fig. 9–15. Hoof wall crack.

may need to be treated medically, and the shoeing modified to treat the underlying cause. (For complete descriptions of hoof crack treatment, read *Equine Lameness,* published by Equine Research, Inc.)

High Heels/Contracted Heels

Feet with high heels have high hoof walls at the heels. This hoof conformation is most often the result of improper trimming: leaving too much heel on the foot. (This is sometimes done purposefully to increase knee/ hock action.) Some horses tend to grow hoof wall at the heel faster than usual, and need to be trimmed more often. High heels can also be caused by lameness. If the horse cannot bear weight on the back part of the foot, the hoof wall at the heel is not worn away naturally. Sometimes high heels are accompanied by upright pasterns, which can lead to hyperextension of the knee (where the knee bends backward) and knee problems.

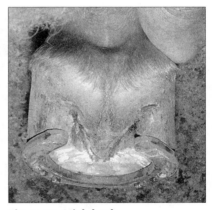

Fig. 9–16. High heels.

High heels inevitably lead to *contracted heels*, where the heel area becomes narrower than normal. But contracted heels does not necessarily involve only the heel—the whole foot can be affected. High

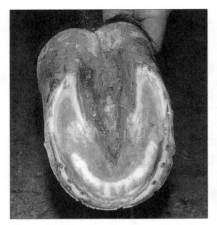

Fig. 9–17. The frog has atrophied due to lack of heel expansion.

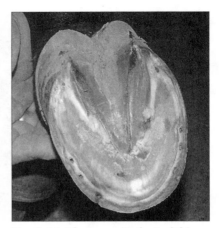

Fig. 9–18. The opposite foot of this horse is normal.

heels lead to contracted heels because high heels are less flexible and do not expand properly when the horse bears weight on the foot. If the heels do not expand, the frog is not activated, and circulation within the foot is reduced. The frog atrophies (shrinks), which creates a narrow, contracted foot.

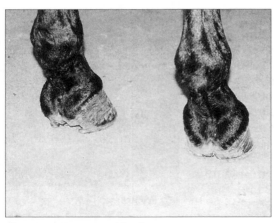

Fig. 9–19. Contracted heels.

A high-heeled, contracted foot does not absorb concussive forces well. Heel and frog expansion are essential to shock absorption. Furthermore, contracted heels have a smaller area through which to absorb concussion.

High heels and contracted heels can be corrected or managed with proper trimming and shoeing.

Low Heels

Feet with low heels have low hoof walls at the heels, sometimes causing the heel bulbs to touch the ground. Excess pressure on the

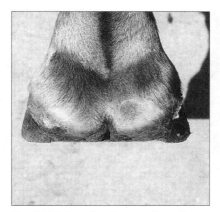

Fig. 9–20. Low heels may allow the heel bulbs to touch the ground. This foot is a poor shock-absorber.

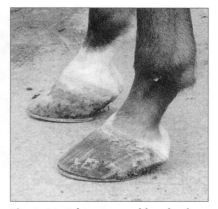

Fig. 9–21. A long toe and low heel stress the structures at the back of the fetlock and foot.

heels increases the risk of lameness. It also causes the hoof wall in that area to wear faster, worsening the problem. Low heels can be caused by lameness or improper trimming and shoeing. However, these faults can also be inherited (and often corrected or managed).

Long Toe–Low Heel

Low heels are frequently accompanied by long toes—a combination often found in Thoroughbreds. *The long toe–low heel* foot conformation develops when the farrier leaves too much toe on the foot, or when the hoof wall grows faster at the toe than at the heel. A long toe and low heel force the horse to bear excess weight on the back of the foot. Concussive forces are no longer directed evenly throughout the foot and up the leg, but are concentrated at the heels. The excess stress contributes to hoof wall cracks and navicular syndrome. A long toe also causes greater strain on the flexor tendons, suspensory ligament, and sesamoid bones.

Under-Run Heels. When the long toe–low heel foot conformation goes untreated, the heels may become *under-run.* This means that the horn tubules (fibers that make up the hoof wall) at the heel grow at a much steeper angle—nearly horizontal—than those at the toe. The horn tubules at the heel are crushed, eliminating any shock absorbing capacity and allowing valuable moisture to escape the hoof wall. Under-run heels can eventually result in quarter cracks, abscesses, and white line disease.

Sheared Heels

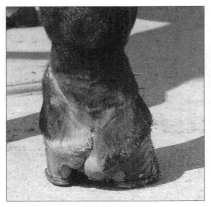

Fig. 9–22. Sheared heels.

Sheared heels occur when the hoof wall at the heel is taller on one side than on the other. The taller heel hits the ground first and takes the initial impact. The heel bulb on that side is pushed upward. As the two heel bulbs are pushed farther apart, the skin between them tears (are sheared). Furthermore, the excess pressure on the taller side of the hoof wall causes it to develop quarter cracks.

Sheared heels are usually caused by poor trimming. It is rarely seen in barefoot horses because the taller heel will wear away naturally. A shoe prevents normal wearing of the extra heel. It is also possible for sheared heels to be caused by uneven weight-bearing due to pain on one side of the foot. Occasionally, it is caused by faster or slower hoof wall growth at one heel. Even if sheared heels is not caused by pain, a horse with untreated sheared heels can become lame.

Flat Feet

In a *flat-footed* horse, the sole is not concave enough, and may touch the shoe or the ground. The horse is more prone to corns and sole bruises. Such feet need a great deal of care to prevent lameness.

Dropped Sole

A sole is *dropped* when it has no concavity at all. It has dropped to the level of the hoof wall, and sometimes below it. This happens when the coffin bone rotates downward, usually due to chronic laminitis or road founder, causing the sole to bulge. X-rays will help the farrier determine the normal angle of the coffin bone, and to match this angle with that of the hoof wall. This is important for proper corrective shoeing.

Sole Bruise

Excessive pressure can cause a reddish *sole bruise.* The pressure may be the result of stepping on a stone, or even stomping the foot

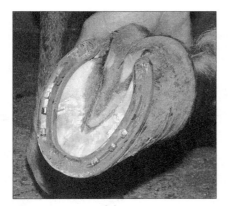

Fig. 9–23. Normal foot.

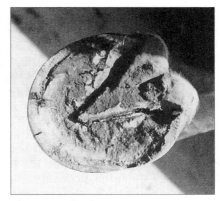

Fig. 9–24. Flat foot.

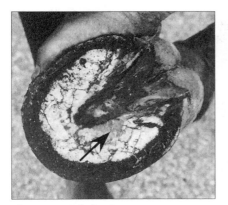

Fig. 9–25. Sole bruise.

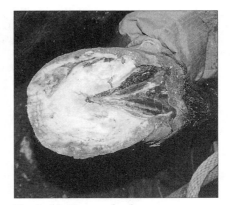

Fig. 9–26. Dropped sole.

on hard ground. It is sometimes several weeks before the bruise can be seen, but the horse is often lame immediately. Sole bruises are common in horses with flat feet, or horses with soles that have been pared too much.

Foot Conformation and Locomotion

Correctly conformed and balanced feet are essential to straight, fluid movement. The point of breakover, foot flight, and foot landing are all influenced by the conformation of the foot and leg.

Foot Breakover

Breakover is the last instant in the stride that the horse's toe is touching the ground. Good conformation causes breakover to occur at the exact center of the toe. Poor conformation causes breakover to occur off-center. When this happens, part of the hoof wall receives excess stress. Good trimming and shoeing will help the horse break over in the center.

Foot Flight and Landing

"Foot flight" is the path the foot travels while in the air. From a front view, if the horse moving straight forward, the foot should also travel straight forward, without deviating inward or outward along the way. The left and right feet should travel in parallel, and no one foot

Normal travel—the foot travels straight forward.

Paddling—the foot deviates outward during travel.

Winging in—the foot deviates inward during travel.

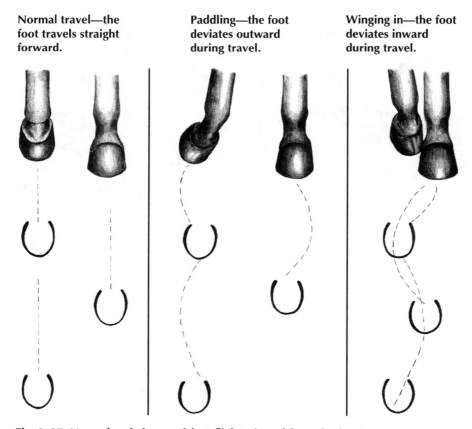

Fig. 9–27. Normal and abnormal foot flight, viewed from the front.

should contact another. Contact of this kind is called "interference."

From a side view, the foot in the air should pass the opposite leg at the height of the arc of travel.

The foot should land on all sides at once. That is, the toe, quarters, and heels should land together.

Altered Foot Flight and Landing

Abnormal foot conformation causes predictable abnormalities in foot flight and landing. This in turn can cause interference and strain of certain structures.

Front View

If the horse is toed-in, the foot deviates outward as it advances. This motion, called "paddling," strains the sides of the joints, although the horse usually does not interfere.

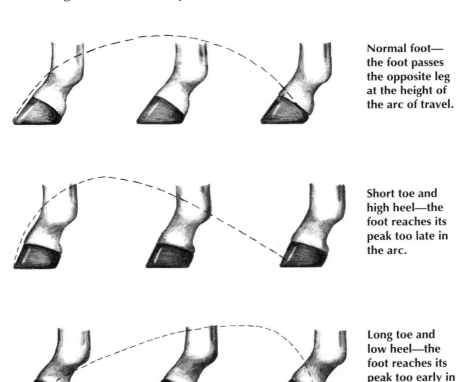

Normal foot— the foot passes the opposite leg at the height of the arc of travel.

Short toe and high heel—the foot reaches its peak too late in the arc.

Long toe and low heel—the foot reaches its peak too early in the arc.

Fig. 9–28. Normal and abnormal foot flight, viewed from the side.

If the horse is toed-out the foot deviates inward as it advances. This "winging in" motion leaves the inside of the opposite foreleg vulnerable to interference.

Side View

A short toe–high heel conformation causes the foot to break over in such a way as to reach its peak too late in the arc. Short toes and high heels land abruptly, increasing concussion and giving a short, choppy ride.

A long toe–low heel conformation causes the foot to break over late, and therefore reach its peak too early in the arc of foot flight. It causes greater trauma to the heels at landing, but does give a smoother ride.

Human Influence on Foot Conformation

Trimming and Shoeing

Just because a foot is not properly conformed does not mean that the farrier should change it to fit the "ideal." If the angles of the hoof wall and pastern match, change only increases the strain on the leg. And even if they do not match, too much change in one trimming can worsen the problem. Corrective changes should be made gradually over several trimmings.

Faults caused by humans can be more easily managed than inherited faults. If contracted heels, flat feet, or brittle hooves are caused by neglect or improper trimming, they can often be corrected by dietary supplements and proper foot care.

Selective Breeding

For centuries, people have tampered with the natural conformation of the horse's feet, in an effort to create a pleasing appearance and smooth ride. The changes have occurred both mechanically and through selective breeding. Every popular breed of horse today has been altered in some way. The feet of Quarter Horses and Thoroughbreds are noticeably smaller, although Appaloosa and Warmblood breeders select for large feet. Thoroughbreds are also known for long toe–low heel foot conformation, which was once believed to produce speed. The feet of Tennessee Walking Horses and American Saddlebreds intended for showing are sometimes grown to extreme length and plastic platforms are added to ensure high action. Even draft horses have had their feet altered, since very large feet are

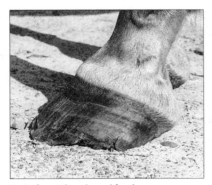

A. Before trimming, side view.

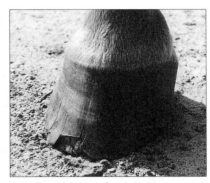

B. Before trimming, front view.

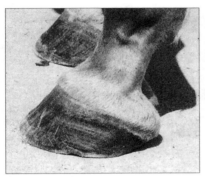

C. After trimming, side view.

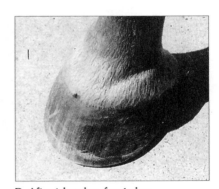

D. After trimming, front view.

Fig. 9–29. Dry, brittle hooves caused by neglect. The farrier will make further improvements gradually over several shoeings.

thought stylish in show circles. Each of these practices creates its own problems, sometimes even lameness. It is unfortunate that only after generations of good horses become unsound do we recognize the harm that is being done.

Continuing research and innovation will help reverse damaging trends in favor of a more natural foot. Trainers and breed associations have the power and the responsibility to educate their clients and members. It is also important to set guidelines and educate judges, ensuring that the problem characteristic is not rewarded in the show ring.

ANATOMY OF THE FOOT

The foot is defined as both the hoof, which is the horny outer covering, and all its internal structures. The primary role of the foot is to protect and support the leg—and ultimately the entire body—while standing and while in motion. It also provides leverage for the leg muscles that produce motion. Many structures within the foot are designed to absorb concussion forces. Another important role of the foot is to squeeze blood back up the veins, returning it to the general circulation. This is why the foot is often called the "second heart." These roles are more thoroughly addressed in later sections as specific parts are introduced.

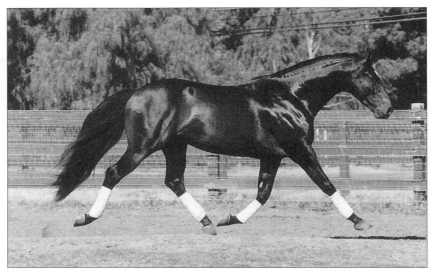

Fig. 9–30. Locomotion helps the foot to act as a "second heart."

The parts of the foot can be grouped into three major structural systems based loosely on their function. Some parts have more than one function, and are therefore listed under more than one category.

- Mechanical structure: bones, joints, tendons, ligaments, bursae, blood vessels, and nerves.
- Insensitive and Sensitive structures: hoof wall, laminae, periople, sole, frog, and the corium which produces them.
- Elastic structure: hoof wall, lateral cartilages, digital cushion, and frog.

Mechanical Structure

The mechanical structure includes the bones, joints, tendons, ligaments, bursa, blood vessels, and nerves. The functions of the mechanical structure are to support the foot and to produce movement.

Bones of the Foot

The bones of the foot include the lower part of the *short pastern bone, navicular bone,* and *coffin bone.* The short pastern bone extends downward from the long pastern bone to just below the coronet. Therefore, half of the short pastern bone is considered part of the pastern area, while the other half is contained within the foot. Here it forms the *coffin joint* with the coffin bone and navicular bone.

Coffin Bone

The coffin bone (also called the third phalanx or pedal bone) is shaped much like the hoof, but is smaller. The small peak in front is called the *extensor process.* The common digital extensor tendon has its final insertion here. At the toe the coffin bone is so perforated with holes that it resembles a hard sponge. The holes allow branches of arteries, veins, and nerves deep within the foot to pass through the bone to supply the active structures nearer the surface.

The underside, or *solar surface* (because it faces the sole), is shaped like a half-moon. The "cup" this forms is called the *semilunar canal.* The deep digital flexor tendon has its final insertion here. The semilunar canal is bisected longitudinally by a small ridge of bone called the *semilunar crest.*

On each side of the coffin bone are the *wings*—small extensions of bone. On their upper surface, each wing gives attachment to a *lateral cartilage.*

Lateral Cartilages

The two lateral cartilages are positioned along the sides of the foot, extending above the coronet towards the heel. They can be easily felt by squeezing above the coronet, as they create the contour of the heel. The lateral cartilages harbor and protect the soft tissues that lie between them.

Navicular Bone

The wedge-shaped navicular bone is also called the distal sesamoid bone. It lies behind the short pastern bone and coffin bone in the coffin joint, across the back of the foot. It has a pulley-like action that

Side View

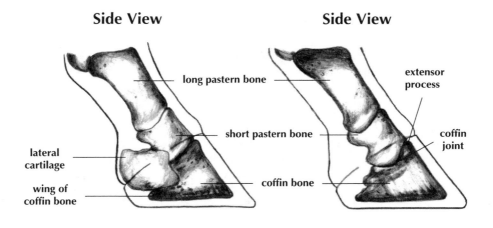

long pastern bone

short pastern bone

lateral cartilage

wing of coffin bone

coffin bone

Side View

extensor process

coffin joint

Front View

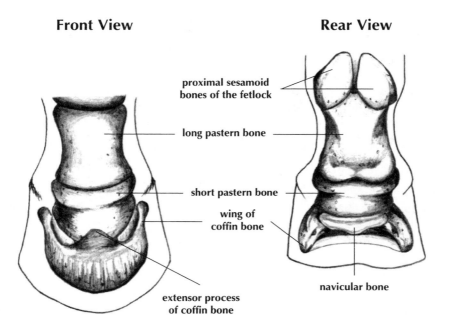

proximal sesamoid bones of the fetlock

long pastern bone

short pastern bone

wing of coffin bone

extensor process of coffin bone

Rear View

navicular bone

Fig. 9–31. Bones of the foot. On the top right drawing, the lateral cartilages have been removed to show the shape of the coffin bone.

changes the direction of pull of the deep digital flexor tendon on the coffin bone. The deep digital flexor tendon passes over the back of the navicular bone, holding it firmly in the joint. The sides of the navicular bone are enclosed by the wings of the coffin bone and the lateral cartilages.

Joints of the Foot

The coffin joint is formed by three bones: the short pastern bone, coffin bone, and navicular bone. Because it is encased within the hoof, the coffin joint is relatively immobile. In a normal standing position it is slightly extended. It has a joint capsule, the lining of which produces synovial fluid, lubricating the joint surfaces.

Tendons of the Foot

Superficial digital flexor tendon—While this structure is not located within the foot, it does help to flex the foot because it acts on the fetlock and pastern joints. It is more thoroughly described in Chapter 6, *Forelegs* or Chapter 8, *Hindlegs.*

Deep digital flexor tendon—This tendon begins as a muscle at the top of the leg. It runs down the back of the cannon, fetlock, and pastern, over the navicular bone, and inserts onto the solar surface of the coffin bone. In the foreleg it functions to extend the elbow, and flex the knee and foot. In the hindleg it functions to flex the stifle and foot, and extend the hock.

Common digital extensor tendon—This tendon runs down the front of the cannon, fetlock, and pastern, finally inserting onto the extensor process of the coffin bone. In the foreleg it functions to flex the elbow, and extend the knee and foot. In the hindleg it functions to extend the stifle and foot, and flex the hock.

(See Figure 9–32 for an illustration of these tendons.)

Ligaments of the Foot

Annular Ligament

An annular ligament is a broad, strong support structure that wraps horizontally around the back of a joint. The *distal digital annular ligament* is located right above the heels. It is attached to each side of the short pastern bone. This ligament covers the deep digital flexor tendon on its way to the coffin bone.

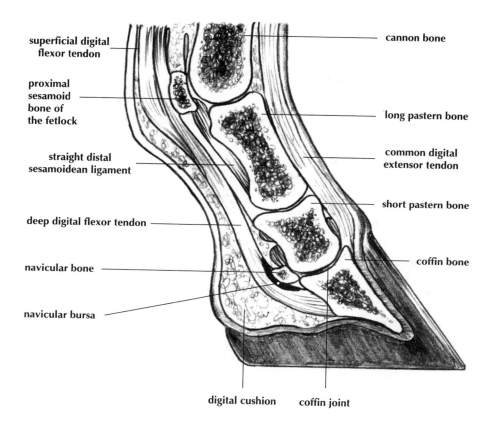

superficial digital
flexor tendon

proximal
sesamoid
bone of
the fetlock

straight distal
sesamoidean ligament

deep digital flexor tendon

navicular bone

navicular bursa

cannon bone

long pastern bone

common digital
extensor tendon

short pastern bone

coffin bone

digital cushion   coffin joint

Fig. 9–32. A cross-section of the horse's foot.

Lateral Cartilage Ligaments

Each lateral cartilage is secured by a set of short ligaments. These ligaments surround the cartilage on three sides, anchoring them to the long pastern bone, short pastern bone, and coffin bone, and the common digital extensor tendon near its insertion in the foot.

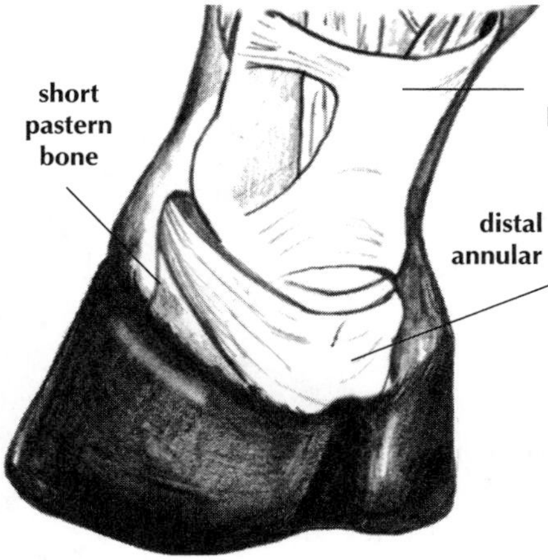

Fig. 9–33. The distal digital annular ligament attaches to the sides of the short pastern bone.

Coffin Joint Ligaments

Like most other joints in the legs, the coffin joint has *collateral ligaments* supporting it on each side. The ligaments run from the bottom of the short pastern bone to the top of the coffin bone, passing underneath the ligaments of the lateral cartilages.

Navicular Ligaments

The navicular bone is suspended and supported by ligaments from both above and below. From above, the two *suspensory ligaments* of the navicular bone originate on each side of the lower end of the long pastern bone, toward the front. They run diagonally across the short pastern bone and insert on the top of the navicular bone. From below, the short *impar ligament* (or distal ligament of the navicular bone) originates on the bottom of the navicular bone and inserts on the underside of the coffin bone.

Bursa of the Foot

A bursa is a fluid-filled protective sac. The *navicular bursa* of the foot lies between the navicular bone and deep digital flexor tendon. The bursa protects the tendon and navicular bone from abrasion as the tendon slides over the bone. It is often this relationship that is disrupted in navicular syndrome.

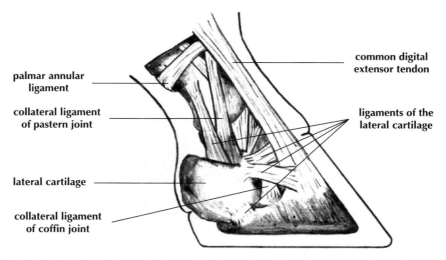

Fig. 9–34. Outside (lateral) view of the lateral cartilage ligaments and nearby ligaments. The bottom of the palmar annular ligament has been removed to show these structures.

Labels for Fig. 9–34:
- palmar annular ligament
- collateral ligament of pastern joint
- lateral cartilage
- collateral ligament of coffin joint
- common digital extensor tendon
- ligaments of the lateral cartilage

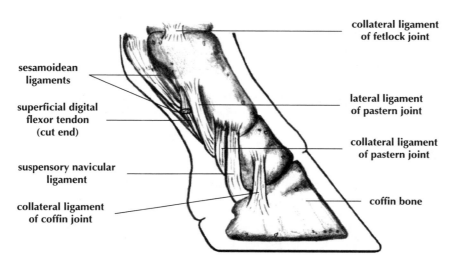

Fig. 9–35. Outside (lateral) view of the coffin joint and navicular ligaments.

Labels for Fig. 9–35:
- sesamoidean ligaments
- superficial digital flexor tendon (cut end)
- suspensory navicular ligament
- collateral ligament of coffin joint
- collateral ligament of fetlock joint
- lateral ligament of pastern joint
- collateral ligament of pastern joint
- coffin bone

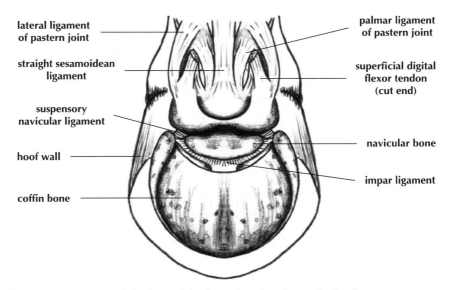

lateral ligament
of pastern joint

straight sesamoidean
ligament

suspensory
navicular ligament

hoof wall

coffin bone

palmar ligament
of pastern joint

superficial digital
flexor tendon
(cut end)

navicular bone

impar ligament

Fig. 9–36. A rear (caudal) view of the foot, showing the navicular ligaments.

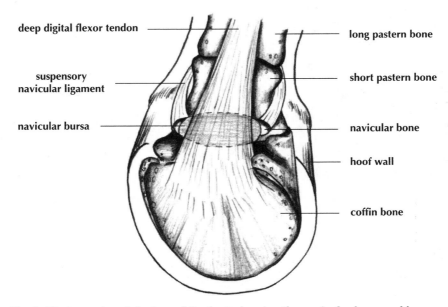

deep digital flexor tendon

suspensory
navicular ligament

navicular bursa

long pastern bone

short pastern bone

navicular bone

hoof wall

coffin bone

Fig. 9–37. A rear (caudal) view of the foot, showing the navicular bone and bursa.

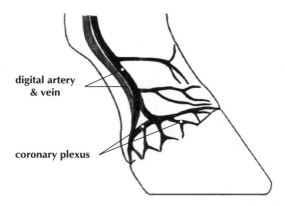

digital artery
& vein

coronary plexus

Fig. 9–38. Outside (lateral) view of the major blood vessels of the foot.

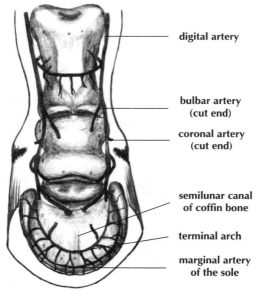

digital artery

bulbar artery
(cut end)

coronal artery
(cut end)

semilunar canal
of coffin bone

terminal arch

marginal artery
of the sole

Fig. 9–39. Rear (caudal) view of the arteries of the foot.

Blood Vessels of the Foot

The feet require a generous blood flow. (Interruption of the blood supply causes the very serious condition, laminitis.) The lateral and medial *palmar digital arteries* (or *plantar digital arteries* in the hind foot) and their many branches supply the foot with blood. These two arteries pass under the coffin bone, and merge together within the semilunar canal. Together they form the *terminal arch.* The terminal arch has many branches radiating outward. Several of these branches pass back up through the holes in the tip of the coffin bone to supply the front of the foot.

Of course, generous blood flow into the foot requires adequate blood drainage out of the foot. There are several networks of veins called plexuses within the foot. The largest is the *coronary plexus,* located at the coronet. This web encircles the upper part of the foot, collecting blood and sending it up to the lateral and medial *palmar/plantar digital veins.*

Nerves of the Foot

The lateral and medial *palmar digital nerves* (or *plantar digital nerves* in the hind foot) run down the back of the pastern, on either side of the deep digital flexor tendon. Each has a dorsal branch that supplies the front of the foot. The main *palmar digital nerve* curls underneath the coffin bone, where it

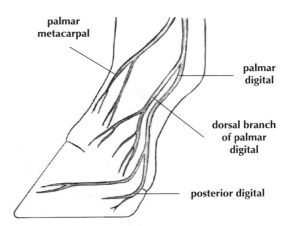

Fig. 9–40. Outside (lateral) view of the nerves of the foot.

becomes the *posterior digital nerve*. It supplies the back of the foot with sensation. A veterinarian may inject local anesthetic to block specific nerves in this region in order to pinpoint lameness.

Insensitive and Sensitive Structures

The insensitive structure of the foot includes the hoof wall, insensitive laminae, periople, sole, and frog. They are called "insensitive" because they have no nerve supply and no blood supply. The insensitive structure is designed to bear weight and dissipate concussive forces.

The sensitive structure of the foot is so named because it does have a nerve supply and a blood supply. The sensitive structure is called the *corium* (also "pododerm"). The corium consists of a highly vascular, inner layer of specialized skin cells that line the inside of the hoof. The cells produce insensitive structures. Therefore, growth of all parts of the hoof originates in the corium. Other functions of the corium include:

- to carry blood which nourishes the horn-producing tissues and keeps the foot warm
- to attach the hoof wall firmly to the mechanical structure
- to dissipate concussion and excess heat

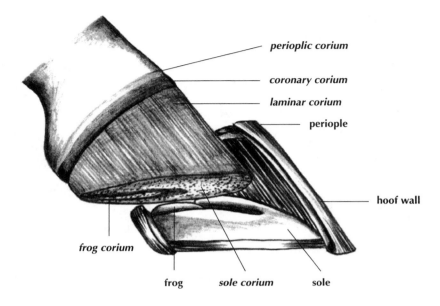

Labels on figure:
perioplic corium
coronary corium
laminar corium
periople
hoof wall
frog corium
frog
sole corium
sole

Fig. 9–41. The sensitive structure, or corium (italics), produces insensitive horn.

The corium is divided into five parts, depending on the type of horn produced. Each part is detailed in the sections to follow.

- The coronary corium encircles the foot beneath the coronet and produces both the horn of the hoof wall and the insensitive laminae.

- The perioplic corium lies just above the coronary corium and produces the periople.

- The laminar corium covers the coffin bone from the coronary corium to the sole, and produces the sensitive laminae.

- The sole corium lines the underside of the coffin bone and produces the horn of the sole.

- The frog corium lies above and produces the horn of the frog.

Hoof Wall

The visible, most familiar part of the foot is the hoof wall—the horny covering, or cornified epithelium. The hoof wall bears most of the horse's weight. The horn grows about ¼ – ½ inch per month, completely replacing itself in 8 – 10 months. It grows evenly downward from the *coronary corium* so that the youngest weight-bearing part of the wall is at the heel, because the foot is shortest there. The wall is thickest at the toe, and gradually reduces in thickness so that the thinnest portion is at the heel. It thickens

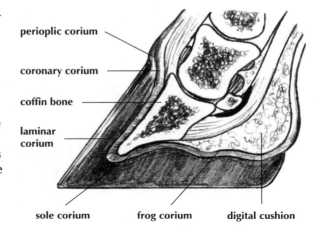

perioplic corium

coronary corium

coffin bone

laminar corium

sole corium   frog corium   digital cushion

Fig. 9–42. Cross-section of the foot showing the corium lining entire inside of the hoof.

slightly, however, at the angles where the bars are formed.

The hoof wall is made up of three layers:

- the periople and tectorial layer on the outermost surface
- the tubular layer, which makes up the bulk of the wall
- the insensitive laminar layer on the innermost surface

Periople and Tectorial Layer of the Hoof Wall

Together the *periople* and *tectorial layer* make up the outermost layer of the hoof. The *perioplic corium* is a narrow ring of tissue located right above the coronary corium, deep to the coronet. It produces both the periople and tectorial layer.

The periople is similar in function to the human cuticle: it protects the seam between the horn and the skin. It is a narrow, whitish band of thin tissue over the upper section of the hoof wall, just below the hairline. It is about ¾ inch wide at the toe and quarter. At the heels it widens to cover the bulbs.

The tectorial layer is a waxy substance that migrates down the surface of the hoof to form a protective coating. It is made up of a thin layer of soft, keratinized cells that coat the hoof wall much like a furniture polish. "Keratinized" simply means that there is keratin—a strong, glue-like material—between the cells. Keratin may be elastic or brittle, depending upon the amount of moisture it contains. It gives the hoof a glossy look and helps to seal in vital moisture. But removing too much of this layer with the rasp during trimming can make the hoof dry and brittle.

Tubular Layer of the Hoof Wall

The coronary corium lies just under the coronet. Since the coronary corium is quite vascular, wounds of this area may bleed heavily. Injuries to the coronary corium may result in a permanent scar or malformation of the hoof wall.

Most of the horny wall consists of *horn tubules* formed by hardened keratin material. These tightly-packed tubules are the fibers of the wall and run parallel to each other as they grow down from the coronary corium to the ground surface. In between tubules is the *intertubular horn*, a cement-like substance that is also produced by the coronary corium.

The outer surface of the coronary corium is covered with villiform papillae (tiny, hair-like projections). These papillae produce the horn tubules. Each tubule emerges from a papilla about as thick as a hair.

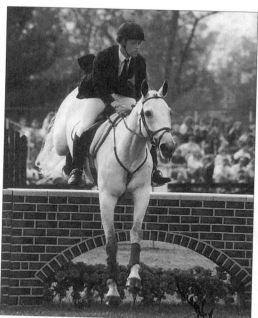

The center of the tubule is hollow and contains its share of the moisture that is so vital to elasticity and shock absorption. The hoof wall contains about 25% water.

Good foot conformation is essential for the hoof wall to retain moisture. This is because the foot's conformation dictates the direction and spacing of the tubules, which determines the hoof's moisture content. For example, the problem with a long toe–low heel foot conformation is that the horn tubules spread apart, allowing moisture to escape from the hoof wall.

Fig. 9–43. The horn tubules contain moisture that is vital to shock absorption.

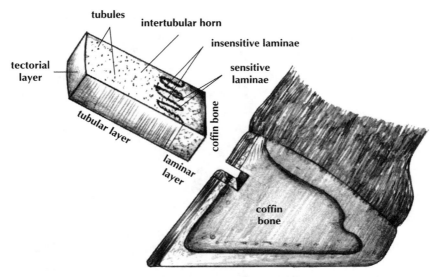

Fig. 9–44. The coronary corium produces the hoof wall and insensitive laminae.

Insensitive Laminar Layer of the Hoof Wall

The inner surface of the coronary corium produces the *insensitive laminae,* which form the laminar layer of the hoof wall. "Laminae" are microscopic projections, similar to the plush of carpet, but formed in rows. About 600 insensitive laminae project outward from the inside surface of the hoof wall. On each of these primary laminae are 100 or more secondary laminae, and each secondary lamina likewise has tertiary laminae. The insensitive laminae grow downward from the coronary corium to the sole. The laminar layer fastens the hoof wall to the coffin bone by interdigitating (interlocking) with matching sensitive laminae on the surface of the coffin bone. These laminae bear most of the horse's weight, since they form the only structural attachment of the hoof wall to the rest of the foot.

Sensitive Laminae

The *sensitive laminae* are produced by the *laminar corium*. The laminar corium is attached to the surface of the coffin bone and lower edges of the lateral cartilages by a membrane of connective tissue. It provides nourishment for the sensitive and insensitive laminae, and the intertubular horn.

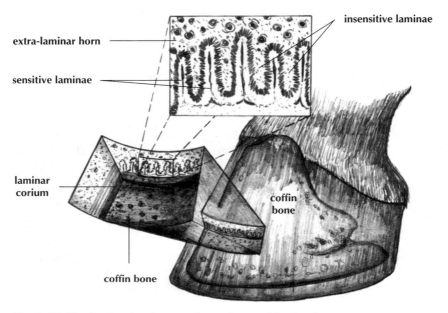

insensitive laminae

extra-laminar horn

sensitive laminae

laminar corium

coffin bone

coffin bone

Fig. 9–45. The laminar corium produces the sensitive laminae.

The laminar corium produces hundreds of primary, secondary, and tertiary sensitive laminae projecting outward. The sensitive laminae firmly mesh with the insensitive laminae of the hoof wall, forming a secure attachment between the hoof wall and coffin bone.

The interlocking of the insensitive and sensitive laminae is visible on the bottom of the foot as the *white line*. Therefore, the white line is a valuable indicator as to the placement of horseshoe nails. Nails must penetrate the bottom of the hoof between the white line and the outside of the hoof wall. If the nail is driven inside the white line, it will pierce the sensitive laminae, causing pain and possibly an abscess. Separation and infection of the hoof wall and sole is called "white line disease" or "seedy toe."

Sole

The sole is a hard plate of horn on the underside of the foot, between the hoof wall and the frog. It is a little thicker on the edges than in the middle, where it is about ¼ inch thick. Its primary function is to protect the vulnerable internal foot structures from injury by hard objects on the ground. Although it is the largest section of

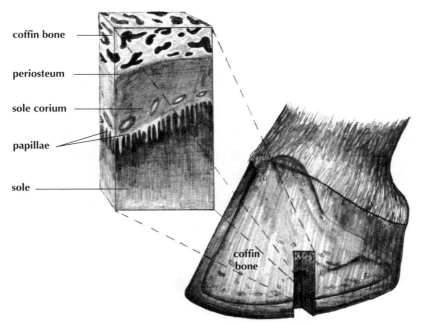

coffin bone

periosteum

sole corium

papillae

sole

coffin bone

Fig. 9–46. The sole corium produces the sensitive sole.

the bottom of the foot, the sole is not intended to bear weight directly. It is slightly concave and bears only a small amount of internal weight. If the sole is allowed to touch the shoe or the ground, lameness from corns or bruises can occur.

The *sole corium* is that part of the sensitive structure which lies underneath the coffin bone and produces the insensitive sole. It is practically indistinguishable from the periosteum (bone covering) of the coffin bone. Like that of the hoof wall, the horn of the sole is produced by numerous villiform papillae (tiny hair-like extensions) and therefore has a similar tubular structure. However, the keratin of the sole is softer—the moisture content of the sole is about 30%. The tubules run vertically, but curl near the ground. This results in self-limiting growth by the constant shedding of flakes of dead horn, making the sole tough and irregular.

Frog

The frog is a V-shaped cushion of soft keratin material located in the ground surface of the foot (the moisture content of the frog is

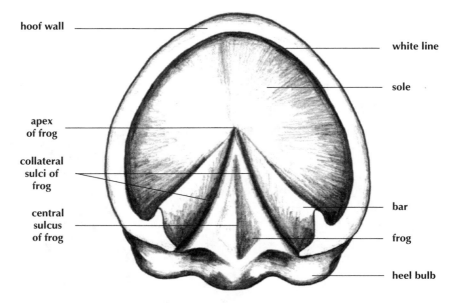

hoof wall

white line

sole

apex
of frog

collateral
sulci of
frog

central
sulcus
of frog

bar

frog

heel bulb

Fig. 9–47. The parts of the bottom of the horse's foot.

about 50%). The point of the frog is called the *apex*. The groove in the middle is called the *central sulcus*. The two grooves on each side are called the *collateral sulci*; they separate the frog from the bars and sole.

The frog has several purposes. One purpose is to give the foot a firmer grip in stopping and turning. Another is to store moisture for the rest of the hoof. The elasticity resulting from this moisture helps it to absorb shock by dissipating concussion forces.

The sensitive structure that lies above and produces the insensitive frog is called the *frog corium*. It is similar in structure to (and continuous with) the sole corium. Its villiform papillae produce the insensitive frog. The frog corium also blends partially with the digital cushion (examined in the next section), working in concert with that structure to absorb shock.

Elastic Structure

The *elastic structure* of the foot refers to the ability of the hoof wall, lateral cartilages, digital cushion, and frog to absorb concussion and help pump blood back up the veins of the leg. The key to absorbing concussion is fluid. Structures with a high moisture content are more flexible, and expand under pressure when the horse bears weight on the foot.

Hoof Wall

The hoof wall has the lowest moisture content of the elastic structures. It is thickest at the toe, and gradually reduces in thickness so that the thinnest portion is at the heel. Since this is also the youngest wall, the heel is the most elastic.

Interestingly, hoof moisture does not come from external sources. It comes from internal water carried through the blood and lymph vessels to the sensitive structures. From there it is transferred to the horn tubules that make up the hoof wall.

Lateral Cartilages

Cartilage is tough, but flexible. So the lateral cartilages are tough enough to protect the soft tissues between them, but flexible enough to expand under pressure. Sometimes they become calcified and bony—this condition is called sidebone. Because calcified cartilages are less flexible, sidebone reduces their shock-absorbing capacity. (For more information on sidebone, read *Equine Lameness*, published by Equine Research, Inc.)

Digital Cushion

The *digital cushion* is a fibrous, fatty, wedge-shaped pad in the back half of the foot. It lies above the frog, between the lateral cartilages and below the short pastern bone and deep digital flexor tendon. The back part of the digital cushion forms the heel bulbs.

Frog

The frog has the highest moisture content of the elastic structures, making it the most flexible. It is also furrowed by the central sulcus and collateral sulci. This arrangement allows the frog to widen and spread when weight is placed on it.

How the Elastic Structure Works

When the horse bears weight on the foot, the frog and digital cushion are squeezed between the coffin bone and the ground. This compression causes them to flatten, which exerts pressure on the lateral cartilages. The normally concave sole also flattens and spreads the

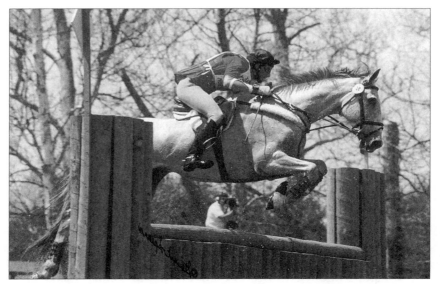

Fig. 9–48. The elastic structure absorbs concussion upon landing. The more intense the activity, the more vital this function becomes.

heels, expanding the bars, hoof wall, and lateral cartilages. These movements occur almost simultaneously, causing the overall height of the hoof to decrease and the heels to expand about $1/16$ inch on each side. The final result is that concussion is dissipated.

In addition to dissipating concussion, the elastic structure helps to move blood around the tissues of the foot, and back up the leg. When the horse bears weight on the foot, the blood vessels within are compressed. This pressure forces blood out of the foot and up the veins of the leg. When weight is lifted from the foot, new blood is allowed to fill the blood vessels. This pumping action is an important means of returning venous blood from the foot back to the general circulation. Lack of motion creates poor circulation within the feet and legs, and is why stalled horses "stock up."

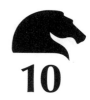

10

COLORS & MARKINGS

While a horse's coat color and markings have little to do with its conformation or anatomy, they are usually among the characteristics that distinguish a breed or type. Some breed enthusiasts prefer certain colors. For example, Clydesdales are usually bay or brown. On the other hand, some colors are very rare within certain breeds: white Thoroughbreds are seldom seen.

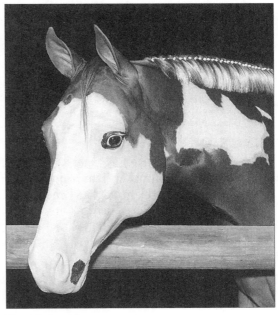

Fig. 10–1.

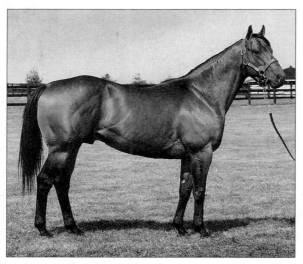

Fig. 10–2. A bay has dark points.

Not having the right markings, or having too much of the wrong markings, can make a horse ineligible for registration or showing. For example, the "high white" rule (no white leg markings allowed above the knee or hock) has been a hot topic in the Quarter Horse community for this reason. And Friesian horses are completely black: a small star is allowed, but no white leg markings are allowed.

COAT COLORS

Bay

A *bay* horse's primary coat color can be anywhere from light yellow-red to red-brown. But it has dark points, meaning its forelock, mane, tail, and lower legs are black.

Black or Brown

A true *black* horse has black skin and all black hair. It has no white face or leg markings and no brown hairs on the muzzle or flanks. If an otherwise black horse has brown or tan hairs on the muzzle and flanks, it is considered *seal-brown*. A *brown* horse may resemble a bay, with a yellow-brown to dark brown coat color and black points.

Chestnut/Sorrel

Like the bay, the *chestnut* or *sorrel* horse can be light yellow, bright red-gold, rich brown, or dark liver. But unlike the bay, the chestnut's points are not black: they echo the primary coat color.

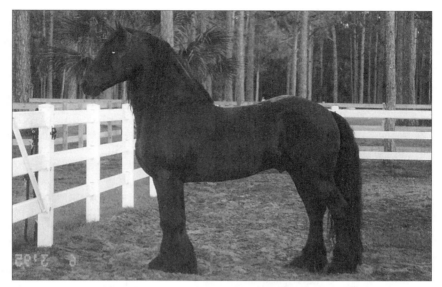

Fig. 10–3. A true black horse has all black hair. This horse is a Friesian.

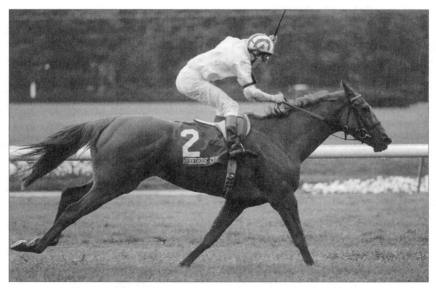

Fig. 10–4. This sorrel has a brown mane and tail, echoing its primary coat color.

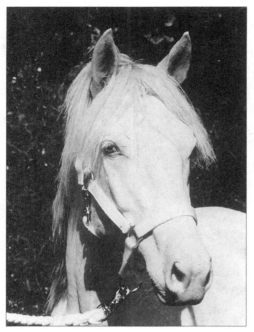

White

A true *white* horse has all white hair and pink skin, although a few dark specks on the skin are acceptable. The horse is born white and does not change color with maturity. Such horses are extremely rare. Contrary to appearances, white horses are not complete albinos (which are even more rare). They do not have pink eyes and do not usually have the other serious congenital health problems that albinos do. Unfortunately, albino foals die shortly after birth.

Fig. 10–5. A cremello horse with pumpkin-colored skin and blue eyes.

Cremello

Cremellos are creamy off-white to a rich cream, but lighter than the palomino. These horses may have the same white face and leg markings as darker horses. Also, their skin appears pink to pumpkin-colored and their eyes are usually amber or blue. The mane and tail can be white, cream, cinnamon, or a mixture of these colors.

Gray

A *gray* horse may have both black and white hairs. It has black skin, even if all the hairs are white. This is the best way to distinguish a gray from a true white (a true white has pink skin). Some gray horses look black at birth, but their coat lightens with maturity.

Within this category are variations of gray. *Flea-bitten grays* have black specks on a white background. *Dapple grays* have rings of darker gray hairs on a black-and-white background.

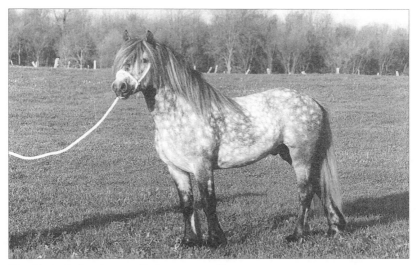

Fig. 10–6. A dapple gray Dales pony stallion.

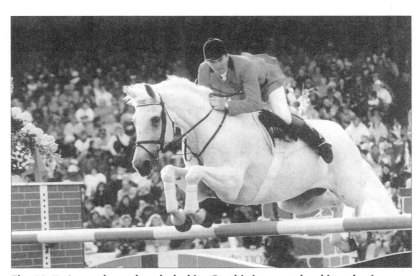

Fig. 10–7. A gray horse has dark skin. On this jumper, the skin color is evident on the muzzle.

Roan

A *roan* horse's coat is an even blend of white and some other color. The head and legs are solid colored. If the other color is black, the horse is called a *"blue roan."* If the horse's hair coat is a blend of white and red-brown, the horse is called a *"red roan"* or *"strawberry roan."* Sometimes these horses have dark colored points.

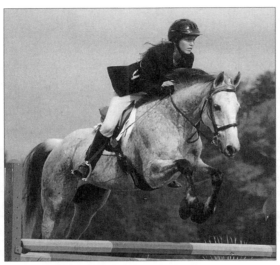

Fig. 10–8. A blue roan with an even blend of white hairs and black hairs.

Appaloosa

Appaloosas have a white or roan coat with black or brown spots, most of which are on the hindquarters. The spots range in size from specks to fist-sized and are rounded or oval. The Appaloosa's other markings include:

- white sclera around the eye
- parti-colored or mottled skin (notably on the muzzle and genitals)
- striped hooves

The mane and tail are sometimes sparse, although this feature is seen less frequently as the breed becomes more refined.

There are three basic Appaloosa spotting patterns. One is the *roan-type* Appaloosa pattern. An Appaloosa roan is distinctive because it has varnish marks (dark areas covering the bony points). Also, it does not have a solid colored head on a roan body: the head is roaned as well. Another is the *blanket* pattern, in which a white blanket, with or without colored spots, covers the hips of a colored horse. A blanket without spots is called a *snowcap*. The third type is the *leopard pattern*. This horse is white with colored spots "from nose to toes." There are also mixed variations of the three patterns listed above.

Leg markings are unusual, but not unheard of. If the horse is to be eligible for registration, leg markings may not be any higher than the

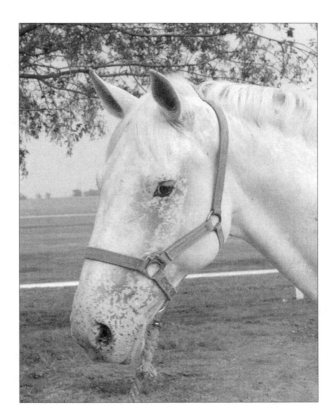

Fig. 10–9. White sclera and parti-colored skin.

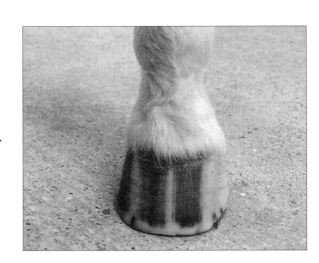

Fig. 10–10. A striped hoof.

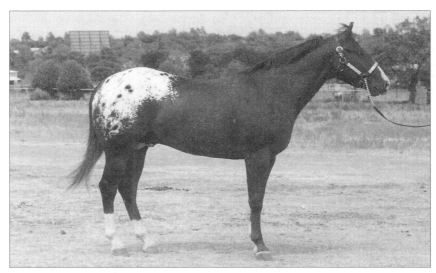

Fig. 10–11. An Appaloosa with a blanket pattern.

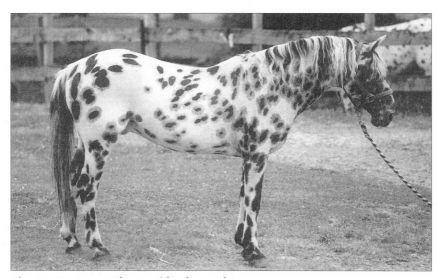

Fig. 10–12. An Appaloosa with a leopard pattern.

horse's knees or hocks. White face markings may not include one or both eyes, the jowls, or the lower lip reaching up to the jowls.

Paint/Pinto

Paint and *pinto* horses have large, irregular patterns of white and dark areas on their bodies. If the horse is black-and-white, it is called *piebald*. If the horse is brown-and-white, it is called *skewbald*. The pattern may be tobiano or overo. *Tobianos* have even, rounded markings, often extending over the back. The legs are usually white. The head is solid-colored but may have regular white face markings. *Overos* have uneven, feathery-edged markings, extending from under the belly but rarely over the back. Usually at least one of the legs is solid-colored. Overos tend to have large white face markings.

Characteristics also associated with the body markings include:

- apron or bald face
- white on the jaws
- blue or white (glass) eyes
- pink skin under the white hair
- parti-colored mane and tail

Blue eyes are common to horses of spotted breeding—especially when the white markings extend over the eye.

(For more information on the difference between a paint and a pinto, see Chapter 11, *Breeds of Horses.*)

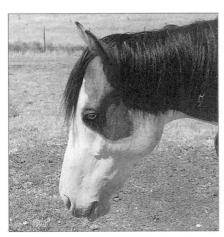

Fig. 10–13. Apron face.

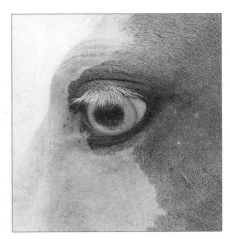

Fig. 10–14. Blue eyes.

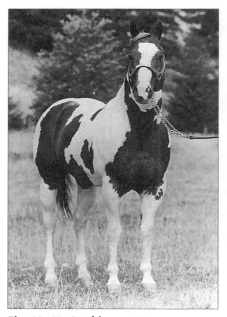

Fig. 10–15. A tobiano pattern.

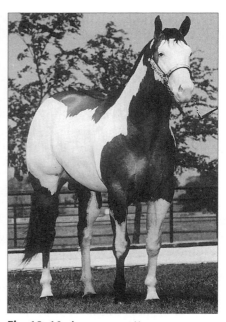

Fig. 10–16. An overo pattern.

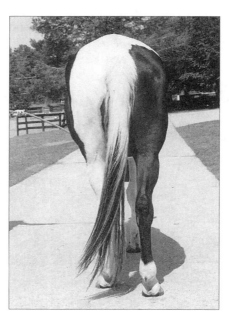

Fig. 10–17. Parti-colored tail.

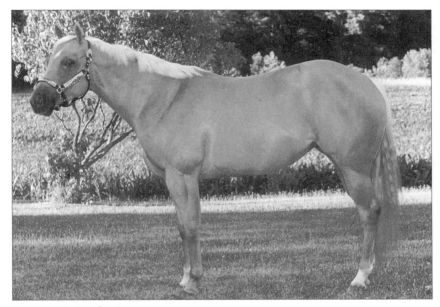

Fig. 10–18. A palomino.

Palomino

A *Palomino's* coat color resembles a newly minted gold coin. (A deep, rich gold is ideal, but the registries accept horses several shades lighter or darker.) The mane and tail are white, ivory, or silver, but may contain no more than 15% black or chestnut colored hair. The eyes are dark, although blue eyes are sometimes found among lighter-colored horses.

Buckskin/Dun/Grulla

Buckskin horses have yellow-brown bodies and dark points (mane, tail, and lower legs), although the exact shades vary. *Dun* horses are similar to buckskins but their coats are more intense and "smutty." A red dun is a chestnut dun with darker red points and dorsal stripe. *Grulla* (pronounced grew-ya) horses are smoky blue, dove, slate, or mousy, with dark points. Buckskin or grulla horses may have a dorsal stripe, shoulder stripes, and/or zebra-like markings on the legs, withers, or ears. White face and leg markings and blue eyes are permitted.

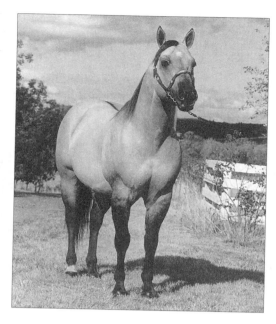

Fig. 10–19. A buckskin horse.

MARKINGS

Markings can be natural or man-made. They are used by breed and type registries to identify individual horses.

Body

Prophet's Thumb—A dent in the flesh, most on the neck or shoulder.

Flesh Mark—A small area of pink skin on an otherwise dark-skinned horse.

Dorsal Stripe—A dark stripe running from the mane to the tail. It is sometimes accompanied by zebra-like stripes on the withers, shoulders, and lower legs.

Whorl—A small area where the hair grows in the opposite direction from the surrounding area. They are usually found on the head, neck, chest, forearm, and gaskin.

Saddle or Girth Mark—A white patch or a hairless patch in the saddle or girth area. Saddle marks often result from saddle sores, caused by poor saddle fit or inadequate padding.

Brand/Freeze Mark—A number or pattern either hot branded or freeze branded permanently into the horse's skin. They are usually found on the shoulders, quarters, neck, or saddle area.

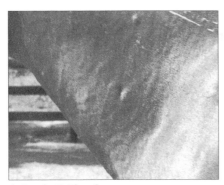

A. Prophet's Thumb.

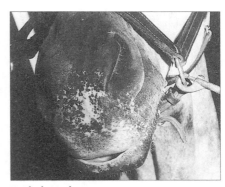

B. Flesh Mark.

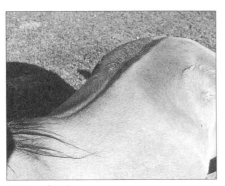

C. Dorsal Stripe.

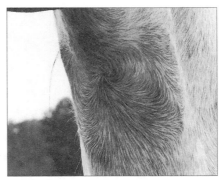

D. Whorl.

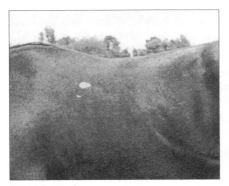

E. Saddle Mark.

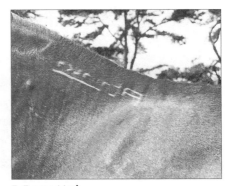

F. Freeze Mark.

Fig. 10–20. Markings on the Body.

Head Markings

Star—A white mark on the forehead.
Strip—A narrow white mark from the forehead to the nose.
Snip—A small white patch between the nostrils.
Blaze—A broad white mark from the forehead to the nose.
Bald Face—A wide blaze that covers most of the face, including the eye area and muzzle.

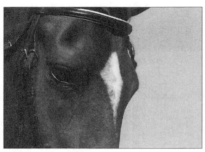

A. Star.

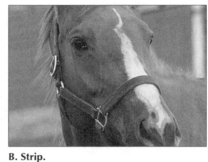

B. Strip.

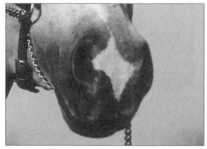

C. Snip.

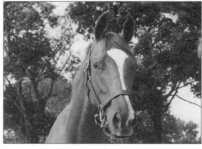

D. Star, Strip, and Snip.

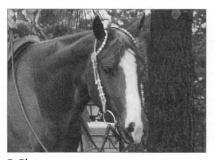

E. Blaze.

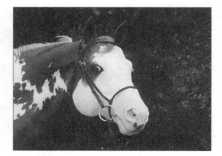

F. Bald Face.

Fig. 10–21. Markings on the Head.

Leg Markings

Coronet—A white strip on the coronet.
Pastern—The hair is white from the coronet to just below the fetlock. Also called a half sock.
Sock—The hair is white from the coronet to above the fetlock.
Half Stocking—The hair is white from the coronet to about halfway up the cannon.

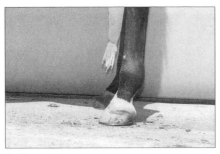

A. Coronet.

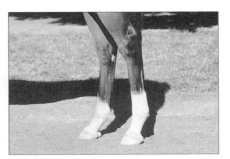

B. Pastern.

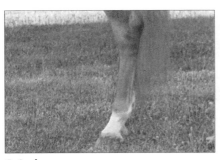

C. Sock.

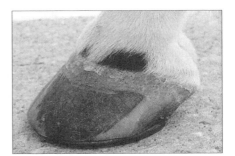

D. Half Stocking.

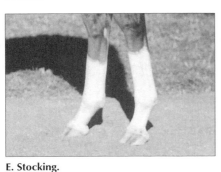

E. Stocking.

F. Ermine Mark.

Fig. 10–22. Markings on the Legs.

Stocking—The hair is white from the coronet to the knee or hock.

Ermine Mark—A small black or brown spot on the coronet.

Chestnut—The patch of soft, horny tissue found on the inside of the leg. Their shape is distinctive and are used to identify an individual.

Ergot—A small, horny structure at the back of the fetlock.

Feather—Long, silky hair on the lower legs and fetlocks. Feathering is heaviest in draft horses.

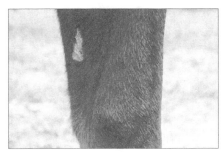

A. Chestnut.

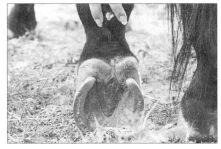

B. Ergot.

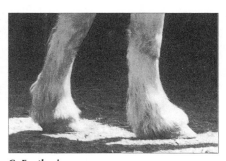

C. Feathering.

Fig. 10–23. Markings on the Legs, continued.

11

BREEDS OF HORSES

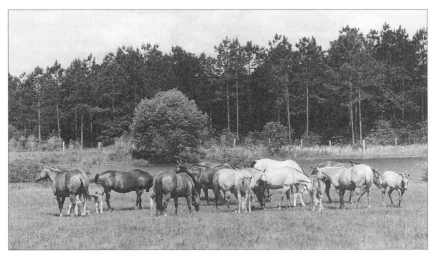

Fig. 11–1.

Abreed is a group of horses with distinctive characteristics that
are transmitted to their offspring. These characteristics may
include conformation, color, performance, intelligence, and
disposition. The different conformational traits of various breeds,
and even of horses within breeds, are generally the result of a combination of natural crosses and artificial selection methods. These
methods are aimed at developing horses to perform specific tasks.

Promoters of some breeds stress certain skills and abilities: Standardbreds, for instance, are bred almost exclusively for speed in harness. Other breeds are touted for their versatility: Arabians, Quarter Horses, and Morgans are excellent all-around performers.

Some breeds developed through centuries of outcrossings with numerous other breeds. On the other hand, several breeds have developed from a single founder—one sire can have a tremendous influence on a breed. Standardbreds, Tennessee Walking Horses, Saddlebreds, and Morgans each have been strongly influenced by one prepotent stallion.

There are more than 300 breeds of horses today. Based on body type and ancestry they are divided into light horse, warmblood, draft horse, and pony breeds. The most popular and influential breeds are discussed in this chapter.

LIGHT HORSE BREEDS

Light horses—unlike draft horses or ponies—are usually lean-legged, athletic animals built for speed and agility. Examples include Arabians, Thoroughbreds, Quarter Horses, and Standardbreds. These horses are suitable for driving, racing, pleasure riding, exhibition, and occasionally light packing. Light horses are also used for showing, jumping, hunting, endurance racing, and general ranch work. They stand between 14.2 and 17 hands and weigh 900 – 1,400 pounds. In the United States, many of the light horse breeds developed when settlers in different regions were faced with certain needs. These breeds may still excel at the purpose for which they were bred. This section mentions the most common uses of each breed, but most are versatile and have been employed in many different activities.

Some horses are bred for certain color characteristics or special gaits. While these horses are also considered light horses, they are grouped within their own sections.

Arabian

The *Arabian* is the oldest breed of light horse and has had a profound influence on the development of most other light horse breeds. Most modern hotblooded breeds trace to the Arabian; even the coldblooded Percherons claim some Arabian ancestors.

Arabians have small, triangular heads, dished profiles, pointed ears, and large eyes. An Arabian's forehead is broad, which sets the

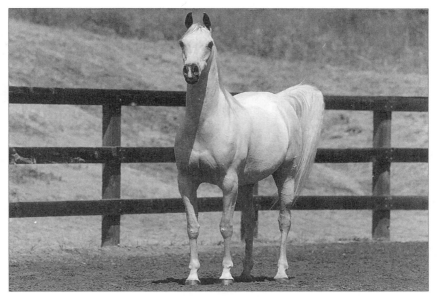

Fig. 11–2. The Arabian is the oldest breed of light horse.

eyes and ears widely apart. The face tapers to a small, fine muzzle with large, flaring nostrils. Its arched neck is moderately long and set high on the shoulder.

The Arabian's back is short and straight with a long, flat croup and a high tail carriage. Some people attribute the Arabian's short back to a reduced number of lumbar vertebrae. But studies show that, like most domestic horses, the Arabian normally has 6 lumbar vertebrae. Some Arabians have one fewer thoracic vertebrae (17 instead of 18) but this seldom affects back length, and the phenomenon often occurs in other breeds.

Arabians usually stand between 14.2 and 15.2 hands, and average 800 – 1,000 pounds. They are used primarily for pleasure and show, although they are also used as stock horses and raced—both flat racing and long distance competition. The breed is noted for docility, intelligence, and stamina.

Thoroughbred

The *Thoroughbred* originated in England when native English mares were crossed with Barb, Turk, and Arabian stallions. Three of

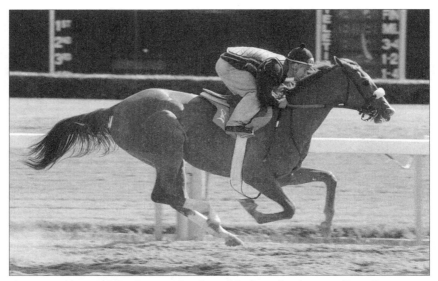

Fig. 11–3. Thoroughbreds were developed for speed at intermediate distances.

these stallions led to the formation of the foundation Thoroughbred lines: the Byerly Turk, the Darley Arabian, and the Godolphin Barb.

The Thoroughbred has served as foundation stock for a number of other breeds and has influenced breeds such as the American Saddlebred, Morgan, Standardbred, and Quarter Horse.

Thoroughbreds, developed primarily for speed at intermediate distances (¾ – 1½ miles), excel at the extended gallop. Their conformation varies somewhat because they have been bred for speed rather than uniformity of appearance. In general, the profile is straight and the nostrils are large and open. The eyes are large and curious, and the ears are medium to long, but not coarse. The neck is long and straight (not as arched as an Arabian's). Most conformationally correct Thoroughbreds have deep chests, medium high withers, short backs, and fairly long forearms and gaskins. They have long, smooth muscling with powerful hindquarters. Common among Thoroughbreds is a long toe–low heel foot conformation. They are also prone to flat feet.

Thoroughbreds range in height from 15 to 17 hands and weigh 900 – 1,200 pounds. They have achieved the most notoriety as racehorses, but they are also used extensively for hunting, jumping, eventing, polo, endurance racing, mounted patrol, and pleasure riding.

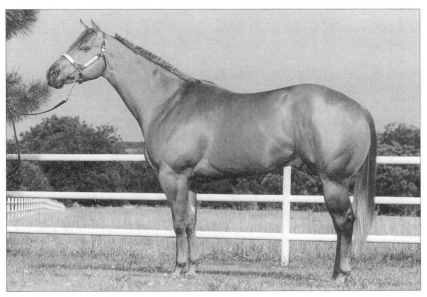

Fig. 11–4. Quarter Horses are heavily muscled.

Quarter Horse

The *Quarter Horse* originated in the United States, and may have developed as a type before the Thoroughbred was established in England. Today, there are more Quarter Horses registered in the world than any other breed.

Quarter Horses were bred for running short distances. Early American settlers raced their horses on streets that were seldom longer than a quarter mile. They came to value the horses' short bursts of speed and ability to navigate rugged courses hewn out of the wilderness.

These horses also became known for their adaptability to ranch life. The Quarter Horse is recognized as the ideal "cow horse." The same attributes that gave it speed and power for shortcourse racing qualified it as a stock horse: a heavily muscled, sturdy body; tremendous drive; and courage. Quarter Horses are powerful enough to pull against roped steers, and fast enough to outrun the speediest calves.

In recent years, increased infusions of Thoroughbred blood have added greater speed and staying power to the running Quarter Horse. The Thoroughbred is also increasing the Quarter Horse's average height.

Quarter Horses are big boned and muscular, yet balanced. The head is short, broad at the forehead, then tapered. The jowls are often large, but the muzzle is small with large, flaring nostrils. The ears are of short to medium length. The neck is straight and muscled, emerging relatively low from the deep shoulder. The chest is wide, and the back is usually short and strong, with well-sprung ribs and muscular loins. The hindquarters are large, rounded, and very muscular. They are sometimes higher at the croup than at the withers (a feature that is not necessarily desirable). The stifles are often higher than other breeds due to a relatively short femur (thigh bone). The legs are strong, being thickly muscled in the forearms and gaskins. The small feet that were once bred for or encouraged through trimming are less popular because of the lameness problems this creates.

The Quarter Horse's height ranges from 14.2 to 16 hands. The average weight is 950 – 1,300 pounds. Quarter Horses are used for pleasure, show, polo, rodeo, ranch work, and racing.

Standardbred

The *Standardbred* is another breed of North American origin. Standardbreds are used primarily for harness racing, and often in roadster classes. In fact, its supremacy in the harness racing world is virtually unchallenged. Once known as the American Trotting Horse, the name "Standardbred" derives from the original performance requirements for registration—if a horse could meet the performance standard, it was admitted to the registry. The current standard is a 2:20 mile at the trot or pace for 2-year-olds and a 2:15 mile for older horses. However, registration on performance alone is no longer granted. Both sire and dam must be registered Standardbreds. If the dam is not a registered Standardbred, other family factors and the performance standard help to determine eligibility.

The performance standard has aided selection for speed. Horses are usually evaluated on their speed over a mile—a fairly objective measurement. Their speed records are less subject to interpretation than those of horses that race under saddle.

Because they were selected for speed rather than conformation, Standardbreds vary somewhat in appearance. Generally, they are less leggy, smaller, and sturdier than Thoroughbreds. The head is less refined than the Thoroughbred's, but has large, open nostrils. The neck is medium to long, well muscled, and set on high. The shoulders are also well muscled, although they are sometimes more upright than the Thoroughbred's. The back is fairly long, as short-

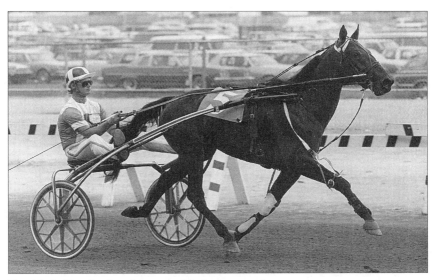

Fig. 11–5. Standardbreds are used in harness racing.

backed horses are more likely to interfere. The croup is usually higher than the withers, often by 1 or 2 inches, and the hindquarters are very powerful.

The Standardbred's average height ranges from 14.2 to 16.2 hands, with 850 – 1,150 pounds as the average weight. Good conformation is more important than size in these horses.

Morgan

The *Morgan* is the only horse breed named after a single horse, Justin Morgan. (The horse was named after his owner.) Every horse in the breed is descended from this stallion. Probably of Arabian and Thoroughbred descent, the horse was compact, spirited, and extremely prepotent. He and his offspring became known for their ability at driving, racing, pleasure riding, and farm work. Until the development of the Standardbred in the mid-1800s, Morgans were desirable as road horses. Morgan blood influenced the Standardbred and has also been instrumental in the development of the American Saddlebred, Tennessee Walking Horse, and Quarter Horse.

Morgans are characterized by a straight or slightly dished profile; prominent eyes set far apart; small, wide-set ears; a prominent jaw, and a small muzzle. They also have an upright, arched neck, great

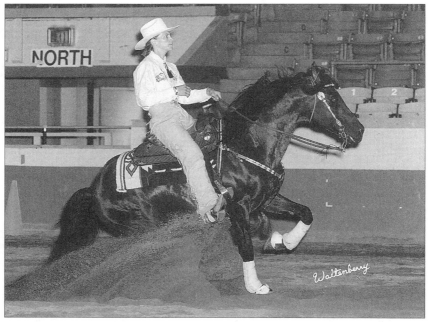
Fig. 11–6. Morgans are versatile horses.

depth and slope to the shoulder, and a short back and loin. The legs are strong and refined. The Morgan has a high-set tail, and gives the overall impression of power in a compact frame.

Morgans average 14.1 – 15.2 hands, and weigh 900 – 1,200 pounds. They are used primarily for pleasure riding, showing in hand and in harness, carriage driving, and distance riding, although they are versatile horses and can be found at almost any performance event.

Andalusian

Andalusians originated in Andalusia, Spain, when invading Moors crossed their Arabs and Barbs with native Spanish horses. The breed has remained relatively pure, while contributing to other breeds.

Andalusians usually have a convex profile (Roman nose), and open, flaring nostrils. The eyes are large and the ears are small to medium sized. The neck is crested, creating a high head carriage. The chest is wide; the back is relatively short, with defined withers. The legs are refined, with short, strong cannons. Andalusians are known for their long, thick, wavy manes and tails.

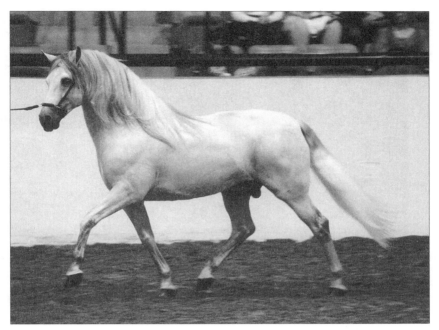

Fig. 11–7. Andalusians originated in Spain.

Andalusians stand 15.1 – 15.3 hands tall. They are used for exhibition, bullfighting, dressage, and jumping.

Lipizzan

Lipizzans have been influenced by many breeds, most significantly those of Spanish ancestry. It also has Arabian, Barb, and many European breeds in its bloodlines. The head of the Lipizzan shows a convex profile, small ears, and large eyes. The crested neck blends into low withers and powerful shoulders. The loin and hindquarters are very strong, which is necessary to the work they do. The feet are sometimes small, but the legs are strong.

Lipizzans stand 14.3 – 15.3 hands tall. They mature slowly and are not fully developed until about age six. They are born with dark coats that lighten as they mature.

The Lipizzan horse is most renowned as the horse used in *Haute Ecole* at the Spanish Riding School in Vienna. It is also popular in circuses, dressage, and driving exhibitions.

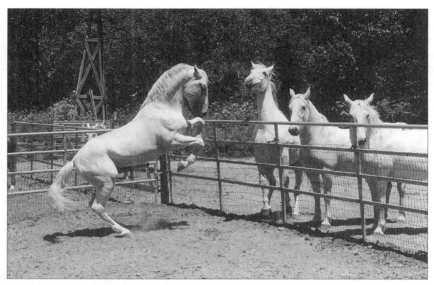

Fig. 11–8. Lipizzan stallion and mares.

Color Breeds

Appaloosa

Although spotted horses existed in prehistoric times, they did not cross the Atlantic to the Americas until the 17th century. The Nez Perce Indian tribe trained these horses and developed them for their own use. The Nez Perce lived along the flat, grassy Palouse River valley in Oregon—hence the name *"Appaloosa."*

To be eligible for registration, an Appaloosa must stand more than 14 hands tall (most are 14.2 – 15.2 hands), and may not be of pony, draft, or pinto ancestry. Otherwise, acceptable markings vary, but must include white sclera around the eye, parti-colored or mottled skin, and striped hooves (see Chapter 10, *Colors & Markings*).

The Appaloosa has an respectable head, and medium, pointed ears. Its neck is medium length, and its back is short and strong. The hindquarters show long, flat muscling. It has sturdy legs and feet, with long, sloping pasterns. Most Appaloosas weigh 950 – 1,250 pounds.

The Nez Perce gelded inferior stallions and selected their best mares to produce a combination war horse, racehorse, hunting horse, and long-distance mount. Today, the Appaloosa possesses the

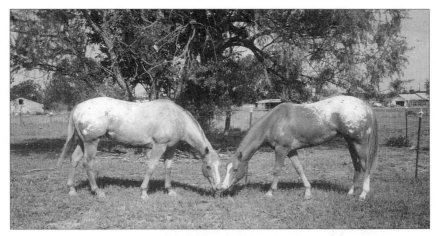

Fig. 11–9. Appaloosa mare and her son, showing variations of the coat pattern.

speed, stamina, and hardiness that adapted it for those purposes. It is therefore extremely versatile, used for dressage, jumping, games, reining, roping, endurance riding, and as a pleasure horse.

Paint/Pinto

Paint or *pinto* horses are colored horses with natural white markings in a tobiano or overo pattern (see Chapter 10, *Colors & Markings,* for definitions). The difference between a paint horse and a pinto horse is mostly one of bloodlines: a paint horse must be registerable with the American Paint Horse Association. Their rules for registration require the horse be of Paint Horse, Thoroughbred, and/or Quarter Horse ancestry. The horse must also have a body marking two inches wide or long with underlying pink skin. Excessive face white and excessive leg white are also acceptable. Solid colored horses can be registered as breeding stock if they have the required bloodlines. Because the markings continue to develop until the horse is about age two, final registration is postponed until then.

If the horse is not registered with the American Paint Horse Association, it is considered a pinto. There are several pinto associations whose color and bloodline requirements vary. For example, the Pinto Horse Association registers horses with 15 square inches of white (with underlying pink skin) on the body, neck, or side of the head. It also registers pinto ponies and miniatures, but not Appaloosa, draft horse, or donkey types.

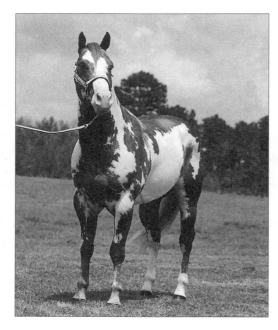

Fig. 11–10. Pinto horses have generous white markings over the entire body.

Because so many types of horses have pinto markings, their conformation (and uses) vary widely. However, the most common conformation is the stock horse type: heavily muscled, sturdy horses of medium height and quick movement.

Buckskin, Dun, and Grulla

Buckskin and *Dun* horses are defined by the registries as being basically yellow-bodied with dark points (mane, tail, and legs). *Grulla,* pronounced "grew-ya," is a smoky blue, light gray, or mousy color. Buckskins, Duns, and Grullas may have a dorsal stripe and/or zebra-like markings on the ears, withers, shoulders, and legs. (See Chapter 10, *Colors & Markings,* for more color information.)

Although the buckskin color is found in a number of breeds, many believe that the color traces to the Spanish Sorraia breed and the Norwegian Dun. These horses probably were crossed with Barb and Arab mares in Spain, and some of the descendants were among the horses brought to America by the Spaniards.

Conformation varies somewhat, although they are sturdy horses with strong feet and legs, known for hardiness and versatility. The horse must stand at least 14 hands. Horses with pony or draft type conformation may not be eligible for registration.

Palomino

The *Palomino* was first recognized as a breed in the United States. A Palomino has a golden body color and light points—the mane and tail are white, ivory, or silver (see Chapter 10, *Colors & Markings,* for more information). The palomino coloring crops up in many breeds of horses, so their conformation and uses vary. In addition to almost any performance event, palominos are popular for show, parades, and circuses.

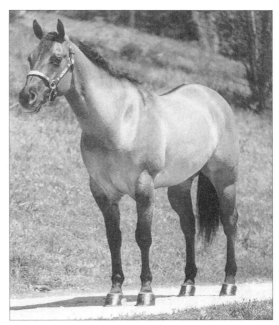

Fig. 11–11. Buckskin with a dorsal stripe.

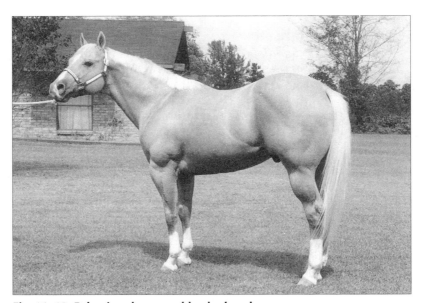

Fig. 11–12. Palominos have a golden body color.

Gaited Horse Breeds

A horse's gait is its way of moving—how the legs move and the feet land during forward motion. Some gaits are natural, in that they are not taught by humans. Natural gaits common to *all* horses include the walk and the gallop. Other gaits are artificial, in that they were taught or encouraged by humans. Examples of these gaits are the pace, running walk, and the rack.

But over centuries of selective breeding for a particular gait, the line between natural and artificial becomes blurred. A gait becomes natural to a certain breed of horses. Most gaited horses can perform their gaits with little or no training.

The gaits discussed are lateral, four-beat gaits. A "lateral" gait means that both feet on one side of the horse move at once. A "four-beat" gait means that one or more of the horse's feet is always on the ground, allowing the horse to move without jarring the rider. So these gaits, as well as the horses' even dispositions, make for very smooth and pleasant riding. Gaited horses originally were developed by landowners to provide comfortable rides over a distance. As more people began riding for pleasure, the popularity of the gaited horses increased. Today they are used as trail horses and show competitors.

Popular gaited breeds include the American Saddlebred, Tennessee Walking Horse, Missouri Fox Trotter, Paso Fino, and Peruvian Paso.

American Saddlebred

The *American Saddlebred* was first bred in the southern and east central United States. It is descended from Thoroughbred, Canadian and Narragansett Pacer, Standardbred, Morgan, Arabian, and Scottish Galloway stock. Settlers wanted quiet horses with good ground-covering strides.

The American Saddlebred has a small, narrow head. The long, arched neck rises from the shoulder at a high angle, giving the horse a high head carriage in extreme collection. Saddlebreds have high withers, sloping shoulders, short backs, and level croups. The legs are fine—sometimes a little too delicate. The elbows are set out away from the body. The pasterns are medium-to-long. Their hind legs are more angulated than the Thoroughbred's, with a preference toward a long hip and short cannon. The average American Saddlebred stands 15 – 16.1 hands and weighs 1,000 – 1,200 pounds.

Depending on its training, a Saddlebred is either three- or five-gaited. If a horse is five-gaited, one of its gaits is a "slow" gait, such as an amble, fox trot, slow pace, or running walk. The other is the rack,

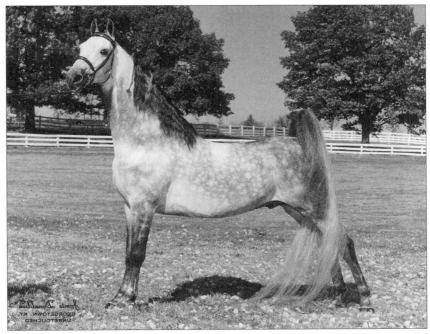

Fig. 11–13. Saddlebreds are used as show competitors.

a flashy, four-beat, nonpacing movement that is faster than the running walk. American Saddlebreds are used extensively as show animals, and some are used as riding and harness horses.

Tennessee Walking Horse

The *Tennessee Walking Horse* was developed from the Thoroughbred, American Saddlebred, Standardbred, Morgan, and Canadian and Narragansett Pacer breeds. It originated in the southern United States more than 100 years ago when plantation owners needed a utility horse, one suitable for riding, driving, and tilling the fields.

Tennessee Walking Horses are larger and stouter than their ancestors. Their heads are average-looking, with long ears, a straight profile, and open nostrils. They have a medium-length neck that emerges high from the slightly narrow chest. The horses have long, sloping shoulders and croup. The back and loin are highly flexible. The tendency to breed Tennessee Walkers to be slightly sickle hocked is no longer dominant. They stand 15.2 – 17 hands high, and weigh 1,000 – 1,250 pounds.

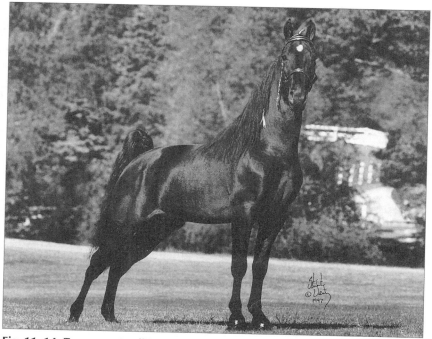

Fig. 11–14. Tennessee Walking Horses are ridden for pleasure and show.

For years, Tennessee Walking Horses were evaluated on the basis of their stamina and comfortable riding qualities. Today, they are ridden primarily for pleasure and show. They are known for their characteristic running walk. The running walk is a fast walk—a four-beat gait in which the hind foot oversteps the forefoot by 12 inches or more. This action makes the horse seem to glide over the ground.

Fox Trotting Horse

The *Missouri Fox Trotting Horse* developed from crosses among Arabians, Thoroughbred, Morgans, Saddlebreds, Standardbreds, and Tennessee Walking Horses. The breed was developed in the Ozark Mountains of Arkansas and Missouri, where farmers needed horses that could cover long distances and rocky terrain at a comfortable gait.

Fox Trotting Horses have a straight profile, long ears, and a square muzzle. The neck is of medium length, emerging low from the chest. The withers are fairly high, sloping into a short back. The legs are strong and clean.

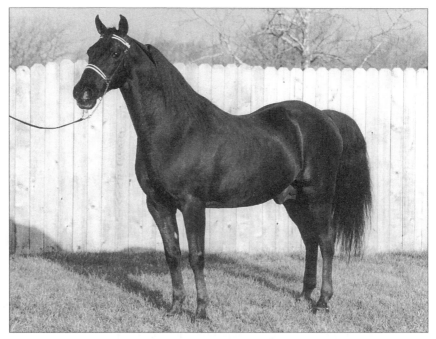

Fig. 11–15. The Missouri Fox Trotter was developed in Arkansas and Missouri.

Fox Trotting Horses stand about 14.2 to 15.3 hands and weigh approximately 950 – 1,200 pounds. They are used primarily for show and pleasure riding, but are sometimes used for endurance racing.

The fox trot is a slow, four-beat, broken diagonal gait; the horse walks with the front feet and trots with the hind feet. The hind foot slides into place to softly contact the ground, making for a very soft ride. This gait is the primary registration requirement.

Paso Horses

Paso horses descended from Andalusian, Spanish Jennett, Barb, and (some say) Friesian horses introduced by the Spanish into South America and the Caribbean. The influence of the smooth-striding Andalusian on the Paso breeds is evident. Also, some people believe that the Narragansett Pacer influenced the developing breeds during the 1600s.

There are two types of Paso horses: *Peruvian Paso* and *Paso Fino.* Peruvian Paso refers only to those Paso horses from Peru or directly

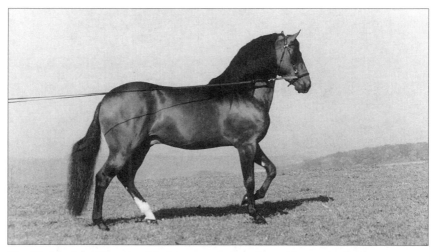

Fig. 11–16. Paso Finos tend to have crested necks and low-set tails.

descended from Peruvian stock. Paso Fino includes Paso horses of Puerto Rican, Colombian, Cuban, and Dominican Republic extraction. Also, the Paso Fino is usually smaller than the Peruvian Paso and the mechanics of the gaits are very slightly different.

The head is medium sized, with a broad forehead, straight or convex profile tapering to a small muzzle, and open nostrils. Pasos tend to have crested necks and medium-high withers. They have short backs, well-rounded croups, and low-set tails. The Peruvian Paso tail is carried "tucked" close to the body. The cannons of the hindlegs may angle forward, making them slightly sickle hocked. They have medium length, sloping pasterns and relatively small feet.

The basic paso gait is similar to a broken pace. The horse moves both lateral legs together, but the hind foot touches the ground a fraction of a second ahead of the front foot. This makes the gait less jarring than a true pace. The paso gait has five forms, ranging from the slow "paso fino" gait to the "paso largo," which can be faster than the canter. The Peruvian Paso's trademark gait is the paso llano with a faster version called sobreandando. Lending flair to this gait is "termino," a distinctive swimming action of the forelegs. Paso Fino breeders select against termino.

Pasos range in weight from 700 to 1,100 pounds, and in height from 13.2 to 15.2 hands. (Full size may not be reached until the horse is five years old.) They are used for pleasure, show, parade, and distance riding.

WARMBLOOD BREEDS

Warmbloods were developed by crossing draft ("coldblooded") types, with "hotblooded" light horses, mostly Thoroughbreds. Within this category of warmbloods, performance enthusiasts have developed recognized breeds. Several warmblood breeds originated in Germany—in fact, almost every province in Germany has its own breed. Other European nations have also developed breeds of warmbloods: Britain, France, the Netherlands, Denmark, Sweden, Poland, and Italy. Not far behind are the United States and Canada, where they are called Sport Horses. Warmbloods can be slow to mature—many are not ready to be ridden until age four or five. But because they are big and tractable, warmbloods are extremely popular in the Olympic sports of dressage, show jumping, eventing, and combined driving.

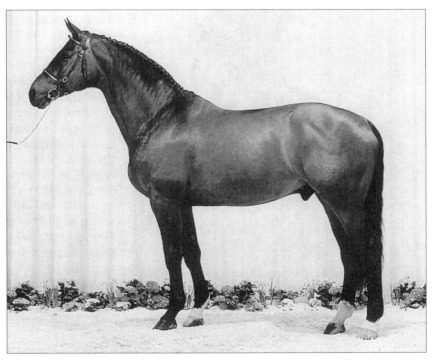

Fig. 11–17. A Danish Warmblood stallion.

Danish Warmblood

The *Danish Warmblood* evolved in Denmark. Native German and Danish horses were crossed with Iberian and Neapolitan horses. Over time, Thoroughbred, Trakehner, and other breeds were added. The profile of the Danish Warmblood is straight. The ears are long but refined, and the eyes are large and prominent. The legs are straight and strong, being well muscled in the forearms and gaskins.

Danish Warmbloods stand 16.1 – 16.2 hands tall. They excel at dressage and show jumping.

Dutch Warmblood

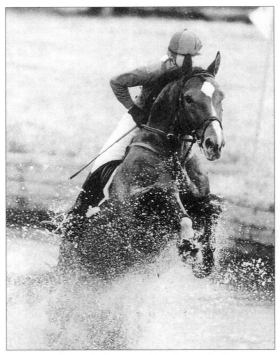

Fig. 11–18. A Dutch Warmblood steeplechaser.

The *Dutch Warmblood* was created in the Netherlands. Many European horses contributed to the breed, especially the Thoroughbred and Holsteiner. It has an average head, with large eyes and medium-length, pointed ears. The neck is light and medium-length to long. The shoulders are angled and the withers fairly high. The back is long, the loins well muscled, and the croup slightly angled. The hindquarters are muscular and deep from hip to stifle.

Dutch Warmbloods stand about 16 – 17 hands tall. They were bred for show jumping, but also make outstanding dressage horses.

Hanoverian

Originating in Germany, the *Hanoverian* is a mixture of many European breeds, including native European ponies, Andalusian, Thoroughbred, Arabian, Holsteiner, and Trakehner. It looks most like a middle- or heavy-weight Thoroughbred.

The head has a straight or slightly convex profile. The eyes are medium to large, and the ears are usually medium-sized. The neck is refined and medium to long, blending into well-defined withers. The back is sometimes long, but the broad, muscular loins and deep hindquarters compensate. The legs have short cannons and angled pasterns. The tail is set on relatively high.

Most Hanoverians stand 16 – 17 hands. They are used for show jumping, dressage, eventing, and combined driving.

Holsteiner

The northernmost province of Germany, Schleswig-Holstein, is home to the *Holsteiner*. The German Marsh Horse was the foundation breed, and over the centuries, many other breeds were added: Andalusian, Neapolitan, Yorkshire Coach Horse, Cleveland Bay, Thoroughbred, and Trakehner. The result is one of the heavier warmblood breeds—the Holsteiner is tall but well-balanced.

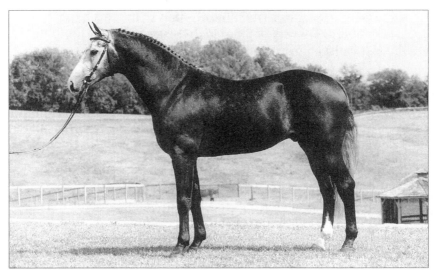

Fig. 11–19. Holsteiners have "self-carriage."

A Holsteiner's head has a straight profile, much like a Thoroughbred's. The eyes are large, and the nostrils flaring. The neck is arched, fairly long, and muscled, blending well into high withers. The shoulders are solid and well angled. The back is sometimes long, and the croup is slightly angled because of its prominent peak. The Holsteiner's elbow is set out away from the body. When viewed from the front, this conformation sets the forelegs squarely at the corners of the body and creates a broad chest. The legs are long and powerful.

Holsteiners stand 16 – 17 hands tall. They excel at show jumping, and are suited for dressage, eventing, and combined driving. In addition to enhancing their abilities in these Olympic events, their "self-carriage" makes them prized as carriage horses and parade animals.

Oldenburg

Another German Warmblood, the *Oldenburg* can trace its origins back further than most. Its founder was Count Anton von Oldenburg who lived from 1603 to 1667. Count von Oldenburg bred stallions from Spain and Italy to Friesian mares. Other breeds have influenced the Oldenburg since its creation, including Thoroughbred, Arabian, Barb, Cleveland Bay, and many other Warmblood breeds.

The Oldenburg's head is medium-to-large, suiting its large frame. The ears are of medium length and pointed. The neck is long and slightly arched. It has a sturdy body with a long, sloping shoulder and clean, strong legs. Oldenbergs stand 16.0 – 16.3 hands.

Oldenbergs are very popular in dressage and show jumping. They are still in use, however, as carriage horses.

Swedish Warmblood

Native Swedish coldblooded horses were crossed with various European breeds to create the *Swedish Warmblood*. It carries Iberian, Friesian, Oriental, and more recently, Thoroughbred, Hanoverian, and Trakehner blood.

These horses resemble Thoroughbreds in the head, with a straight profile, medium-to-long ears, and refined features. The neck is long, arched, and very slightly crested. The shoulders display the conformation of all good riding horses: long and angled. The back is of medium length, while the legs are long and leanly muscled.

Most Swedish Warmbloods stand 16 – 17 hands tall. Bred exclusively for riding, they excel at dressage, show jumping, and eventing.

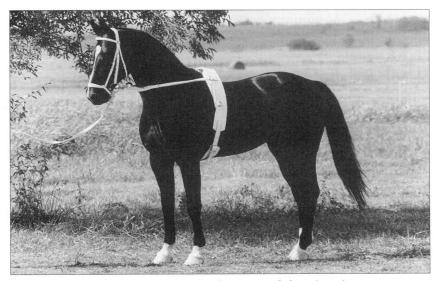

Fig. 11–20. Oldenburgs are popular in dressage and show jumping.

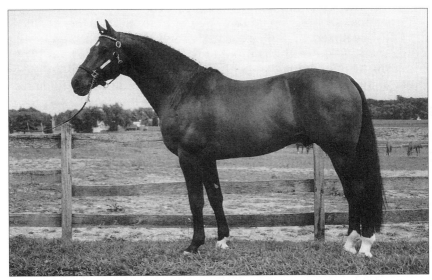

Fig. 11–21. The Swedish Warmblood strongly resembles the Thoroughbred.

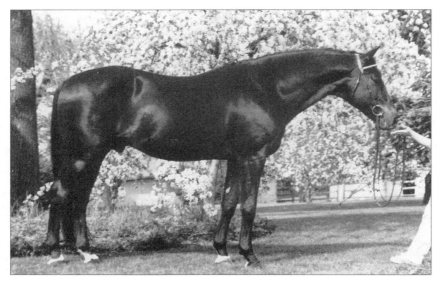

Fig. 11–22. Trakehners are used in eventing and dressage.

Trakehner

The *Trakehner* originated in East Prussia, currently in Poland, although its registration is controlled by a German society. Its bloodlines are mixed, including the native Schweiken, Thoroughbred, and Arabian. Of these, the Thoroughbred has been the most influential.

The head of the Trakehner is similar to the Thoroughbred's, with a straight or slightly concave profile, small muzzle, and refined features. The forehead is broad, which sets the large eyes apart. The ears are long but delicate. The neck is long and set on relatively high. The shoulders are angled, and the withers are fairly high. The back is moderately long, and the long croup angles slightly. The hindquarters are heavily muscled, and the hind leg is more angled than the traditional Thoroughbred's. The long, sloping pasterns complement strong, straight legs and heavy joints.

Trakehners stand about 16 – 17 hands tall. They were used extensively as a cavalry horse. Their military background makes them ideal for the Olympic sports of eventing and dressage. Moreover, they are considered to be the elite among Warmbloods and are often used to improve other breeds.

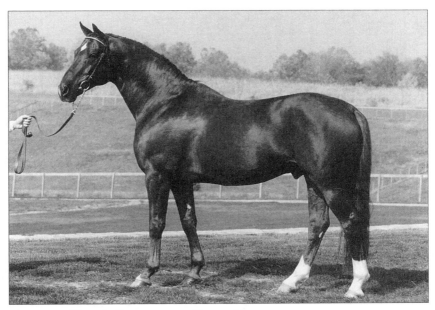

Fig. 11–23. Westphalians are versatile sport horses.

Westphalian

Native German horses were crossed with Thoroughbreds to create the *Westphalian.* Added to the blood mix are Hanoverians and Arabians. The head is average-looking, with a straight profile, medium-sized eyes, and medium-length ears. The neck is medium to long. The withers are prominent, the back is neither long nor short. The hindquarters are muscular and deep from hip to stifle.

The Westphalians are not as large as some other warmblood breeds, standing 15.2 – 16.2 hands tall. They are used primarily for show jumping and dressage. Some are also used for eventing. But these horses also make good pleasure riding horses and harness horses.

DRAFT BREEDS

Draft horses were once common all over the world, but since the introduction of mechanized agriculture their numbers have decreased. There has been a resurgence of interest in the animals for exhibition and show during recent years.

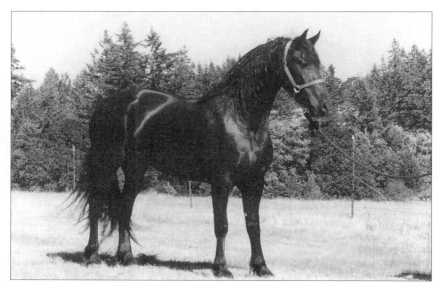

Fig. 11–24. A champion Friesian mare.

Draft animals are proportionately wider than light horses, with straighter shoulders and massive necks. Draft horses have round, heavily muscled hindquarters and large feet.

Draft horses were domesticated during the first century, when they were trained to pull plows, heavy carts, and chariots. Their bulk and more upright foreleg conformation made them more efficient than light horses at pulling heavy weights at slow speeds. During medieval times, these sturdy horses were selectively bred to develop an ideal war horse. They carried knights who often weighed more than 400 pounds in armor, and the horse also wore protective armor. Later some breeds were adapted to road work, pulling lighter carts and carriages. Hard pavement and slippery streets demanded sound horses with more sloping shoulders and pasterns, and strong feet.

Draft horses stand 15 – 19 hands and weigh 1,400 – 2,800 pounds.

Friesian

The *Friesian* originated in the Netherlands when breeders combined primitive heavy draft horses with more refined breeds such as Orientals and Andalusians. Its Dutch name, Harddravers, means "good trotter" and it is no coincidence that this breed has influenced most of the world's trotting horses.

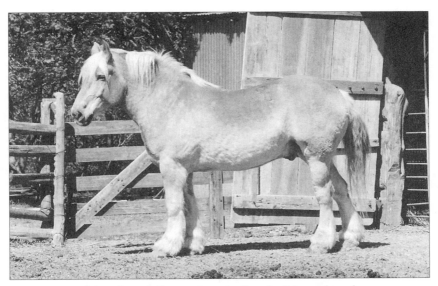

Fig. 11–25. Belgians have influenced most other draft horse breeds.

The head of the Friesian is long but refined, with small, curled ears, and flaring nostrils. It has a long, arched neck, sloping shoulder, and a compact body. The hindquarters are round and the tail is set on low. The fetlocks and pasterns are feathered with long, silky hair on the lower legs. The mane and tail are very long (trimming is not allowed!), and the coat is always black.

Friesians stand 15 – 16 hands tall. They have a high action, which creates a showy gait. They are favored as carriage, circus, and parade horses, and also participate in dressage and combined driving.

Belgian

The *Belgian*, or Brabant, is a popular modern breed that developed in Belgium. This breed has influenced most of the other draft breeds, and is often crossed with Thoroughbreds to produce quality Warmbloods/Sport Horses.

The head of the Belgian is medium sized and typical for a draft horse, with relatively small ears and eyes, and a large jaw. The neck is short but muscled and heavily crested. It arches smoothly into the withers and sloping, muscular shoulders. The body and hindquarters are typical of a draft horse: large, rounded, and strong. They have short cannons and large feet with feathering at the fetlocks and pasterns.

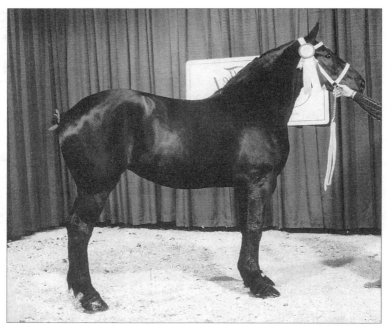

Fig. 11–26. Percherons originated in France.

Belgians stand 16 – 17 hands tall, and weigh about 2,000 pounds. They are preferred not only for their size and strength, but for their high knee and hock action. They are used for hauling, showing, and pulling competitions.

Percheron

The *Percheron* originated in the La Perche region, near Normandy in France. Arabian blood contributed to the Percheron's refinement.

Percherons are tall and heavy boned. They have a head much like a large Thoroughbred's: straight profile, broad forehead, large eyes, and short to medium-length ears. Their thick, arched necks are of medium length, and they carry their heads up instead of out. The shoulders are sloping and the withers fairly high—lighter Percherons make good riding horses. They have deep hindquarters, heavily muscled in the lower thigh and gaskin. Percherons do not have much feathering at the fetlock.

Most Percherons stand 16.2 – 17.3 hands high and weigh about 1,900 pounds. They are popular for hayrides, sleighrides, and parades.

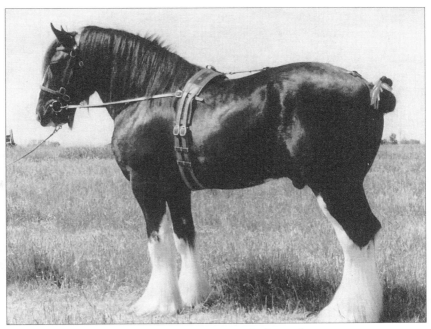

Fig. 11–27. Shires have profuse feathering on the lower legs.

Percherons are favorites at draft horse shows because they have attractive, snappy trots. They are sometimes crossed with Thoroughbreds to create good warmbloods/sport horses.

Shire

Shires originated in 18th century England, and were mixed with German and Flemish horses. They were not as popular in America for farm work horses as some other draft breeds because of their straight shoulders and pasterns, feathering, and undeserved reputation for sluggishness. However, Shire stallions were often used on lighter mares to produce good farm horses.

The Shire has a "noble" head with a slightly Roman nose, long ears, and deep-set, gentle eyes. The neck is thick, long, and arched. The back is short, with a long loin and angled croup. The legs are long and strong, with long cannons and short pasterns. The points of the hocks are set close together. If they also turn inward the horse is cow hocked, although it rarely leads to lameness in these horses. Shires have feathering on the lower legs, and their feet are large and tough.

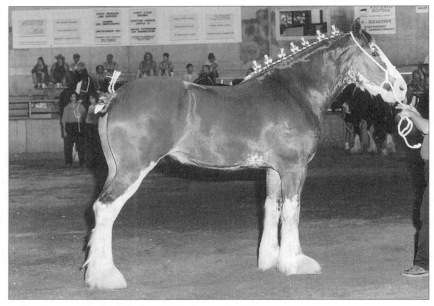

Fig. 11–28. Clydesdales are very refined for their size.

Shires stand 17 hands tall (or more—sometimes as tall as 19 hands) and weigh as much as 2,400 pounds. They are used for exhibition and show, and to make short-haul deliveries for breweries in England. Their excellent action (due to their being bred as war horses) make them popular in Warmblood/Sport Horse breeding programs.

Clydesdale

The *Clydesdale* developed in the Lancaster region of Scotland. Outcrosses with the Cleveland Bay horse added style and action to the Clydesdale's size. It is known among draft breeds for being the most refined, and for its lively action.

In the Clydesdale, the forehead is broad with large eyes and ears. The muzzle is also broad with large nostrils. The neck is long and arched, merging into high withers. The body is deep, with short, flat ribs. The back and loin are long. The forelegs fall straight from the sloping shoulders, but the hindlegs are planted closely together. If the points of the hocks turn inward the horse is cow hocked. Clydesdales have short, thick cannons and straight, silky feathers on the back of the fetlocks and pasterns.

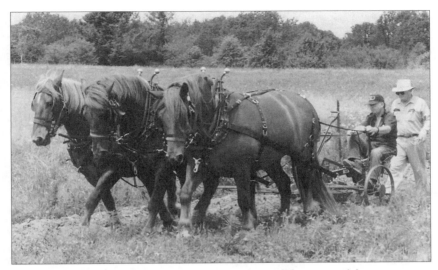

Fig. 11–29. The Suffolk Punch is comparatively small but powerful.

The average Clydesdale stallion stands 17 – 19 hands; mares are a little shorter. They weigh 1,600 – 2,200 pounds; again, mares may weigh 200 pounds less. They are used for farming and ranching, as well as for exhibition in harness and show.

Suffolk

The *Suffolk* horse developed in Norfolk and Suffolk, England. It is comparatively small (15.3 – 16.1 hands), however, it is heavily muscled and powerful. The compact, "punched up" appearance encouraged its common name, the Suffolk Punch.

The head is fairly large, with a straight or convex profile. The forehead is broad, and the eyes are large and kind. The neck is thick and arched. The Suffolk's shoulders tend to be upright, denoting power under harness. The back is short, and the flank area is as deep as the girth. The tail is set on relatively high. The Suffolk's legs, while appearing short, are clean, straight, and heavily muscled in the forearms and gaskins. They have little, if any, feathering. The feet are medium sized and strong.

Because it is more compact and efficient at feed conversion than other draft breeds, the Suffolk traditionally has been popular as a farm work horse in England. In the United States, however, some farmers thought the Suffolk too small to cross with American light

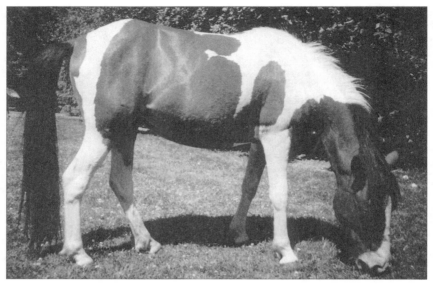

Fig. 11–30. Chincoteague pony.

horses to produce a drafter they considered large enough to work in the fields. This was unrealistic, because the Suffolk is a game worker and an economical keeper. Suffolk Punches are used for show, and by breweries in England for hauling.

PONY BREEDS

Ponies by definition stand less than 14.2 hands (58 inches) at the withers when fully mature. They are used for a variety of activities and differ widely in conformation according to their primary purpose. Depending on the breed, ponies may resemble either light horses or draft horses in build. Ponies are known to be long-lived: many live well into their thirties. Because they often developed in harsh climates, they are sturdy and easy keepers.

Chincoteague

The *Chincoteague* (pronounced chin-co-teak) pony developed in the Chincoteague Islands off the coast of Virginia. Legend has it that they are the descendants of horses that were shipwrecked on Assateague Island around the year 1600. These hardy horses stand 14 hands and under, with an average of 12 hands. However, they do not always display stereotypical pony characteristics—they resemble small, sturdy horses. Chincoteague ponies often have pinto markings, although some are bay.

Connemara

Connemaras developed in Ireland, but over the centuries they have been mixed with many other breeds. The head reveals its Arab and Thoroughbred blood: it has a straight profile, small ears, and large, open nostrils. Their long necks and sloping shoulders make them excellent riding mounts. The legs are short and strong, but not coarse.

Connemaras stand 13 – 14.2 hands tall. In America, Connemaras have been increasing in size—the average Connemara stands over 15 hands—and they are now one of the largest pony breeds. Connemaras make good hunting and jumping horses.

Dartmoor

The *Dartmoor* developed in Devon, England from crosses between the Celtic pony and Welsh Cob, Arab, and Thoroughbred horses.

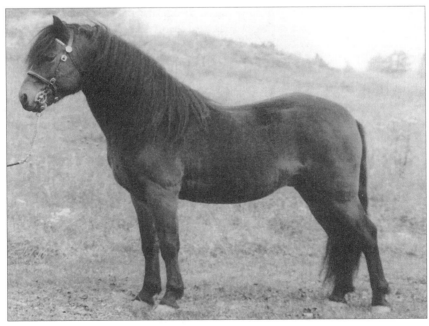

Fig. 11–31. The Dartmoor has typical pony conformation.

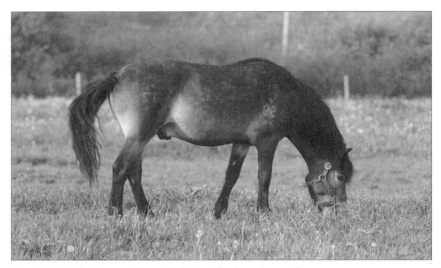
Fig. 11–32. The Exmoor has a light tan flank and muzzle.

This breed and its cousin the Exmoor have been carefully bred back from near extinction after World War II.

Dartmoors have typical pony conformation—stocky and strong, but balanced, with straight legs and good feet. It has a small head and small ears, with large, curious eyes. The crested neck is of medium length; the shoulder sloping and the withers low. The tail is set fairly high onto well-muscled hindquarters.

The Dartmoor stands 11.2 – 12.2 hands tall. Its movement is long and low, with almost no knee action. It is used as a child's mount for pleasure riding and hunting/jumping, and also for carriage driving.

Exmoor

The *Exmoor* is the oldest of the pony breeds, and today is still a very pure breed. It evolved on the wild moors of Devon and Somerset in prehistoric England, responding to the rugged environment by developing extreme hardiness. For that reason, the Exmoor has been influential in many other pony breeds.

Exmoor ponies are stocky animals with slender but strong legs. Their heads are distinctive, with short, thick ears and "toad eyes" (fleshy eyelids). They have a thick, arched neck of medium length and full, wiry mane and tail.

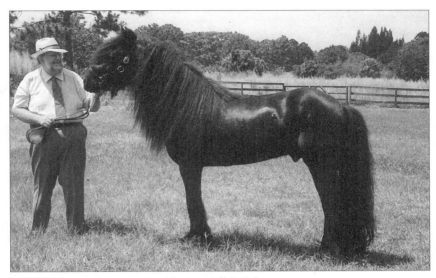

Fig. 11–33. A Fell pony resembles a small Friesian.

Exmoors are born with light tan ("mealy") flank, muzzle, and ring around the eyes. They stand about 12 hands tall. Exmoor ponies are used for pleasure riding, jumping, endurance racing, and driving.

Fell

The *Fell* pony is native to the Cumberland and Westmoreland areas of England. The Romans introduced Friesian blood, which accounts for the strong resemblance to that breed. It was also influenced by the Scottish Galloway, an extinct breed.

The Fell pony's head is refined for a pony breed, with a broad forehead and prominent, intelligent eyes. The profile is straight or slightly convex. The neck is fairly long, blending smoothly into a sloping shoulder. The barrel is rounded with well-sprung ribs. The hindquarters are powerful. The Fell pony usually has clean, strong legs with short cannons and tough feet. The feathering may extend up to the knees. The mane and tail are long and thick.

Fell ponies have a smooth stride and showy action. They average 13 – 14 hands in height. They are used for pleasure riding, in harness, and even still as working animals on sheep farms. Like Friesians, Fell ponies excel at trotting long distances.

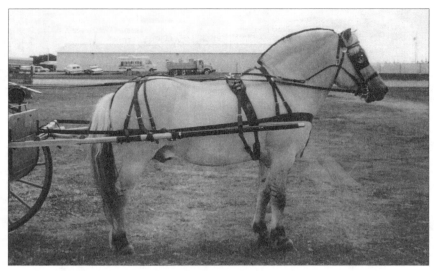
Fig. 11–34. Fjord ponies resemble Przewalski's horse.

Fjord

The *Fjord* pony, or Vestland, originated in Norway. Other breeds have been introduced, but none have changed its unique characteristics. An ancient breed, it was used as a war horse and fighting horse by the Vikings.

The Fjord pony bears great resemblance to Przewalski's horse. Most are yellow or cream-colored dun with a dorsal stripe from the poll, through the middle of the mane, down the back, and through the tail. Some Fjords have zebra stripes on the upper legs.

The head is of pony-type, broad with short ears, large eyes, and short muzzle. The neck is muscular and heavily crested. The body and legs are also characteristic of pony breeds: round body, short-coupling, sturdy legs, and tough feet. Fjord ponies typically stand 13 – 15 hands. They are used for trekking, and have even been seen on show jumping courses and in reining and dressage arenas. They are even still used for farming.

Galiceno

The *Galiceno* descended from the same Spanish stock as the Paso Fino horse of Central and South America, but is of pony size. The American Mustangs have Galiceno blood.

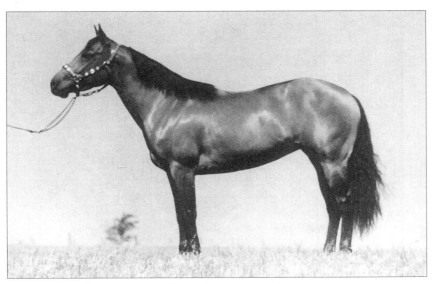

Fig. 11–35. Galicenos are popular performance ponies.

The Galiceno's head is refined with a broad forehead and prominent eyes. The medium-sized ears are pointed, with the tips curving inward. The rather arched neck blends into moderate withers. The back is short and straight, flowing to a sloping croup and fairly high tail carriage. The well muscled hindlegs are placed slightly under the body. The pasterns are medium long.

Galicenos usually stand 12 – 13.2 hands high, weighing 625 – 700 pounds. Their smooth gaits make them popular performance ponies for young or small adults, participating in Pleasure classes, jumping, barrel racing, and cutting.

Gotland

The *Gotland* originated on the island of Gotland off the coast of Sweden before the Stone Age. It has influenced other breeds, but remains relatively pure itself, with only a little Syrian and Welsh blood introduced.

Gotlands are built like small, primitive horses without the stereotypical pony characteristics. They have a small head with a straight or concave profile, broad forehead, and rounded, prominent jaws. The ears are wide and the eyes large. The neck is muscular and rather short. The back is of medium length, and the croup rounded.

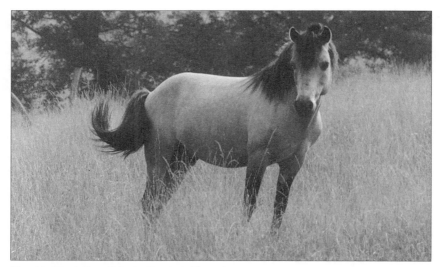

Fig. 11–36. A Swedish Gotland stallion.

The tail is closely carried. The legs are refined, but sturdy and sound. Chestnuts are often absent on the hindlegs. The feet are small but very tough.

Gotlands stand 12 – 13 hands high. They are used as riding ponies and jumpers for children, and participate in trotting races and endurance rides. They are occasionally used in light harness.

Hackney

Hackney ponies are pony-sized versions of the Hackney Horse, which has become increasingly rare as the ponies become more popular. Hackneys developed in Norfolk, England, descending from Thor-

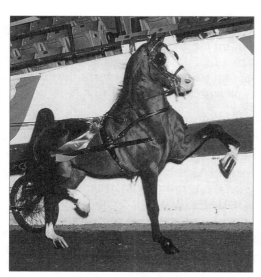

Fig. 11–37. Hackney ponies have high, flashy action.

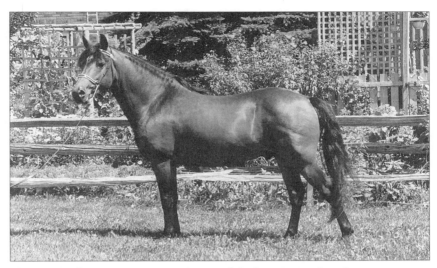

Fig. 11–38. The New Forest Pony is one of the larger pony breeds.

oughbred, Arabian, Norfolk Trotter, and Welsh Pony ancestry. They have infusions of Fell and Welsh Mountain Pony blood as well.

They have refined features, with short muzzles, convex profiles, and pointed ears set close together. Their arched necks lend hauteur to their high head carriage. The back is straight and the croup flat, with the tail set on high. The legs are straight with a long forearm and gaskin, and short cannons. They are 11 – 14.2 hands tall. Hackney ponies are bred almost exclusively for showing under saddle and in harness: they are best known for high, flashy knee and hock action.

New Forest

The *New Forest Pony* originated in Hampshire, southern England. The Celtic ponies and most other native British ponies were mixed with Arab, Barb, and Thoroughbred horses. This has produced what is now one of the largest pony breeds.

The New Forest Pony resembles a small warmblood. The head is a typical pony-type head, with a broad forehead, large eyes, and open nostrils. The body is deep, with well-sloped shoulders. The legs are slender and straight, with strong feet.

The average New Forest pony stands 12 – 14.2 hands tall. They are used for pleasure riding and driving, and as hunters, jumpers, and dressage horses for young or small adults.

Pony of the Americas

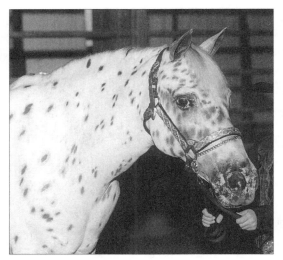

Fig. 11–39. The Pony of the Americas is a versatile mount with Appaloosa markings.

The *Pony of the Americas* (POA) developed from Black Hand #1, its foundation sire, a cross between an Appaloosa mare and a Shetland pony stallion. These animals are intended to be child-size working ponies. POAs today have conformational characteristics of both Quarter Horses and Arabians, with Appaloosa markings. The head and neck are refined like the Arabian. The shoulder is sloping, the back straight and muscled. The forelegs and hindlegs are heavily muscled like the Quarter Horse.

These ponies stand 11.2 – 14 hands high. They are used for all kinds of events, including jumping, endurance racing, and even flat racing for ponies.

Shetland

The *Shetland,* one of the smallest ponies, evolved on the inclement Shetland Islands. Its isolation prevented outcrossing with other breeds and, combined with scanty food supplies,

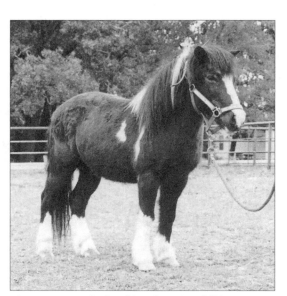

Fig. 11–40. A Shetland is a favorite child's mount.

led to the pony's diminutive size (9 – 11 hands; 250 – 500 pounds). The Shetland possess amazing strength for its size. It derives most of its power from a short back, deep girth, and well-sprung ribs.

Two basic types exist. The native British type has a short, stocky, round-barreled build. There is also a more slender, fine-boned Oriental version.

The Shetland's mane and tail are long and thick. The nostrils are small, as are the ears. The legs are short, with relatively short forearms that create a slightly choppy stride. It may have some feathering at the fetlocks.

Shetlands are used for pleasure riding, as companion animals for other horses, and in harness at exhibitions and circuses. Well-trained ponies are used as mounts for children in every event from gymkhana to hunting and jumping.

Welsh

Welsh ponies developed in the rugged hills of Wales. They are often crossed with larger saddle horses to produce intermediate-sized riding horses or small hunters. The Welsh Pony Society classifies the breed into four divisions, or "Sections":

- Section A—the small Welsh Mountain Pony
- Section B—the Welsh Pony, a slightly larger riding pony
- Section C—the Welsh Pony of Cob Type
- Section D—the Welsh Cob, the largest, with both jumping ability and stamina

Cob type horses are stocky and compact, with big, round bodies and short, sturdy legs. They average about 15 hands tall. The Welsh Cob and Welsh Pony of Cob Type are two of the few actual breeds of Cob horses.

Welsh Mountain Pony

The *Welsh Mountain Pony's* head resembles the Arabian's. It has a dished face, a small muzzle, and flaring nostrils. The forehead is broad, which sets the large, expressive eyes and short ears widely apart. The neck is medium-length and arching. The pony's back is short with strong loins. The barrel has a deep heartgirth and well-curved ribs. The legs are straight and strong with short cannons and well-muscled forearms and gaskins. The feet are relatively small. The tail is set on high. The Welsh Mountain Pony's maximum height is 12.2 hands. They are known for a natural jumping ability, but are also used in harness.

Welsh Pony

During the 1800s native Welsh Mountain Ponies were crossed with Arabians, Hackneys, and Thoroughbreds, which lent the breed action, height, and speed. The *Welsh Pony's* head resembles the Thoroughbred more than the Arabian, although the face is slightly dished. The neck is moderately long, blending into high withers and sloping shoulders. The loins are strong and somewhat arched. Like the Welsh Mountain Pony, the upper legs are well muscled and the cannons are short. The Welsh Pony stands at a maximum height of 14.2 hands and weighs 700 – 1,000 pounds. It is used for pleasure riding and most junior performance events.

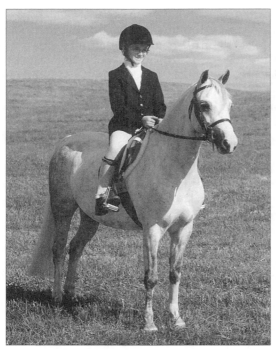

Fig. 11–41. Welsh Pony.

Welsh Pony of Cob Type

The *Welsh Pony of Cob Type* has a straight profile and clean-cut features. The ears are relatively small, the forehead is broad, and the eyes are widely spaced. The neck is long and arched. The pony has medium-high withers and long, sloping shoulders. The loins dip slightly before blending into the croup and deep hindquarters. The legs are strong, and the feet are medium-sized with dense hooves. The fetlocks are lightly feathered. It stands at a maximum height of 13.2 hands.

Welsh Ponies of Cob Type make good riding horses for small and young adults, and disabled riders. They are popular in harness and are used for combined driving events. They are also found in the show ring.

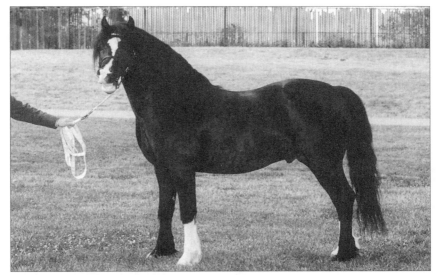

Fig. 11–42. Welsh Pony of Cob Type.

Welsh Cob

The only difference between the *Welsh Cob* and the Welsh Pony of Cob Type is height. Welsh Cobs must be over 13.2 hands, and most are 14.1 – 15 hands tall. They are used in combined driving, hunting, jumping, dressage, and cross-country events.

Miniature Horses

Miniature horses stand less than 34 inches at the shoulders when fully mature. The tiny horses are rare, but are becoming popular as family pets. They have been bred down from full-size horses and ponies.

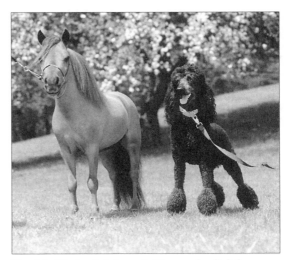

Fig. 11–43. A miniature stallion, only slightly bigger than the standard poodle.

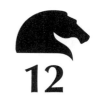

12

TYPES OF HORSES

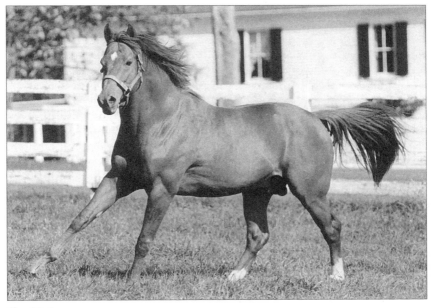

Fig. 12–1.

A horse's type refers to its activity, and not to its breed. Certain types of horses have conformational features that enhance their ability to perform specific activities. For example, show jumping horses are leggy and lean, while reining horses are stocky and muscular. Draft horses are stout and heavy, but most long distance competitors, while muscled, are relatively small and slender.

351

SHOW HORSES

The ideal *show horse* possesses beauty, impeccable manners, and a smooth, stylish way of going, along with animation and spirit. The

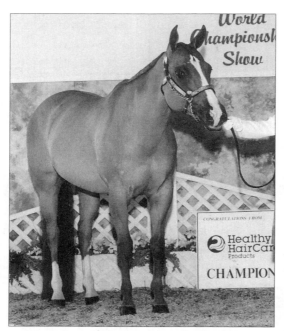

horse should display a high degree of poise and execute its maneuvers willingly and in a manner that appears effortless.

A show horse that is judged on conformation must excel in that area, but it must also adhere closely to breed standards. It should have those specific conformational characteristics that distinguish its class or event.

Two horses may have essentially the same conformational traits, but if one has been better conditioned than the other, this fact often influences the judges.

Fig. 12–2. A show horse should display the ideal description of its breed.

Color may also be a factor: it should be representative of the breed, both in shade and intensity. In some breeds, "flashy" colors and markings are desirable, while in others, subdued colors win more show classes.

RACEHORSES
Flat Racing

Conformation, to a great extent, determines a *racehorse's* performance. Certain conformational traits are associated with staying power while others are representative of speed. Generally, a "stayer" has a long stride and easy action, and is usually taller than it is long.

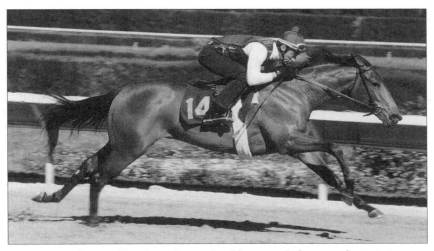

Fig. 12–3. A Thoroughbred racehorse should possess balance and symmetry.

The horse tends to have a long, well-shaped neck; long forearms; a short croup; and a long pelvis. The "sprinter," on the other hand, has a shorter back, but more length than height due to extra length in the croup. It has a strong loin, powerful hindquarters, and straight legs.

Size and Soundness

Conformation also relates closely to soundness. While size is usually a secondary consideration in selecting a racehorse, excessive height or heaviness may hurt performance. Heavy horses will overstress their legs and feet and are more predisposed to lameness. They mature slower and are more difficult to keep sound as youngsters. Small horses are at somewhat of a disadvantage because their strides are shorter and other horses bump them, especially at the gate. (This is one reason why fillies do not usually run with colts.)

General Conformation

Overall, the racehorse should possess balance and symmetry. The head should be clean-cut and reflect intelligence and good breeding. The horse should have a long, tapering neck that emerges relatively low from the chest, blending into a flat, sloping shoulder. A horse with an overly thin neck may be too delicate, or may lack sufficient room for air intake. A horse with a thick neck may not be able to extend itself fully.

Legs

Foreleg conformation should be as faultless as possible, because a young racehorse will sustain tremendous concussion before its bones are set. Any deviation from the ideal straight column of support subjects the leg to excessive stress. Also, a racehorse must have considerable freedom of movement. The horse should have a sloping shoulder for great stride length, a long, well-muscled forearm, and a short cannon with definitive creases between the bone and tendons. It should be lean-legged: horses with round, thick legs seldom remain sound.

The knees of a good runner should be large and flat, and perfectly aligned when viewed from both front and side. Calf kneed horses are often slow breaking out of the gate, because their weight rests toward the rear of their feet. Their knees are subject to fatigue, and these horses often suffer from bone chips in the knee. Some excellent Thoroughbred racehorses are actually buck kneed, and their knees generally remain sound.

Freedom of movement behind means that the hindquarters must straighten out as far as possible, to allow the greatest amount of "ground gain" with each stride. So a successful racehorse usually has a relatively straight and level croup, with an angle of about 25° – 30° with the ground. The femur (thigh bone) should be short and turned slightly outward at the hip. This angles the horse's hocks almost imperceptibly inward, enabling the horse to collect itself more easily and work with the hocks closer together. The angles formed by the hip joint and stifle are as straight or "open" as possible. From behind, the hindlegs should be straight, with a muscled, medium-length gaskin that places the hocks fairly low and straight. They should be wide and strong, and should taper to slender cannons.

The pasterns on the forelegs should slope at about a 47° to 54° angle, with the hind pasterns being slightly steeper. The pasterns may be shorter and more upright in sprinters than in distance horses.

Feet

Like the legs, the feet should be set on straight, with no outward or inward deviation. The feet should be sufficiently large, with healthy frogs and well-built bars.

A common conformational defect in Thoroughbreds is toed-out hind feet. Horses that toe-out in front are especially subject to fracture of the inside sesamoid bone. Toeing-in subjects them to injury

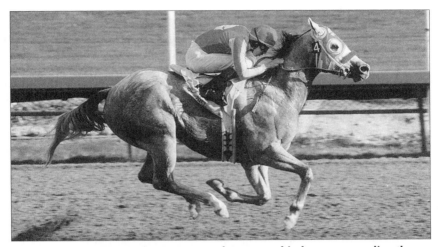

Fig. 12–4. A Quarter Racing Horse may have more hindquarter muscling than the Thoroughbred racehorse.

of the outside sesamoid bone or suspensory ligament. They may also develop splints.

An even more common conformational defect in Thoroughbreds occurs in the feet: long toes and low heels. In the past this foot shape was mistakenly believed to encourage speed. It affects the biomechanics of the entire leg, and is responsible for many racing injuries, such as bowed tendons.

Body

The withers should have good definition, the back should be short and strong, and the loin should be well-muscled. A deep heartgirth and well-sprung ribs provide space for the heart and lung capacity essential to the racehorse.

Quarter Racing Horses

Racing Quarter Horses sprint over shorter distances than Thoroughbred racehorses, so they need heavier muscling for quick power and short bursts of speed. They tend to have a short femur, placing the stifle high. The gaskin is fairly long and well muscled. Strong, straight, clean hocks are essential, set on neither high nor low. Their pasterns might be slightly shorter or more upright and their hindquarters more powerful than the Thoroughbred.

Harness Racing

Virtually every *harness racehorse* on the track today is a registered Standardbred—this breed has come to be synonymous with harness racing. (It is possible for a horse of another breed to be registered with the United States Trotting Association "for racing purposes only.") These horses have been selectively bred for more than 100 years to perform on the track.

Harness racehorses fall into two categories: trotters and pacers. Some Standardbreds perform well at both gaits—these horses are called "double-gaited." But generally a young horse shows a tendency toward one gait, and its training is directed accordingly. One in five Standardbreds are trotters; the rest are pacers.

While a trotter's legs move diagonally, a pacer's legs move laterally: the two nearside legs move forward in unison, followed by the two offside legs. This creates the pacer's characteristic rolling motion. The pace is an efficient gait—for a set distance, the speed records of pacers are faster than trotters.

The Standardbred may have certain characteristics that would be undesirable in riding horses, although many make a successful transition to pleasure riding horses after their racing careers. The trotter or pacer has a distinctive higher head and neck set, a longer back, and a more sloping croup. A harness horse may have a comparatively upright shoulder: unlike a riding horse, its primary purpose is not to provide a comfortable ride or a springy step.

The harness racer requires adequate air intake. It should have wide, open nostrils; considerable width between the jaws; and a long, graceful neck.

Legs

A harness horse's conformation must allow a clean gait, without interference. Such free movement requires straight legs with good width between them. The forelegs, when viewed from the front and side, should ideally be straight, with the toes pointing forward. If a horse toes out, especially at the pace, its knees may hit. If the horse toes in, it may hit its cannons or fetlocks. That being said, several top pacers have raced well despite toeing out. Toeing in seems to be more difficult to overcome.

The knees should be broad across the front but not excessively thick. Knee action is important, and to test it the trainer should pick up the front foot, bend the leg at the knee and make sure the hoof

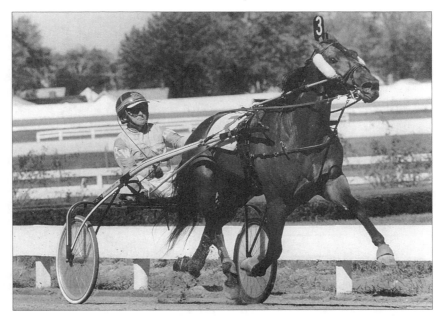

Fig. 12–5. Ambro Iliad, a record-breaking trotter.

can touch the elbow. Splints on the front legs might be acceptable if they do not extend into the knee, but their presence could indicate poor flexion. Splints on the back of the splint bone can also be harmful if their location causes them to irritate the suspensory ligament.

Most trainers find slightly buck kneed horses acceptable, but they discriminate strongly against the weaker calf knees. A horse's legs tend to bend back at the knee when it is fatigued. If the horse is already calf kneed, it may develop bone chips when raced.

Properly conformed hindlegs should have a moderate amount of angulation when viewed from the side. Sickle hocks in a Standardbred could be acceptable if the horse's action is unimpaired and if it has not developed curbs. The pasterns may be straighter than those of a flat-racing horse because the Standardbred does not need as smooth a stride. Pasterns that are too straight, however, absorb little concussion and lead to development of osselets and sesamoid problems. Too much slope strains the suspensory ligaments and leads to the development of bowed tendons. In all, a moderately sloped pastern is best. (For more information on these conditions, read *Equine Lameness* published by Equine Research, Inc.)

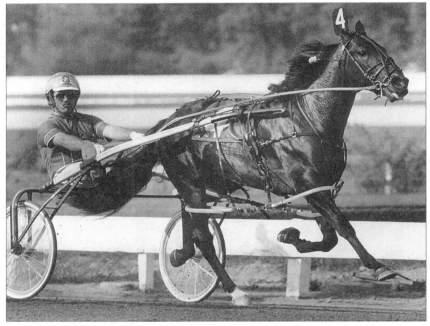

Fig. 12–6. World Champion pacer Tooter Scooter.

Feet

The feet, one of the racehorse's major structural components, should be moderately large and rounded at the toes with square, wide heels. Generous heels help to protect a horse from painful problems. The hoof wall should be thick and strong to withstand frequent reshoeings. Feet that are badly dished (concave) can also lead to lameness by exerting pressure against the short pastern and coffin bones.

Body

The horse needs a wide chest and heartgirth to provide adequate room for heart and lung expansion. The barrel should be wide and long, especially in the trotter. Short-barreled trotters tend to hit their hind shins with their front feet when they travel. A Standardbred needs a powerful shoulder for a long, bold stride, but the slope can be less than that desired of a riding horse. When viewed from behind, the hindquarters should appear muscular and the hips level. A horse with one hip down will travel crooked.

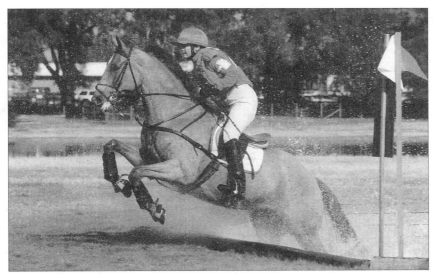

Fig. 12–7. A steeplechaser needs good jumping ability.

Hurdling & Steeplechasing

Hurdlers and *steeplechasers* race cross-country races over obstacles. Steeplechase obstacles are higher and sometimes more numerous than those in hurdle races. Also, steeplechases include water hazards, while hurdle races do not.

Hurdlers and steeplechasers, like flat racing and harness horses, need considerable strength and staying ability to cover courses as long as 2 miles at racing speed. A steeplechaser also needs good jumping ability, as well as size and substance to meet the challenge of rigorous courses. Even a 2-mile steeplechase (the minimum distance) contains at least 12 fences which measure 4½ ft or higher, and at least 8 hurdles that are 3½ ft high. These horses need a deep chest, prominent muscles, and solid bones to help it withstand the frequent concussion that the forelegs are subjected to upon landing.

HUNTERS & JUMPERS

Both *hunters* and *jumpers* need jumping ability, but power and boldness are more important in the jumper because the obstacles are higher. The hunter is scored on conformation, style, and manners as well as performance over jumps (which rarely exceed 4½ feet).

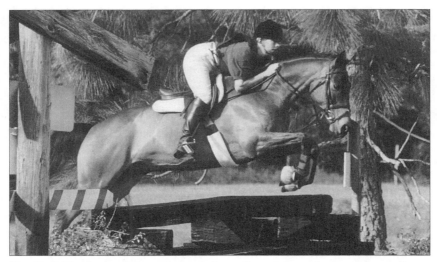

Fig. 12–8. The hunter is scored on conformation, style, and manners as well as performance.

Whether selecting a hunter or a jumper, the most important characteristic to look for overall balance. The front half of the body should be proportional in power to the back half, because a horse uses its head and neck for jumping balance and propels itself with the hindquarters. The chest, shoulders, and forelegs are especially important because they bear the horse's weight upon landing. A wide, powerful chest; a strong, medium-length back; and well-built forelegs indicate that a horse has weight-carrying ability and can withstand the impact of landing. A long back makes collection for jumping easier, but it tires more rapidly. A hunter/jumper should stand straight and not stand toed-out nor toed-in.

Small horses (or those with choppy strides) have difficulty pacing themselves on courses designed for lanky Thoroughbred types. Most successful hunter/jumpers measure 16 – 16.2 hands at the withers. A smaller horse may be willing and able to jump amazingly high, but it usually jumps with less grace and style than a larger horse. Taller horses have efficient, ground-covering strides to carry them across the course; obstacles are less imposing to them. A horse with an effortless stride subjects its legs to less impact-related stress that can lead to unsoundness.

Hunters

Hunters need sturdiness and strength to carry their riders across fields and streams during a hunt. To follow a pack of hounds across the countryside, a horse needs staying power, endurance, and the ability to leap fences and ditches. In the show ring, hunters receive points for conformation and/or performance.

Most hunters are of Thoroughbred breeding because Thoroughbreds have the size, speed, and athletic ability to carry riders of various weights across the country during a season's hunting. Many people favor some cold (draft horse) blood in their hunters, because they believe it contributes to size and stamina and exerts a calming influence on the more volatile Thoroughbred temperament. Some of the world's best hunters and jumpers are predominantly Thoroughbred, but have some Shire or Irish draft horses in their pedigrees. These crosses are called heavy hunters. Thoroughbred matings with the German Holsteiner and Trakehner horses have also become popular, because the horses produced by such warmblood crosses seem to have increased endurance and strength.

Jumpers

Show jumpers must be powerful enough to carry a rider over a prescribed series of jumps, with enough stamina to do so at the canter and gallop. Thoroughbred blood dominates in jumpers, and includes warmblood crosses. Many powerfully built, leggy Quarter Horses have also become excellent stadium jumpers.

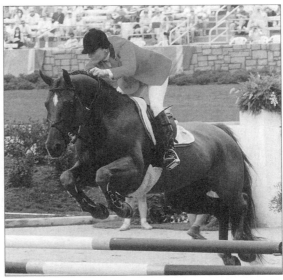

Fig. 12–9. Show jumping is an Olympic event requiring power and stamina.

The jumper should be a substantial-looking athlete with a long, sloping shoulder leading to laid-back but high withers, a well-defined elbow, and a muscular forearm. The hindquarters should also be very powerful in order to push off cleanly. It also should have a high hip and thick stifle. Many trainers prefer a long loin in a jumper, and point out that animals geared for jumping, such as cats, have that trait. The croup should have a slightly more downward angle. A steeply angled croup and a low tail set would be considered faults in many show horses. But these characteristics help a jumper by enabling it to draw its legs under its body and clear jumps more efficiently. The femur is relatively long and more sloping, closing the angle of the hip and stifle joint—also an aid in pushing. As with most athletes, short cannons and clean joints are essential to soundness.

DRESSAGE HORSES

A *dressage horse* is required to perform certain maneuvers in sequence, and each movement occurs at an assigned point in the dressage arena. The movements include the piaffe, passage, pirouette, and transitions within gaits. The horse should ideally be so controlled that it performs without visible cues from the rider.

A horse used for dressage should have sound limbs, free movement of the joints, and powerful hindquarters. The neck should not be set on too low, or collection will be difficult. Some dressage enthusiasts prefer crested necks because they enhance the horse's collected appearance. However, the throatlatch must be clean and not thick, or flexion at the poll will be impaired. A long, sloping shoulder

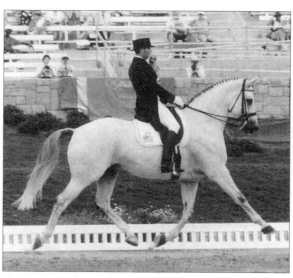

Fig. 12–10. A long, sloping shoulder allows a dressage horse full extension of the forelegs.

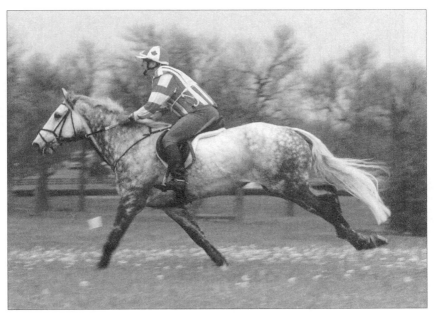

Fig. 12–11. An eventer has strong hindquarters and a deep chest.

allows full extension of the forelegs, while a relatively flat croup allows the horse to work with the hindquarters under itself, creating impulsion (forward, driving motion).

EVENTERS

Eventing, also called combined training, is a demanding sport originally designed to test the speed and fitness of cavalry mounts. Today, *eventers* need suppleness and discipline for dressage, endurance and speed for cross-country work, and jumping ability. They need an inherent natural balance and impulsion that training alone cannot provide.

A good prospect is one with strong hindquarters, a maneuverable forehand and the general conformation of a good hunter/jumper. The shoulder should be long and sloping; the legs, clean and straight. The horse needs excellent heart and wind, so it should have room across the chest and depth through the heartgirth. The horse should have a short loin. While a long back is acceptable, a short back usually is not. A back that is too short gives a horse little room to collect

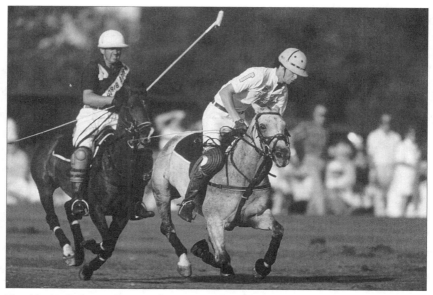

Fig. 12–12. Polo ponies must be strong and agile.

its hindlegs for a jump. The horse should have long gaskin muscles, strong, clean-cut hocks, and short cannons.

The horse's size affects both speed over a course and timing between jumps. A horse that is too tall may have trouble handling tricky distances between obstacles. A good choice might stand about 16 hands tall, and should have good bone and substance.

POLO PONIES

A polo match consists of six periods or chukkers (also called chukkas), each lasting 7 minutes (indoor) or 7½ minutes (outdoor). Often a *polo pony* plays for only one period, but occasionally it plays more than one, especially if it is the rider's best athlete. The pony must be very fast and responsive. It also must be very well conditioned and agile, able to perform quick stops and starts and sudden turns.

Although they are called "ponies," most horses participating in the sport of polo stand taller than 14.2 hands. Polo ponies usually stand 15 – 16 hands: short enough to be nimble, but large enough that being bumped by another horse will not hurt. A medium-long neck enables the horse to balance and maneuver. The throatlatch should be wide but fine, able to flex at the poll and jaw. The shoulders should be well-laid back and muscled. In the body, the ribs should be well curved and spacious; the back short and strong for agility. In the forelegs, the elbow should be set away from the body, increasing the horse's flexibility. The cannon should be short for strength. The quick starts and stops require well-muscled hindquarters and strong gaskins. Some people believe a cow-hocked horse has greater hind-quarter maneuverability. But in the performance horse, this conformational fault creates more problems than it solves. As with all athletic horses, straight legs and good feet are essential.

That being said, the enthusiastic polo pony can make up for conformational problems. A pony that loves the game will learn to compensate for any faults.

Most polo ponies are Thoroughbreds or Thoroughbred crosses. Quarter Horses are gaining popularity, especially for indoor polo or polocrosse (a combination of polo and lacrosse).

WESTERN HORSES
Stock Horses

The multi-talented *stock horse* still performs many jobs on modern ranches. It helps the rider to herd cattle, cut individual animals from the herd, and rope them for branding or doctoring. A good stock horse is versatile and possesses both innate ability and trainability.

Various breeds (including the Morgan, Appaloosa, Arabian, and Paint Horse) are successful stock horses, but it is the Quarter Horse that has emerged as the ideal. This is because of its short coupling, agility, speed, and reputation for having "cow sense."

A person selecting for this type should look for a horse with an excellent heart and respiratory system, evidenced by a deep heartgirth and well-sprung ribs. Cutting, roping, and carrying a rider for long periods place heavy demands on a horse. The horse needs:

- considerable athletic ability to endure the strain
- speed, to overtake fast calves
- weight, to brace itself against the pull of a heavy steer
- endurance, to withstand long hours under the saddle

Short coupling gives a stock horse greater weight-carrying ability. Short, strong cannons combined with clean joints and straight legs reduce the chances for lameness. The forearms should be well

365

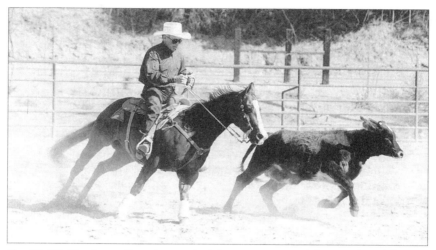

Fig. 12–13. Short coupling gives a stock horse greater weight-carrying ability.

muscled, but not excessively heavy or too wide through the chest since the forehand should be light for maneuverability. Perhaps most important, the stock horse needs good muscling in the stifle, gaskin, and loin. The horse "works off" the hindquarters and is provided propulsion by them. To balance these powerful hindquarters, the horse needs a good head and a fairly long neck.

Cutting Horses

A *cutting* horse wades into a herd, "cuts" a calf from the herd, and then prevents it from returning. It needs speed, agility, and strength, not to mention "cow sense." Well-developed, powerful hindquarters give the cutting horse a point of balance over which it can pivot and spin. They also provide power for short bursts of speed the horse needs to keep from losing the calf. The cutting horse needs fairly prominent withers to anchor the saddle. Size preferences vary: some people prefer large, strong horses, but others argue that smaller horses (less than 15 hands) are more maneuverable.

Roping Horses

Like cutting horses, *roping* horses need strong hindquarters for bursts of speed, but they also need to execute sliding stops. The roping horse chasing a calf at full speed must slide to a stop on cue, then

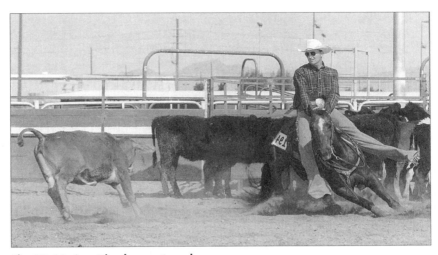

Fig. 12–14. A cutting horse at work.

hold the rope taut while the calf is tied. The horse must have power for quick starts and speed over short distances, and be able to get its hindlegs well under its body to stop. Traditional roping competitions are judged on speed. There are also "ranch roping" competitions where the horse/rider team is judged on style and skill rather than speed.

Steer roping horses need considerable strength and weight to brace themselves against the pull of heavier steers. Small, quick

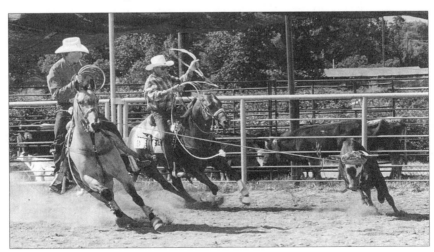

Fig. 12–15. Roping horses should be solidly built.

horses (less than 15 hands) may be maneuverable, but generally taller, stouter horses make better roping horses because they have a height advantage (and usually weight advantage) over cattle.

Competitors in team roping need two kinds of horses. The head horse is for the rider who ropes the steer's horns. The heel horse is for the rider who ropes the steer's hind feet. A good header is usually tall (about 15.2 hands) and normally weighs 1,200 – 1,350 pounds. It is a big-boned, solid horse with considerable substance. A heeler can be somewhat lighter, because it needs agility to maneuver into position for a follow-up throw. Most heelers stand about 15 hands tall and weigh about 1,100 pounds.

Barrel Racing Horses

A *barrel racing* horse must be both extremely fast and agile. The horse and rider sprint to the barrels, circling each of three barrels in a cloverleaf pattern, and then sprint back to the gate.

Like all athletes, the barrel racing horse should be balanced and symmetrical. This horse is a sprinter, and therefore needs large nostrils and a clean throatlatch to allow plenty of oxygen.

The barrel horse needs a strong, sloping shoulder to help it turn smoothly and to ensure a long stride. A short back helps the horse turn smoothly, as do short loins, which enable the horse to get its hindlegs under it to drive around the turns. Because of the tremendous forces placed on them, it is vital that the horse has straight, clean legs. Short cannons are preferred because long cannons, or "high hocks," reduce the horse's ability to get its legs under it for power. The hindquarters should be long and deep, allowing room for smooth, powerful muscles which drive the barrel horse.

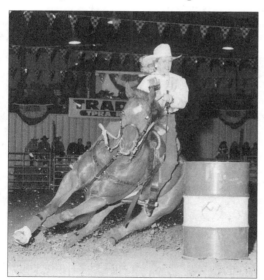

Fig. 12–16. A barrel racing horse is a top-notch athlete.

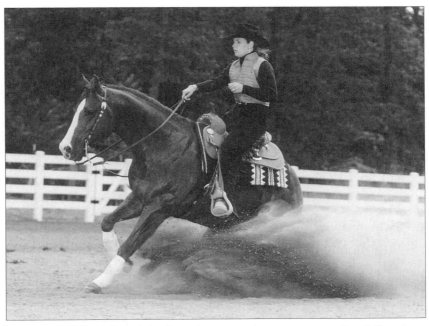

Fig. 12–17. One of the reining horse's spectacular maneuvers—the sliding stop.

Reining Horses

The Olympic sport of *reining* demonstrates the responsiveness and skill of a ranch horse. The horse is ridden on a loose rein in one of nine precise patterns at speed. The pattern includes all of the following maneuvers:

- galloping full-out in a straight line
- halting in a rollback—the horse lifts its front feet and pivots 180 degrees, then gallops in the other direction
- sliding stop
- backing up fast and straight
- loping small, slow circles and galloping large, fast circles with flying lead changes at the centers of figure eights
- transitions within circles from fast to slow, and back to fast
- spinning in circles very quickly with one hindleg planted

Some good reining horses are slightly sickle hocked. Riders believe this conformation helps the horse get its hocks "up under it" for hindquarter collection.

LONG DISTANCE HORSES

Long distance horses must carry weight over rough terrain. They endure temperature extremes that may vary from below freezing to 120°F—all on one ride.

There are basically two types of long distance trail rides: *endurance rides* and *competitive trail rides.* Typical ride lengths are 50 – 100 miles. Endurance rides are actually races, and the first horse across the finish line wins provided that it remains sound and in good condition. Horses in competitive trail rides are scored on condition and not speed, although they must complete each day's riding within a specific time limit.

Certain breeds have proven especially suited to long distance competition. Favored is the Arabian for its smaller size, dense bone, low feed consumption, and reputation for remaining sound into old age. Also popular is the Thoroughbred for its courage and lengthy stride.

Conformation of Distance Horses

Large nostrils are a sign of good oxygen-carrying capacity. A trim throatlatch and long, relatively thin neck indicate maneuverability. High, muscular withers hold the saddle in place. Because weight-carrying ability is so important, a trail horse needs a short back, a strong loin, and a long underline.

A deep, wide chest and well-sprung ribs provide sufficient room for the expansion of heart and lungs. This is necessary for the horse to cover great distances at speed and to recover for the vet checks.

The legs should be straight from both front and rear views. Any deviation or minor unsoundness will lead to serious problems when pushed over a 100-mile course. The pasterns should be sloping, the cannon bones short, and the forearms long to allow a swinging gait and effortless stride. All the bones should be dense and flat, and the joints should be large (but not puffy). Well-defined tendons, with deep grooves separating them, indicate healthy tendons.

The hooves should be large but not disproportional. A relatively thick hoof wall can tolerate the frequent reshoeing necessary. The heels should be open, and should be examined for interference marks that could indicate that the horse is over-reaching and injuring itself. The hoof horn should be dense, and the bars firm. The frog

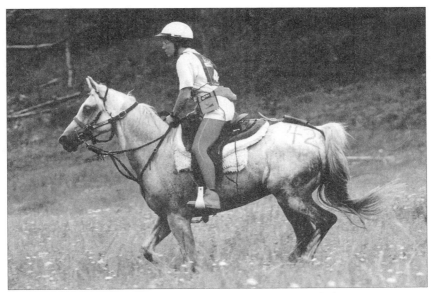

Fig. 12–18. Distance horses should be lean and lightly muscled.

should be elastic and untrimmed. (Trimming the frog improves its appearance but may reduce the hoof's ability to absorb shock.)

Muscling

A lean, lightly muscled horse will fare better than a heavily muscled animal. Heavy muscles do not shed heat effectively. Also, heavy muscle or excessive fat requires the horse to carry additional weight, and the horse will tire more readily. Endurance comes from long, slim muscles.

Size

The size of a trail horse is a definite consideration. Small horses (around 15 hands) sometimes have the advantage because they shed heat more effectively than larger horses. A small horse has proportionately more body area for evaporation than a bulky horse. Since evaporation of sweat cools the body, a small horse can shed excess heat more efficiently. A small horse may also be a better feed converter and have greater weight-carrying capacity in proportion to its size.

DRAFT HORSES

Draft horses are shown at fairs, pulling contests, and other exhibitions. However, they are still used for farm work and drafting, and are essential in warmblood/sport horse breeding programs to produce world-class dressage, show jumping, and competitive trail athletes.

Conformation of Draft Types

Overall, working animals should be deep, broad, and muscular. They should have the rugged construction, size, and substance necessary to pull heavy loads at a walk. Most draft horses weigh more than 1,600 pounds, and stand 16 – 19 hands tall.

Body and Legs

The ideal build should be powerful and compact. The draft horse has a deep, wide chest, a massive neck, and a heavy forehand. Weight in the forehand is especially important, since the draft horse pulls loads greater than its own weight by pushing its heavy neck, shoulder, and chest against the collar. (However, a chest that is too wide increases concussion and predisposes the horse to ringbone.) The loin and topline should be strong, the back short, with ribs springing high from the spine to create the rounded barrel. The belly and flanks are deep: long from top to bottom. A well-muscled croup and gaskin, a thick stifle, and a heavy forearm—accompanied by a strong, flat cannon bone—gives the horse pulling power.

Certain conformational traits that would normally be undesirable in a riding horse may be acceptable in a draft horse. The shoulder, for example, may be straighter, the croup more vertical, and the withers less prominent. The horse also has more power if its legs are short in proportion to body height. Several draft breeds stand close behind, which means their hocks are placed close together. This trait has been encouraged through breeding under the assumption that it gave the horse a firmer column of support and enabled it to keep power under its body. Although the assumption is questionable, cow hocks are common in those breeds. Most of these horses are lightly worked and remain sound.

Ideally, the body length should be several inches more than its height at the withers. The body depth from withers to underline should be several inches more than the distance from the belly to the

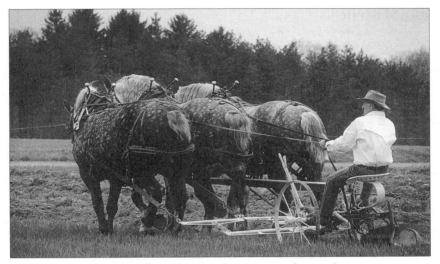

Fig. 12–19. An ideal draft horse is muscular, stout, and rugged.

ground. The draft horse needs a good foundation for support, and its short, straight legs should taper down to lean ankles and adequately angled pasterns. Again, draft horse owners will tolerate a more vertical angle here than is found in a riding horse. However, short, very upright pasterns should be discriminated against. Such conformation accounts for a high incidence of sidebone in draft animals.

Feathering

On Shires, the leg *feathers* extend from the hock to the ground. They should be long, flowing, and silky but not excessively abundant. Clydesdales have less feathering than Shires. Profuse feathering on the fetlocks and pasterns makes skin care on the legs a constant concern for the owner.

Feet

The feet should be large and rounded, full at the toe and quarters, and wide and deep at the heel. Wide heels expand when the foot hits the ground, absorbing the concussion. Flat soles, contracted heels, and other problems, especially of the front feet, should be discriminated against.

Refinement

Strength in the body and legs is vital, but it is not necessary to sacrifice quality. A draft horse should be balanced and possess style and refinement: the head should be well shaped (not coarse), the eyes large and bright, the ears alert, and the face intelligent. Small heads in foals and yearlings often indicate early maturity and an ultimate lack of size, so they should be discriminated against.

Action

The draft horse's action should be swift and elastic—power is not necessarily accompanied by sluggishness. The Clydesdale, for example, has considerable animation and high action. Its springy gaits stem from longer than average pasterns, and its collected appearance from being slightly cow-hocked. The Shire has excellent balance and attractive movement valued in dressage.

13

TEETH & AGING

The horse's front teeth are called the *incisors*. They are used to grasp and nip food when grazing. The *cheek teeth* are called the *premolars* and *molars.* They grind the food into small particles while it is mixed with saliva. The teeth are longer than many people imagine, consisting mostly of crown with short roots. In a young horse, most of the tooth is still embedded in the jaw. The tooth erupts continuously as the horse

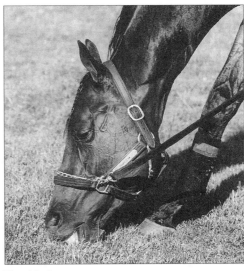

Fig. 13–1.

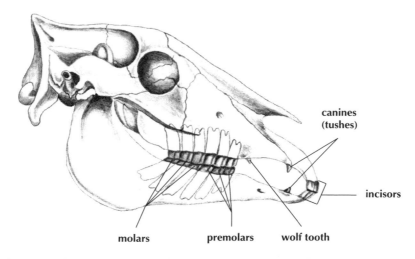

Fig. 13–2. The teeth are embedded in the skull and mandible of a young horse.

ages to compensate for wear. By the time the horse is about 20, there is very little tooth embedded.

The incisors can be used fairly accurately to determine a horse's age until about nine years. After this, age can only be estimated. (The cheek teeth can be used to age the horse but they are difficult to examine.)

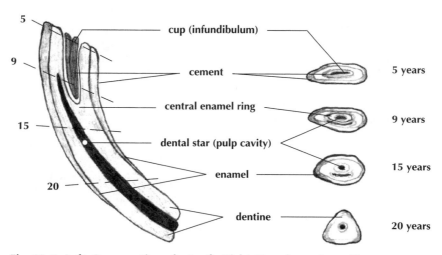

Fig. 13–3. Left: Cross-section of a tooth. Right: Top views at specific ages.

Temporary Teeth

Young horses have *temporary milk teeth*. These teeth are smaller, whiter, and smoother than permanent teeth (which are strong and yellowish). Also, milk teeth have an indentation, or "neck" at the gum line, which permanent teeth do not have.

One-Year-Old

By the time the horse is 1 year old, it has a complete set of 24 teeth. They include 12 temporary incisors, 12 permanent premolars, and 4 permanent molars.

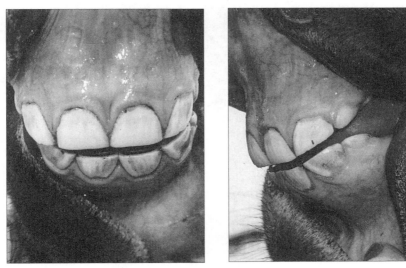

Fig. 13–4. One year old—complete set of milk teeth.

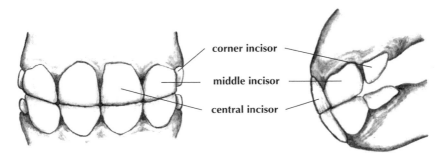

corner incisor

middle incisor

central incisor

Fig. 13–5. The upper and lower milk teeth are erupted, but not all are touching.

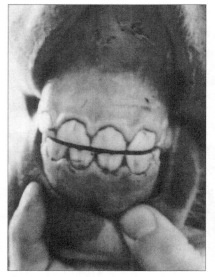

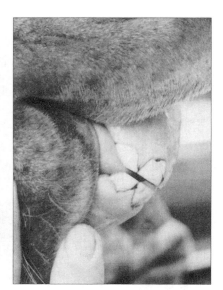

Fig. 13–6. Age two—mature milk teeth.

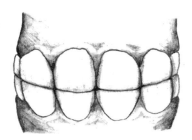

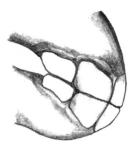

Fig. 13–7. Upper and lower temporary incisors are fully erupted and touching.

Two-Year-Old

At two, all of the horse's milk teeth are more fully erupted. The upper and lower sets of incisors are touching. Because they are touching, they will begin to show wear, beginning with the central incisors.

Permanent Teeth

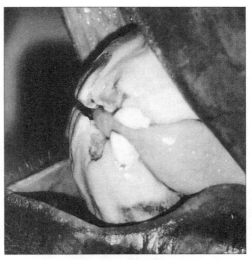

Permanent adult teeth begin to replace the temporary milk teeth when the horse is about 2½ years old. (Teeth are shed in autumn.) The two *central incisors* are fully erupted by age 3. The two *middle incisors* appear at about age 3½, and are fully erupted by age 4. In males, the four *canine teeth*, or tushes, on either side of the corner incisors appear at this age. (Females do not usually have canine teeth, and if they do, the teeth are small.) The *corner incisors* erupt

Fig. 13–8. About 3$^1/_2$ years old. The central incisor is permanent, the middle incisor is shed, and the corner incisor is temporary.

at age 4½, and are fully erupted by age 5. At this time, the horse also has a complete set of 24 permanent premolars and molars.

Wolf Teeth

Some horses develop another set of premolars, called *wolf teeth,* just in front of the cheek teeth *(see Figure 13–2).* They have been known to appear as early as six months, but they usually appear by age 2. Those horses that develop them are usually males. Sometimes the lower wolf teeth develop but do not erupt above the gumline. If they do erupt, they are small and have relatively short roots. They are easily lost when the horse chews on hard objects—they can even be lost due to bit pressure. These teeth should be removed if present because they may interfere with bitting.

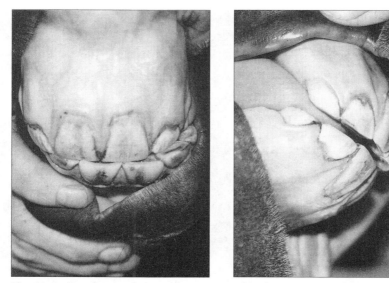

Fig. 13–9. Age three—the permanent central incisors are erupted.

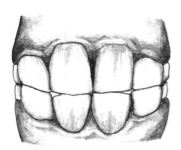 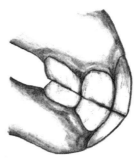

Fig. 13–10. The permanent central incisors are larger and darker than the temporary incisors.

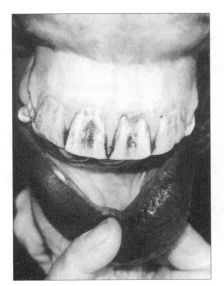
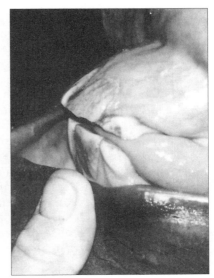

Fig. 13–11. Age four—the permanent middle incisors are erupted.

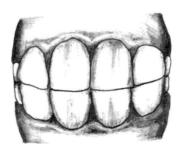
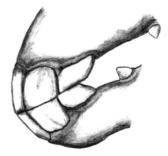

Fig. 13–12. The horse has two sets of permanent incisors, but the corner incisors are still temporary. The canine teeth have erupted.

Dental Care

The cheek teeth require regular dental care because they do not mesh perfectly. The lower jaw is more narrow than the upper jaw. Therefore, the lower arcades (rows) are closer to each other than are the upper arcades. This means that the outside edge of the upper teeth and the inside edge of the lower teeth do not touch the opposite teeth. Furthermore, the horse chews on only one side of its mouth at a time, and applies pressure to the jaw only when it is moving on the path of least resistance: upward and inward, in a side-to-side grinding motion.

As a result, the outside edge of the upper teeth and the inside edge of the lower teeth are not worn away by chewing, but become sharp ridges. The ridges can cut the inside of the mouth or cause incomplete chewing of feed, either of which can lead to further complications. Regular dental care by rasping away the ridges, called "floating" the teeth, helps to avoid dentition problems.

Fig. 13–13. The cheek teeth wear unevenly, which creates sharp ridges. Regularly floating the teeth with a rasp will prevent chewing difficulties.

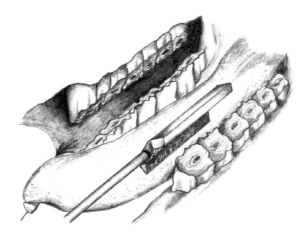

Estimating Age After 5 Years

Beyond 5 years old, the horse's age is estimated by:

- the amount of wear on the cups of the incisors
- the shape and inclination of the incisors
- the groove that appears in the upper corner incisors

Cups

The *"cups"* are the pits in the center of the teeth. They are filled with cement and surrounded by a ring of enamel. Feed causes the cups to blacken. As the horse ages and the tooth wears, the cups gradually disappear. The cups of the lower incisors disappear at the following ages:

- Central incisors—6th year
- Middle incisors—7th year
- Corner incisors—8th year

Similarly, the cups of the upper incisors disappear during the 9th, 10th, and 11th years. (**Note:** These ages are approximate. Changes are gradual, and each horse is a little different depending on its diet and state of health.) The remnant of the enamel surrounding the cup after it has worn away is called the *"mark."*

Shape and Inclination

The teeth change shape as the horse ages. When they erupt, the chewing surfaces (table) are oval. At about age 12, the central incisors become round. At age 17, all incisors are round. When the horse is 18, the central incisors are triangular. By the time the horse is 23 years old, all incisors are triangular. From age 24 to age 29, the horse's teeth once again become oval, but elongate in toward the back of the mouth. Also, a 6-year-old's teeth are more-or-less perpendicular when viewed from the side, while a 20-year-old horse's teeth slant sharply forward.

Galvayne's Groove

At about age 10, *Galvayne's groove* develops. It first appears at the gum line of the upper corner incisors. As the horse ages, the groove extends downward and is stained yellow-brown. By the time the horse is 20, the groove extends all the way down the surface of the tooth. After this age, the groove starts to disappear, again from the gum line down. By the age of 30, Galvayne's groove has disappeared completely.

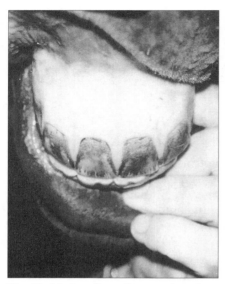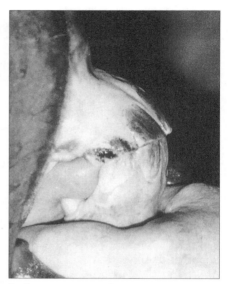

Fig. 13–14. Age five—the permanent corner incisors are erupted.

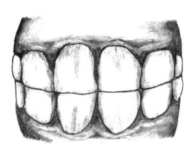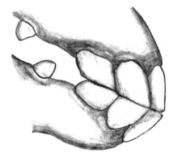

Fig. 13–15. The horse has three sets of permanent incisors.

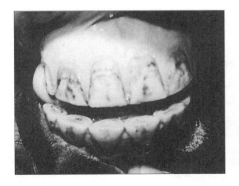

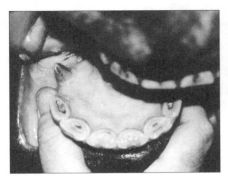

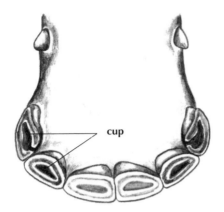

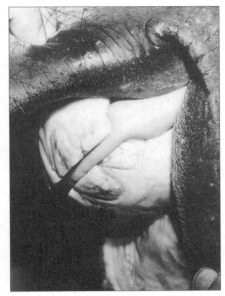

Fig. 13–16. About age six—the incisors are beginning to show wear.

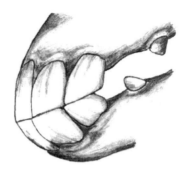

Fig. 13–17. Between the ages of 6 and 7, the cups of the central incisors disappear.

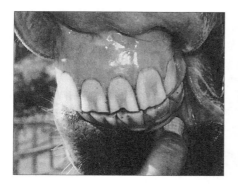

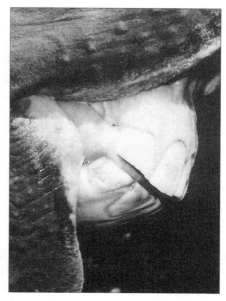

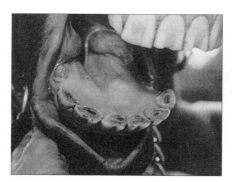

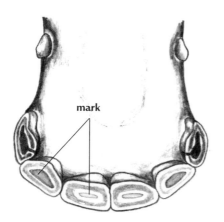

Fig. 13–18. About age seven.

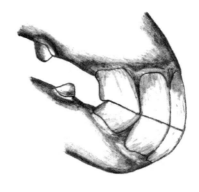

mark

Fig. 13–19. Between the ages of 7 and 8, the cups of the middle incisors disappear.

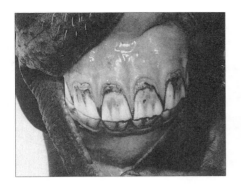

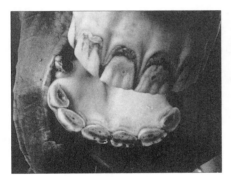

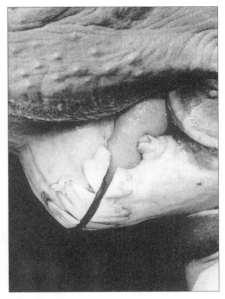

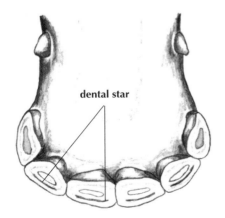

Fig. 13–20. About age eight.

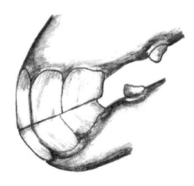

dental star

Fig. 13–21. Between the ages of 8 and 9, the cups of the corner incisors disappear.

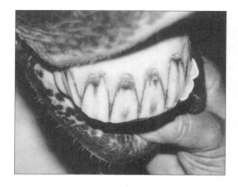

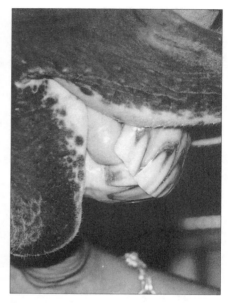

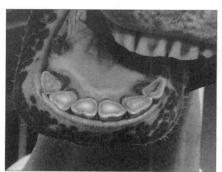

Fig. 13–22. About age 12—The teeth are larger and darker. Galvayne's groove is showing near the gumline of the upper corner incisor.

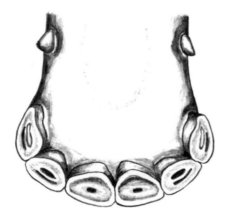

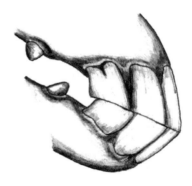

Fig. 13–23. The central incisors are becoming rounded.

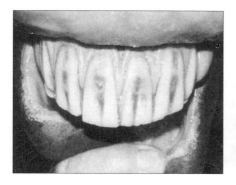

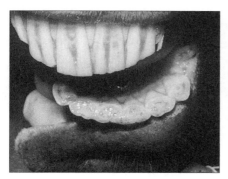

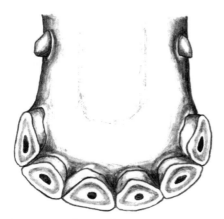

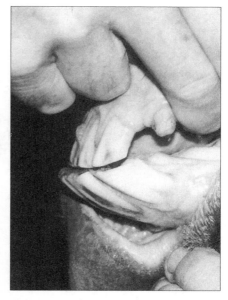

Fig. 13–24. About age 15—The teeth are longer.

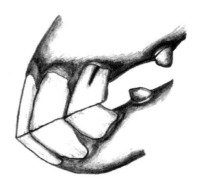

Fig. 13–25. The middle incisors are becoming more rounded. From the side, the teeth slant forward noticeably.

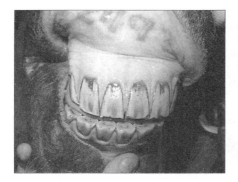

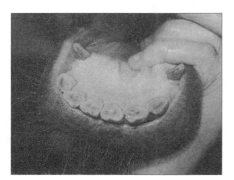

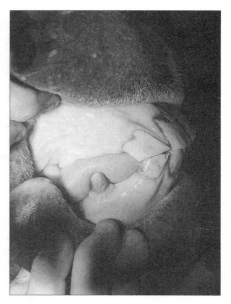

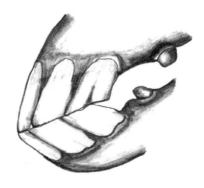

Fig. 13–26. About age 22—the teeth slant forward markedly. Galvayne's groove is disappearing from the gum line down. By age 30 it will be gone.

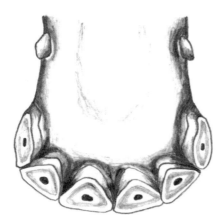

Fig. 13–27. The central and middle incisors are triangular. From age 23 to 29, the incisors will regain an oval shape, but this time they elongate in toward the back of the mouth.

Premature Aging of Teeth

Horses that live in dry, sandy areas wear their teeth faster than other horses. Likewise, horses with stable vices such as cribbing and wood chewing wear down the incisors quickly. Horses with an overbite (parrot mouth) or underbite (bulldog mouth) also wear their teeth unevenly.

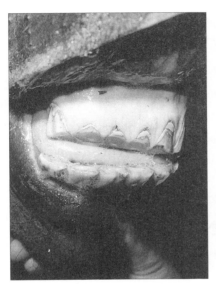 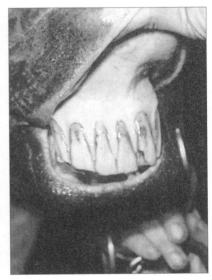

Fig. 13–28. The horse on the left is a cribber—the incisors are worn to virtually nothing. Compare this 22-year-old to the 38-year-old horse's teeth on the right. The older horse has very long and yellowed teeth.

All of these factors make determining the horse's age more difficult. Also, these horses usually require dental care more often.

14

BODY SYSTEMS

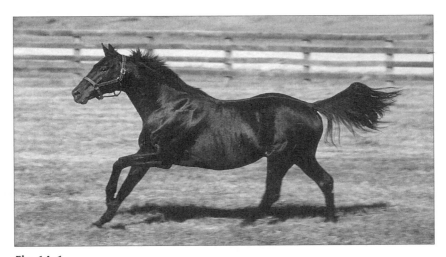

Fig. 14–1.

The internal body systems of the horse include the respiratory, circulatory, nervous, digestive, urinary, and reproductive systems. A basic knowledge of the anatomy and functions of these systems will lend a greater understanding of the horse both as a species and as an individual—its welfare, contentment, abilities, and limitations.

(These sections are a general overview of equine anatomy. For more information read *The Illustrated Veterinary Encyclopedia for Horsemen* published by Equine Research, Inc.)

RESPIRATORY SYSTEM

Respiration is the process by which the horse takes in oxygen, and rids its body of carbon dioxide. The initial step in respiration in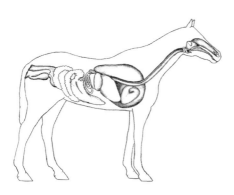volves the body making this exchange with the atmosphere. Air enters the horse's nasal passages through the nostrils, travels through the larynx to the trachea (windpipe), and then to the lungs.

But in a final sense, this process takes place in every part of the horse's body. That is, the living cells take oxygen from the blood, and give back carbon dioxide.

(More information on the nasal passages, pharynx, larynx, and trachea can be found Chapter 2, *Head*, and Chapter 3, *Neck*.)

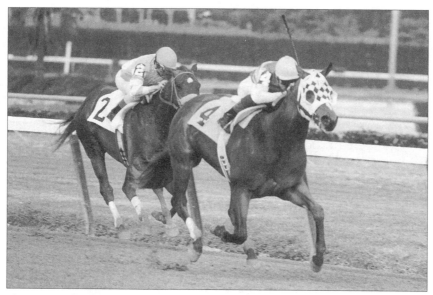

Fig. 14–2. A healthy respiratory system is vital to a racehorse.

Secondary functions of the respiratory system include temperature control, vocal communication, and facilitation of the sense of smell.

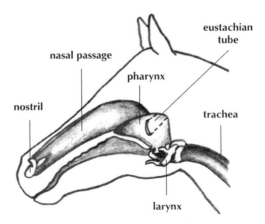

Fig. 14–3. Parts of the upper respiratory system.

Nasal Passages

The *nasal passages* conduct air from the outside to the throat. The openings of the nasal passages—the *nostrils*—are built around crescent-shaped cartilages. These cartilages are flexible and allow the nostrils to be flared to take in more air when needed during exercise. The nasal septum is a strip of cartilage that separates the left and right nasal passages.

Pharynx

The *pharynx* is a muscular sac between the nasal passages and the larynx in the throat. It is also built around cartilage. The function of the pharynx is to direct air and food properly. It is therefore a vital part of both the respiratory and digestive systems. Unless the horse is swallowing, the *epiglottis* of the larynx overlaps the pharynx. This separates it from the mouth and allows air to flow from the pharynx into the larynx.

The pharynx has small slits in the side that open into the *eustachian tubes*. These tubes lead to the middle ear: their function is to equalize air pressure on both sides of the eardrum.

A blind sac (open only on one end) called a *guttural pouch* communicates via each eustachian tube with the pharynx. With each breath, air moves in and out of each guttural pouch. (See Chapter 2, *Head*, for more information and an illustration.)

Larynx

The *larynx* serves as a tubular valve between the pharynx and the trachea. It is made of nine cartilages that together create a cavity.

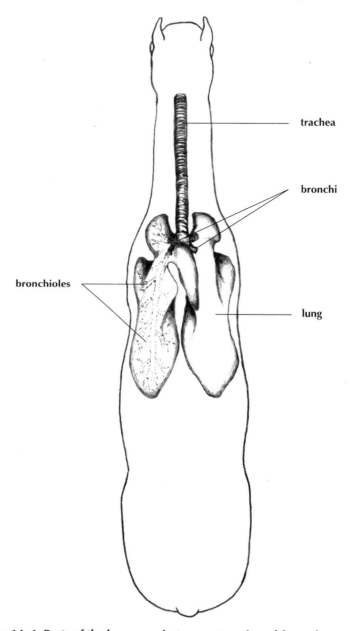

trachea

bronchi

bronchioles

lung

Fig. 14–4. Parts of the lower respiratory system viewed from above.

The two *vocal cords* stretch over the lower opening of the larynx. These ligaments give the horse its voice. If one or both of the muscles that move the cords are paralyzed, the horse shows symptoms of roaring syndrome, a respiratory condition characterized by noisy breathing.

Trachea

The *trachea* (windpipe) is a tube that conducts air from the larynx to the lungs. The tube is about 2 inches in diameter, built around rings of cartilage, and lined with a mucous membrane. The membrane contains cilia (tiny hair-like structures). Motion of the cilia create a constant flow of mucus up the throat. Foreign matter is trapped by the mucus, driven up to the top of the trachea, and then swallowed. This mechanism helps to prevent respiratory infection.

The trachea branches just after it reaches the thorax into two tubes called *bronchi*. These bronchi are the passageways to the left and right lobes of the lungs.

Lungs

The horse's *lungs* are shaped roughly like arrowheads from the side, but they are contoured to accommodate the organs around them. Oxygen-containing air enters each lung via the bronchi. After the bronchi enter the left and right lobes of the lungs, they branch further into *bronchioles*. The bronchioles end in *alveoli*—microscopic sacs that resemble bunches of grapes. Blood flows from small capillaries into thin membranes of the alveoli. It is here that oxygen in the lung is exchanged for carbon dioxide in the blood.

Diaphragm

The *diaphragm* is a dome-shaped muscle that lies behind the lungs. Contraction of the diaphragm causes inhalation. Exhalation does not require muscular effort in the resting horse. It occurs automatically due to the difference in air pressure between the outside and inside of the horse, and the natural rebound of the flexible ribs. During exercise, the abdominal muscles contract to help force the diaphragm forward. This allows more air to enter and leave the lungs with each breath. (See Chapter 7, *Body* for illustrations of the diaphragm and abdominal muscles.)

CIRCULATORY SYSTEM

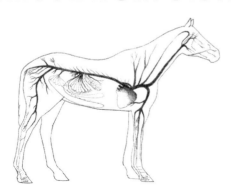

The circulatory system is responsible for carrying blood to and from the body tissues, delivering nutrients and oxygen, and picking up waste products and carbon dioxide. The blood also carries hormones that act as chemical messages, and cells that activate the immune system to defend the body against invaders. The vessels through which the blood travels are the arteries and veins. The powerful driving force behind the circulatory system is the heart.

Heart

The *heart* is a hollow, cone-shaped, muscular organ located in the center of the chest, between the right and left lungs opposite the third

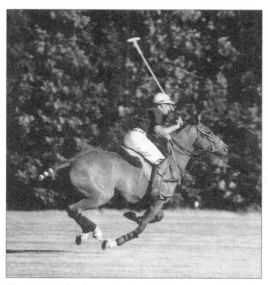

Fig. 14–5. The heart is the driving force behind the circulatory system.

to sixth ribs. Through muscular contraction, it forces blood through the blood vessels.

The heart is divided into left and right sides. Each side contains two chambers, an *atrium* and a *ventricle.*

The right atrium receives blood from the *vena cava* and passes it to the right ventricle. The right ventricle pumps blood out of the heart, through the *pulmonary artery* to the lungs for oxygenation. The left atrium receives oxygen-rich blood from

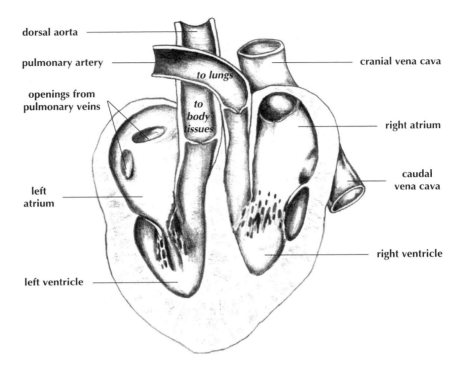

dorsal aorta

pulmonary artery

to lungs

openings from
pulmonary veins

to body tissues

cranial vena cava

right atrium

caudal vena cava

left atrium

right ventricle

left ventricle

Fig. 14–6. Cross-section showing the chambers of the heart.

the lungs via the *pulmonary veins* and forces it into the left ventricle.
The left ventricle pumps the blood through the *dorsal aorta*, which
eventually supplies all body tissues. The muscle tissue of the heart
itself is supplied by the coronary vessels on its surface.

Blood Vessels

A system of *blood vessels* carries blood to and from the body tissues
in a continuous, circular path. *Arteries* are thick, muscular vessels
that carry blood from the heart. The major artery that leaves the
heart is the *dorsal aorta*. It divides into smaller and smaller branches,
becoming *arterioles* and eventually *capillaries* as it progresses
through the body.

Capillaries are found at the tissue level. Their walls are very thin,
allowing fluid, nutrients, and other molecules to escape. Therefore it
is here that the oxygen and nutrients in the blood are delivered to the

tissues. The arterial capillaries join with venous capillaries, whose function is just the opposite: to pick up waste products and fluid. These capillaries enlarge to form *venules,* and eventually *veins,* which transport blood back to the heart.

The walls of the veins are not as thick or muscular as those of the arteries. Veins are often larger and more numerous, and closer to the skin surface than arteries. Very little arterial blood pressure is transmitted through the capillary beds to help return blood to the heart. So the veins are equipped with one-way valves, which prevent blood from flowing back toward the capillary beds. Most veins are situated between masses of muscles so that muscular contractions of normal movement squeezes them and forces blood back to the heart.

Lymphatic System

Lymphatic circulation is made up of lymph fluid, lymph vessels, lymph ducts, and lymph nodes. The lymph vessels, ducts, and nodes form a series of channels throughout the body to supplement the return function of the veins. Also, the lymphatic system aids in filtering out and destroying substances that may be harmful.

Lymph

When nutrients and oxygen leave the bloodstream in the capillary beds, fluid also escapes. Most of this fluid is reabsorbed by the venous capillaries, but some remains out in the extracellular spaces. This excess fluid is collected by lymph vessels, and is called *lymph* as soon as it enters the vessels. Lymph is a clear liquid similar to blood plasma. After being filtered by lymph nodes along the courses of the vessels, lymph is channeled into the venous circulation at the cranial vena cava. In this way it is returned to the bloodstream.

Lymph Vessels

The *lymph vessels* form a system of one-way channels and have valves (like veins), allowing lymph to flow only toward the heart. Lymph moves along the lymph vessels driven not by the heart, but by movement of the leg muscles. Like arteries and veins, lymph vessels converge, becoming larger and larger until they finally empty into the *cranial vena cava.*

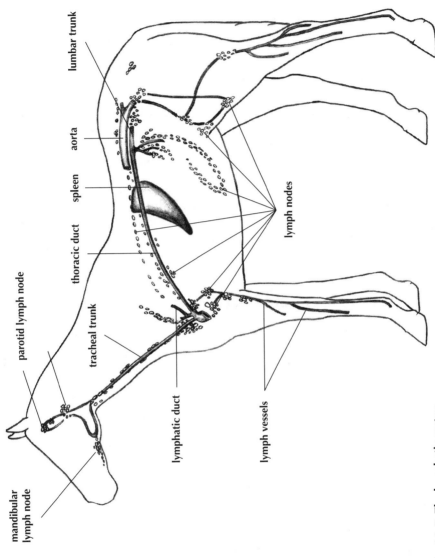

Fig. 14–7. The lymphatic system.

Lymph Ducts and Lymph Nodes

Lymph ducts are the gateways into and out of lymph nodes. *Lymph nodes* are masses scattered throughout the body, along the paths of most blood vessels. Lymph nodes serve as one of the first barriers against infection because they produce immune system cells and antibodies. They act to filter the lymph that passes through them, trapping harmful substances and destroying them. The tonsils and spleen are specialized lymph nodes.

The tonsils are unique because they are the only lymph nodes exposed to the outside environment. Inhaled air passes directly over the tonsils on its way to the pharynx.

The comma-shaped spleen is located in the upper part of the abdomen between the stomach and diaphragm. This sponge-like organ serves as a storage area for blood and is filled with lymph nodules (a node is a cluster of nodules). It varies in size according to the amount of blood it contains. As a general guide, though, the spleen is about 20 inches long and 8 inches wide, weighing about 2½ lbs. The spleen is more properly called a "hemyl node" because it filters the blood directly, not just the lymph, and has no lymph ducts.

NERVOUS SYSTEM

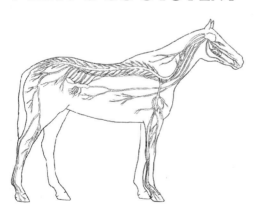

The nervous system is basically a complex biological guidance system. It provides the horse with information about its internal and external environment, and it activates the body's response to that information. Because of its complexity, it is divided into two parts—the central nervous system and the peripheral nervous system.

Central Nervous System

The central nervous system consists of the brain and spinal cord. Information regarding the horse's environment comes to one or

Side View—Cross-Section

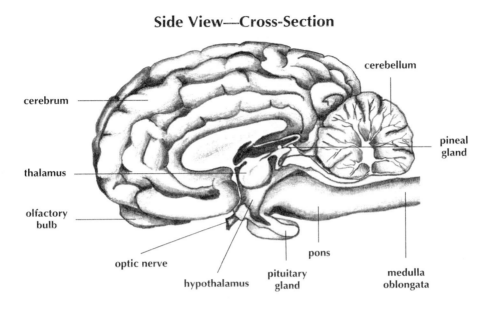

Top View

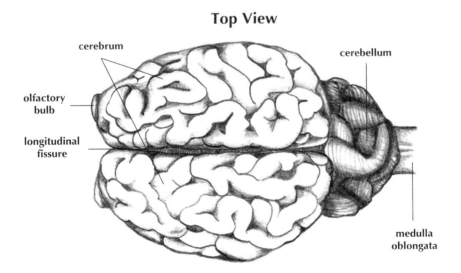

Fig. 14–8. Parts of the brain.

both of these structures. The signal that activates the body's response to that information also originates here.

Both the brain and the spinal cord are surrounded and protected by bone. The brain is encased by the skull. The spinal cord is enclosed within the spinal column.

Brain

The *brain* has three sections, each with a specific responsibility. The *cerebrum* is the largest part of the brain. It controls intelligence, memory, emotion, and the senses. The *cerebellum* is located behind and beneath the cerebrum. It controls muscle coordination and balance. The brainstem, or *medulla oblongata,* is the upper end of the spinal cord. It controls involuntary actions such as the heartbeat and circulation, respiration, and body temperature. (See Chapter 2, *Head,* for more information on the skull and brain.)

Spinal Cord

For purposes of description, the *spinal cord* is divided into five sections: cervical, thoracic, lumbar, sacral, and coccygeal. These sections are named for the corresponding vertebrae of the spinal column.

The spinal cord is capable of many responses to the environment in which the brain is not necessarily involved. One example of an "unconscious" adjustment is when the horse jerks away from a needle prick. This reflex action is involuntary; the brain is not involved. (Flattened ears and an open-mouthed lunge afterward, are, however, completely voluntary.) The spinal cord also serves as an intermediary between the brain and the rest of the body.

Peripheral Nervous System

The *peripheral nervous system* consists of the *nerves* branching off of the brain and spinal cord. Nerves are bundles of fibers that emerge from the brain and spinal column. They transmit information between the brain and body tissues. *Motor nerves* are concerned with movement, such as contracting a specific muscle to flex a joint. *Sensory nerves* relay sensation, such as pressure or pain. Motor nerves and sensory nerves often run together within the same bundle. If a nerve is damaged, the part it supplies no longer functions correctly.

Generally speaking, nerves are named for their locations. For example, 12 pairs of *cranial nerves* emerge from the brain. They are

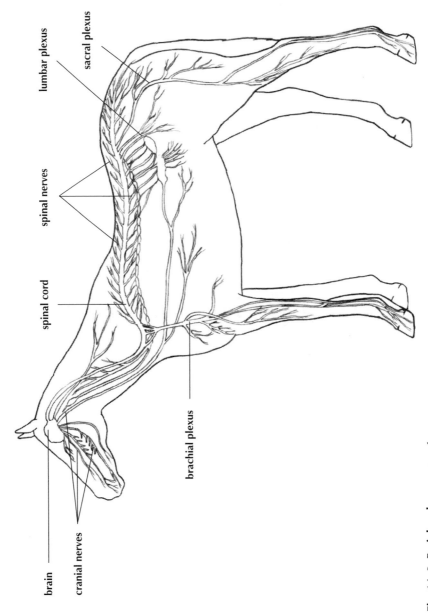

Fig. 14–9. Peripheral nervous system.

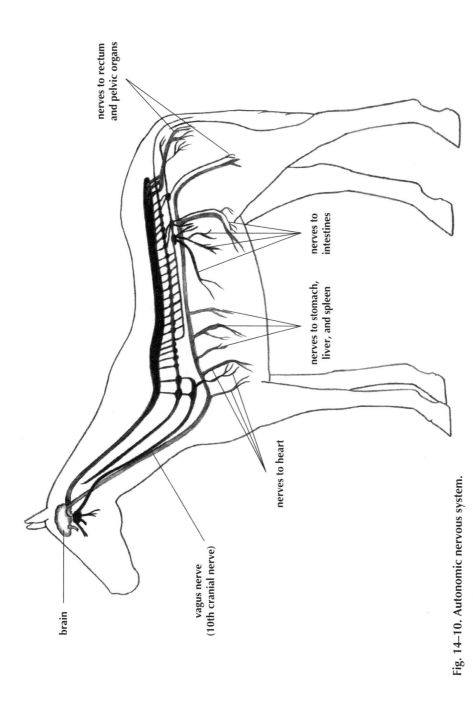

nerves to rectum
and pelvic organs

nerves to
intestines

nerves to stomach,
liver, and spleen

nerves to heart

vagus nerve
(10th cranial nerve)

brain

Fig. 14–10. Autonomic nervous system.

responsible for sight, smell, hearing, taste, eye movement, facial expression, movement of the pharynx and larynx, and some neck and shoulder muscle activation.

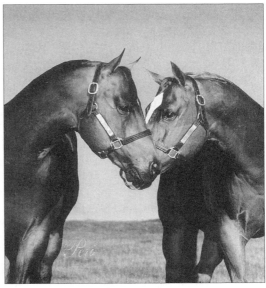

As the spinal cord travels the spinal column, *spinal nerves* branch off of each side, emerging from between the vertebrae. There are 42 pairs of spinal nerves. Specifically, cervical nerves emerge from the cervical section of the spinal cord, thoracic nerves emerge from the thoracic section, etc.

Fig. 14–11. Cranial nerves control sight, smell, hearing, eye movement, and facial expression.

As the nerves travel further from their origin, and branch into new territory, they receive new names. For example, the last few cervical nerves and the first few thoracic nerves combine to form the *brachial plexus*. The brachial plexus supplies motion and sensation to the foreleg. One of its branches is the radial nerve. The radial nerve travels near the radius (forearm bone), activating the muscles at the front of the forearm. (See Chapter 6, *Forelegs*, for more information.)

Autonomic Nervous System

The *autonomic nervous system* is a division of the peripheral nervous system. It is responsible for the activities of the heart, blood vessels, body temperature, glands, and digestive and urinary systems. Its regulatory function becomes critically important in stressful situations. When the horse senses danger, the autonomic nervous system launches a systemic response. The *adrenal gland* pours adrenaline into the bloodstream. The heart rate increases and the blood vessels dilate. Meanwhile, blood is shunted away from the digestive system, slowing it to a virtual standstill. All of these events instantaneously prepare the horse for "flight or fight."

DIGESTIVE SYSTEM

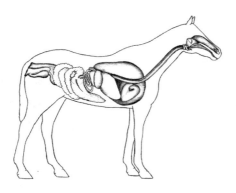

The digestive system is responsible for the intake (ingestion and grinding) and subsequent breakdown (digestion and absorption) of foods. The horse's body uses the nutrients contained in food for energy, tissue repair, and growth. Digestion takes place through muscular action, enzyme action, and bacterial fermentation. The process is complete when usable nutrients are absorbed and undigested food residues and waste products are excreted.

The *digestive tract,* or alimentary canal, consists of a muscular tube, which begins at the lips, and ends at the anus (and several associated organs). Between the mouth and the anus are the pharynx, esophagus, stomach, small intestine, cecum, small colon, large colon, and rectum. Associated organs that aid the digestive process are the teeth, tongue, salivary glands, liver, and pancreas.

The digestive tract is about 100 feet long in the mature horse. It changes diameter abruptly in several places, enlarging at the stomach, narrowing at the small intestine and enlarging again at the cecum.

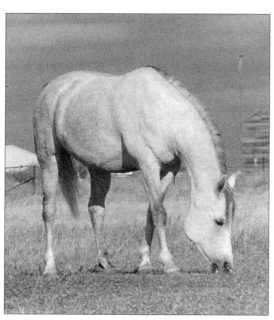

Fig. 14–12. The horse's body uses the nutrients contained in food for energy.

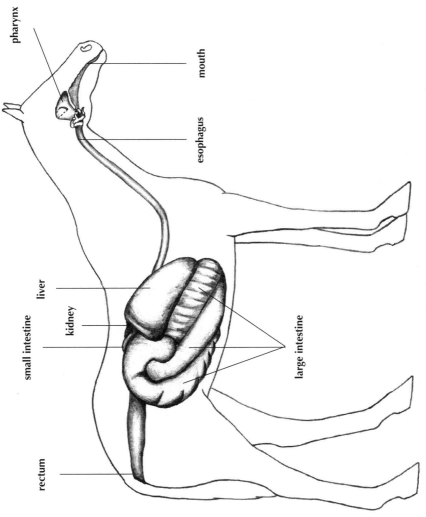

Fig. 14–13. The digestive tract from the right side.

pharynx

mouth

esophagus

liver

kidney

small intestine

large intestine

rectum

The tract is lined with mucous membranes, most of which contain glands that secrete digestive fluids.

Mouth

The *mouth* is the beginning of the digestive tract. The lips grasp food, passing it back to the teeth. The teeth grind the food in preparation for digestion. Meanwhile, three sets of *salivary glands* secrete saliva to moisten the food. The great amount of saliva mixed with the food increases its volume to nearly twice what was measured out as the feed ration. This should be considered when deciding how much to feed a horse at each meal. The saliva contains small amounts of digestive enzymes, which begins the digestive process.

The tongue passes the food back to the pharynx—gateway to the esophagus. In drinking, the horse uses its tongue like a piston on a suction pump to draw water back, just as a person does in drinking from a straw. Each swallow takes in about ½ pint. The horse's ears draw forward as a reflex action at each suction and fall back during the swallowing phase of each gulp.

(See Chapter 2, *Head*, for more information on the mouth. See Chapter 13, *Teeth*, for more information on the teeth.)

Pharynx

The *pharynx* is a passage between the mouth and esophagus. Food moves by muscular action through the pharynx. Being part of both the respiratory and digestive systems, the pharynx also provides an air passage between the nostrils and larynx. The *soft palate*, at the back of the mouth, acts as a trap to prevent food, water, and air from returning to the mouth from the pharynx. For this reason, the horse can neither breathe nor vomit through the mouth. Any food unable to pass down the esophagus due to obstruction or illness will return through the nostrils rather than through the mouth.

Esophagus

The *esophagus* is a tube about 5 feet long, connecting the pharynx to the stomach. It passes down the neck, through the thorax (chest cavity), and then through an opening in the diaphragm. The circular muscles of the esophagus force food and water down by waves of constriction called *peristalsis*.

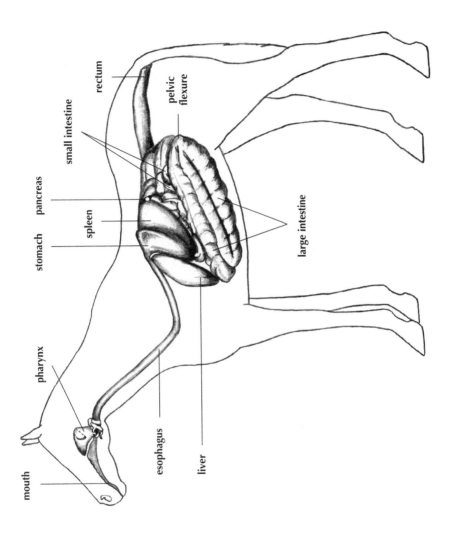

mouth

pharynx

esophagus

liver

stomach

pancreas

spleen

small intestine

rectum

pelvic
flexure

large intestine

Fig. 14–14. The digestive tract from the left side.

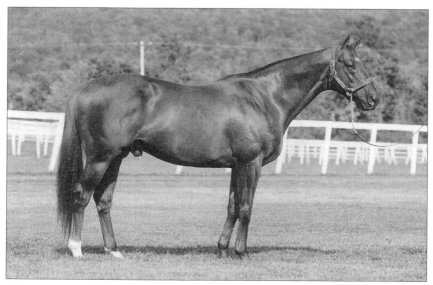

Fig. 14–15. A healthy horse's digestive system operates most efficiently on small, frequent meals.

This muscular action cannot work in reverse. This is because the esophagus enters the stomach at a very acute angle. Therefore, excessive gastric pressure—which in other species would push food back up the esophagus—closes the membrane flaps of the cardia (orifice where the esophagus enters the stomach). This action prevents vomiting, except on rare occasions involving certain severe forms of colic. In fact, stomach distension may cause the stomach to burst before it causes the horse to vomit.

Stomach

The *stomach* is a J-shaped muscular sac in the front of the abdomen close to the diaphragm and liver. The opening from the esophagus is called the *cardia;* the opening to the small intestine is called the *pylorus.*

Considering the horse's size, the stomach is relatively small. It can hold up to 4 gallons, but the first stage of digestion is more efficient when it is filled to about 2½ gallons rather than full capacity. Therefore, it is best that food be given in small amounts at frequent intervals.

The stomach lining secretes hydrochloric acid and digestive enzymes. Digestion begins as soon as food enters the stomach. Then a

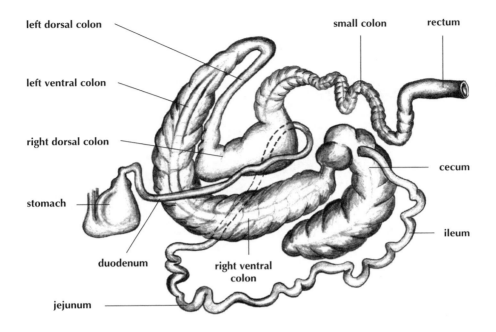

Fig. 14–16. Diagram of the digestive tract.

steady stream begins to pass out of the stomach into the small intestine. At this point the semi-digested food is called *chyme*.

Small Intestine

The *small intestine* is a muscular tube that runs from the stomach to the large intestine. It is about 70 feet long, has a diameter of 2 – 3 inches, and holds approximately 12 gallons.

The small intestine is located mainly in the upper part of the left abdomen, although much of it has no fixed position. Most of it is suspended from the top of the abdomen by a wide, fan-shaped fold of tissue called the great mesentery. The mesentery carries nerves and blood vessels that supply the intestines.

For purposes of description, the small intestine is divided into three parts. The first 3 feet is the *duodenum*. The liver and pancreas secrete digestive juices into this section via a common duct. The next 60 feet of the small intestine is called the *jejunum*. The final 6 feet is called the *ileum*.

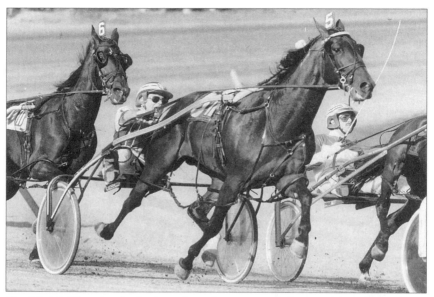

Fig. 14–17. Digestion in the large intestine occurs via bacterial fermentation. Intense exercise can disrupt the resident bacterial population, causing colic or other digestive disorders.

The major enzymatic breakdown of food occurs in the small intestine. Proteins, sugars, and fats are absorbed and enter the bloodstream through the intestinal walls. The remaining food matter, consisting mostly of fiber, moves on to the cecum and colon.

Large Intestine

The *large intestine* extends from the ileum to the anus. It is 25 – 28 feet long and consists of four parts:

- cecum
- large colon
- small colon
- rectum

The horse eats large amounts of cellulose, which normal enzymes cannot digest. But the horse's gut contains bacteria, which use fermentation to break down the cellulose into substances that the intestines can absorb. Because the resident bacteria need time to act, the cecum and the large colon are enlarged in order to hold more chyme. Food, therefore, moves very slowly in the large intestine.

Cecum

The *cecum* is comma-shaped, having an apex, body, and base. It is about 4 feet long and holds 7 – 10 gallons. It extends from the right flank forward and downward to near the diaphragm. Its openings from the small intestine *(ileocalceal valve)* and to the colon are close together.

Since its contents are mostly liquid, the cecum is sometimes called the water gut. Chyme from the small intestine and much of the water drunk by the horse spend a long time in the cecum. There they are mixed well together by contraction and relaxation of four longitudinal muscle bands called *taeniae coli.* This causes the cecum to form into saccules and then smooth out. During this process the resident bacteria in the cecum further breaks down the chyme, resulting in the formation of fatty acids and some vitamins that are absorbed from the cecum and the large colon.

Large Colon

The *large colon,* between the cecum and small colon, is 10 – 12 feet long and 8 – 18 inches in diameter. It can hold about 20 gallons of material. It is usually distended with relatively fibrous contents that are liquefied, but not as much as in the cecum. Some food digestion, mostly by bacterial fermentation and absorption, takes place here. The large colon has only one taenia coli in some parts, while three and four of these muscles are present in other parts. It is folded into four sections, in the following order:

1. *right ventral colon*   2. *left ventral colon*
3. *left dorsal colon*   4. *right dorsal colon*

Between the left ventral colon and left dorsal colon is a sharp, narrow turn called the *pelvic flexure.* This is often the location of the blockage in impaction colic.

Small Colon

The *small colon* is 10 – 12 feet in length and 3 – 4 inches in diameter. It extends from the large colon to the rectum. Since most of the moisture of the digested food is absorbed in the cecum and large colon, the remaining food residue is relatively solid. The small colon forms it into balls of manure. The fecal balls are formed by muscular action of the small colon, which has two taeniae coli for this purpose.

The *rectum* is a foot-long tract that reaches from the small colon through the pelvis to the anus. It holds the solid waste material until it is passed out of the horse's body through the anus during a bowel movement. The *anus* is composed of the *external anal sphincter muscle.* (Sphincter means "ring-like.") It prevents continuous leakage of solid waste. Associated muscles are the *coccygeus* and *levator ani.* These muscles help prevent herniation of the intestines during defecation and birthing. They extend from the os coxae (pelvis) to the sacrum and coccygeal vertebrae of the tail.

Liver

The *liver* is the largest gland of the horse's body and weighs 10 – 20 pounds. It has three lobes and is a relatively flattened organ located at the front and top of the abdomen. It lies against the ribs and diaphragm.

The liver is the chemical processing plant for the body. It manufactures bile, which it secretes into the duodenum of the small intestine to aid digestion. The liver also processes the digested proteins, sugars, minerals, and other food products. The food-enriched blood from the stomach, spleen, pancreas, and intestines is conducted to the liver via the large *portal vein.*

Once processed, the liver's regulatory abilities allow it to either put these products to immediate use, or to store them. Blood leaves the liver through the short *hepatic veins,* which empty into the *caudal vena cava.*

The liver itself receives nutrient blood from the *hepatic artery,* a branch of the *celiac artery.*

Pancreas

The *pancreas* is another flattened organ that lies at the central top of the abdomen just beneath and in front of the kidneys. It is formed of many lobules and ducts for the manufacture and secretion of digestive enzymes. The pancreas manufactures a hormone called *insulin,* which is involved in the metabolism of sugar that has already been absorbed into the bloodstream.

URINARY SYSTEM

The urinary system is responsible for collecting and removing fluid waste material from the horse's body. It is composed of two kidneys, each with a ureter that leads to the urinary bladder. There is also a urethra that leads from the bladder to an external opening.

Kidneys

The two kidneys are located in the loin area, one on each side of the spinal column. The right kidney is heart-shaped and lies near the last two ribs. The left kidney is bean-shaped and lies further back. They weigh about 1½ pounds each.

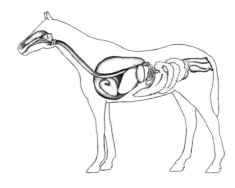

The kidneys filter the blood to eliminate fluid wastes from the body. They also help regulate the amount of certain substances in the body, maintaining its natural balance of salts, sugars, and fluid. Blood enters the kidney through the renal artery. After processing, the blood exits the kidney through the renal vein.

Ureters

Fluid waste, or urine, gradually drains from the kidneys into the bladder via two tubes called ureters. Urine is composed of water, urea (the final waste product of protein foods), uric acid, and salts.

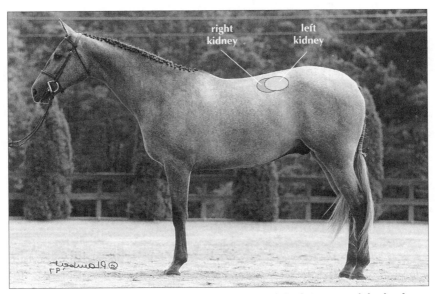

Fig. 14–18. The kidneys are located on each side of the loin area of the back.

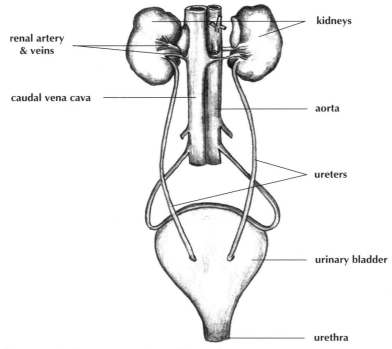

renal artery & veins

caudal vena cava

kidneys

aorta

ureters

urinary bladder

urethra

Fig. 14–19. Urinary system viewed from above.

Urinary Bladder

The *urinary bladder* is a hollow, pear-shaped, muscular organ. It is located in the lower pelvic region. The bladder serves as a storage chamber for urine with a normal capacity of 3 – 4 quarts. As the bladder fills with urine and expands, the thick walls become thinner.

Urethra

When the bladder is full, its walls contract and urine exits the body through the *urethra*. The urethra is surrounded by the *urethralis muscle* for this purpose. This muscle is served by the *pudendal nerve*. It has both longitudinal and transverse fibers. In the mare, urine exits via the vulva, and in the stallion it exits via the penis.

REPRODUCTIVE SYSTEM
Mare

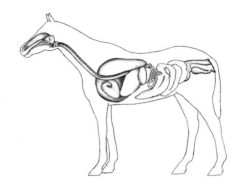

The mare's reproductive system is comprised of two ovaries, two oviducts (also called Fallopian tubes), a uterus, a vagina, and a vulva. The ovaries are called primary sex organs because they produce the ovum, or egg. The oviducts, uterus, vagina, and vulva are called secondary sex organs because they facilitate transport and fertilization of the egg, development of the fetus, and birth of the new foal.

Ovaries

The *ovaries* are two bean-shaped glands located below and behind each kidney. They are suspended from the "roof" of the abdomen in a fold of peritoneum (a membrane lining the abdomen) along with the oviducts, uterus, and vagina. This fold of peritoneum is called the *broad ligament.*

The ovaries have two main functions. The first function is to produce an ovum. But they also produce hormones necessary for normal reproductive function. Estrogen and progesterone are two hormones that are secreted by the ovary and absorbed directly into the mare's bloodstream.

The ovaries of a normal mare vary in size, shrinking as the mare ages. They measure from about 1½ x 3 inches in a young mare to about 1 x 1½ inches in an old mare.

During each estrus cycle, a follicle on the ovary matures, softening and then rupturing. This process, called ovulation, releases an ovum from the ovary. Ovulation corresponds with certain behavioral changes in the mare which indicate that she is in heat. (For more information, read *Breeding Management & Foal Development* published by Equine Research, Inc.)

The *ovarian artery* supplies blood to the ovaries. The *renal* and *aortic plexus* provides the nerve supply.

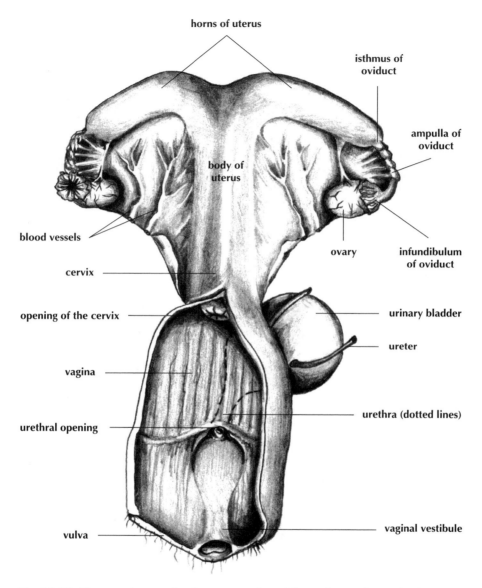

horns of uterus

isthmus of oviduct

ampulla of oviduct

body of uterus

blood vessels

ovary

infundibulum of oviduct

cervix

opening of the cervix

urinary bladder

ureter

vagina

urethra (dotted lines)

urethral opening

vaginal vestibule

vulva

Fig. 14–20. The mare's reproductive system viewed from above. The vagina has been cut lengthwise to show the opening of the cervix and the urethral opening.

Oviducts

The *oviducts* are small tubes that extend from each ovary to the uterus. The function of an oviduct (or Fallopian tube) is to transport ova from the ovary to the uterus. It is also the site of fertilization.

The oviduct has three parts. The funnel-shaped end of the oviduct near the ovary is called the *infundibulum*. It guides the ovum into the oviduct. This end of the oviduct is not completely attached to the ovary, but hooked only on one side. The second, tube-shaped part of the oviduct is the *ampulla*. The third part is the *isthmus*—the junction between the oviduct and the uterus.

Both circular and longitudinal layers of muscles make up the wall of the oviduct. These muscular layers help to transport ova through the length of the oviduct. It usually takes 6 – 8 days for an ovum to travel through the oviduct.

Uterus

The *uterus* is a hollow, muscular organ that accommodates the developing fetus. It has three parts: the body, horns, and cervix. In a nonpregnant mare, the *body* of the uterus is usually about 10 inches long and 4 inches in diameter. It is located partly in the abdomen and partly in the pelvis. The two *horns* are about 7 – 8 inches long, fairly straight, and blunted on the ends. They are located in the abdomen.

To support the developing fetus, the uterus is well supplied with blood via three arteries:

- *uterine artery*
- uterine branch of the *pudendal artery*
- uterine branch of the *ovarian artery*

It is supplied with nerve function via the *uterine* and *pelvic plexus.*

Cervix

The *cervix* (literally meaning "neck") is a strong, smooth, sphincter muscle. It is 2 – 3 inches thick and projects into the vagina 1 – 2 inches. It functions to separate the vagina from the uterus. Most of the time it remains tightly closed, only relaxing during heat and birth. During pregnancy the cervix secretes mucus, which forms a plug to seal off the uterus from the vagina. This mucous plug guards against infection.

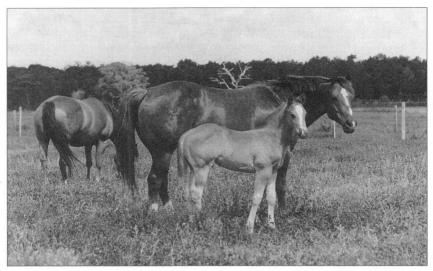

Fig. 14–21. The mammary glands within the udder produce milk for the foal.

Vagina

The *vagina* is the part of the birth canal between the uterus and the vulva. It is 6 – 8 inches long and 4 – 5 inches in diameter. The walls are constructed of an inner, circular layer of smooth muscle and an outer, longitudinal layer of smooth muscle.

The vagina is supplied with blood by the *pudendal arteries*. It is supplied with nerve function via the *pelvic plexus*.

Vulva

The *vulva* extends from the vagina to the exterior of the mare, forming the external opening of the reproductive and urinary systems. It is 4 – 5 inches long. The external lips of the vulva are called *labia*. Between the labia, the slit which forms the opening to the vagina is 5 – 6 inches long.

Together the vagina and vulva form a passageway for sperm at the time of breeding and for the foal at the time of birth.

Movement of the vulva is accomplished by the action of the *vestibular constrictor* and *vulvar constrictor muscles*. Both muscles originate on the *ventral sacrococcygeal muscle* and run vertically the length of the vulva.

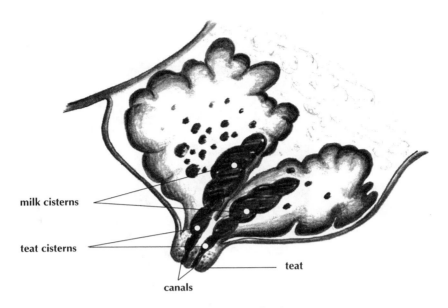

milk cisterns

teat cisterns

teat

canals

Fig. 14–22. A cross-section of the mammary gland.

Mammary Glands

The *mammary glands* are contained within the *udder*. They produce milk to nourish the foal. Within the gland is a system of channels that collect milk and direct it to the *milk cistern* just above the *teat*. From there the milk flows into the *teat cistern*. Each of the two teats has at least two passageways from the teat cistern to the outside orifice.

Blood supply to the udder is accomplished via the *external pudendal artery* and the *caudal mesenteric plexus*. The *inguinal nerve* provides the nerve supply.

Stallion

The genital organs of the male horse include two testicles (testes), each with an epididymis, a ductus deferens, and a spermatic cord. There are also various unpaired accessory sex glands and the penis.

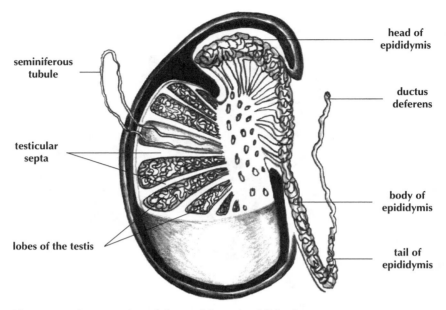

seminiferous tubule

head of epididymis

ductus deferens

testicular septa

body of epididymis

lobes of the testis

tail of epididymis

Fig. 14–23. Cross-section of the testicle and epididymis.

Testicles

The *testicles* are specialized glands that produce *spermatozoa* (sperm) and testosterone (male sex hormone). A normal testicle is egg-shaped, 3 – 5 inches long, and weighs about 10 ounces in the adult stallion. The relative size of each testicle varies from stallion to stallion, but usually the left is larger than the right.

Each testicle is suspended within the scrotum by its *spermatic cord.* The spermatic cord consists of the *testicular artery* and *testicular veins, external cremaster muscle, testicular plexus,* and ductus deferens. All of these structures are surrounded by a thin membrane, which is an extension of the abdominal peritoneum.

Epididymis

The *epididymis* is a storage area and transport tube for sperm. It is a long, winding tube that connects the testicle to the ductus deferens. It is divided into three sections: the head, body, and tail. The head, attached to the top of the testicle, is composed of multiple coiled tubules. The tubules unite to form a single tube or "duct," which is the body and tail. The body runs the length of the testicle, then the tail terminates in the ductus deferens.

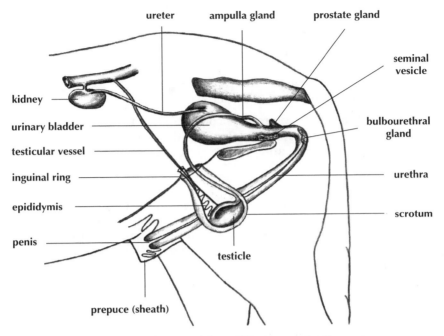

ureter   ampulla gland   prostate gland

seminal
vesicle

kidney

urinary bladder

bulbourethral
gland

testicular vessel

inguinal ring

urethra

epididymis

scrotum

penis

testicle

prepuce (sheath)

Fig. 14–24. Outside (lateral) view of the stallion's reproductive system.

Ductus Deferens

The *ductus deferens* (also called the vas deferens) is another muscular tube that extends from the tail of the epididymis to the urethra. On its way it passes through the *inguinal canal,* which is a passage from the abdomen to the exterior. The function of the ductus deferens is to propel the spermatozoa from the epididymis to the urethra during ejaculation.

Cremaster Muscle

The *cremaster muscle* holds the other structures of the spermatic cord together. It is also capable of lifting the testes from the scrotum into the lower part of the inguinal canal.

Urethra

The *urethra* is a long tube extending from the bladder to the end of the penis. It receives openings from the accessory sex glands and is enclosed by the *urethralis muscle,* which aids in the ejaculation of semen as well as in the expulsion of urine.

Accessory Sex Glands

The male accessory sex glands include:

- ampullae of the ductus deferens
- two *seminal vesicles*
- one *prostate gland*
- two *bulbourethral* (Cowper's) glands

Their function is to produce components of semen. Semen provides nutrition to the spermatozoa, aids its transport through the mare's genital tract, and protects it from the acid environment there.

Scrotum

The *scrotum* is composed of thin, relatively hairless skin. It is pliable so as to conform in size, shape, and location to the testes within. The *external cremaster muscle* can draw the scrotum up toward the abdomen for protection or when exposed to cold. The scrotum is supplied with blood by the *external pudendal artery.* Nerve supply is accomplished via branches of the second and third *lumbar nerves.*

Penis

The penis, located between the thighs, is the male organ of copulation. In the stallion it is about 20 inches long when relaxed, and more-or-less cylindrical. It is divided into three parts: glans, body, and root.

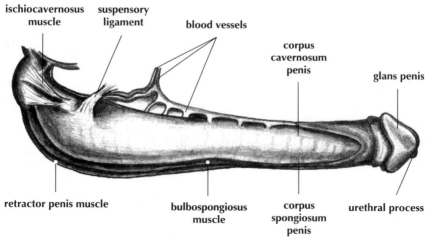

Fig. 14–25. Parts of the penis.

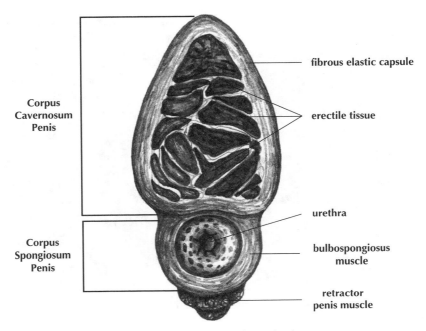

Corpus Cavernosum Penis

fibrous elastic capsule

erectile tissue

Corpus Spongiosum Penis

urethra

bulbospongiosus muscle

retractor penis muscle

Fig. 14–26. Cross-section of the penis viewed from the front.

The *glans penis* is the enlarged free end of the penis. The horse has a free portion of the urethra called the *urethral process* projecting beyond the glans. Just deep to the urethral process is a small fold of tissue called the diverticulum of the fossa glandis. This area is where smegma (secreted by the sebaceous glands of the sheath) collects, forming what is called a "bean." The bean should regularly be removed as part of the hygienic maintenance of the penis of the stallion or gelding.

The *body* of the penis is divided lengthwise into upper and lower parts. The upper part is called the *corpus cavernosum penis*. It is a tube that contains most of the erectile tissue, and carries nerves and blood vessels. (Erectile tissue is made of blood channels separated by connective tissue; it fills with blood during an erection.) The tube is surrounded by a thick fibrous elastic capsule, making the corpus cavernosum penis the larger of the two parts.

The lower part of the body of the penis is called the *corpus spongiosum penis*. This part contains the urethra and a lesser amount of erectile tissue.

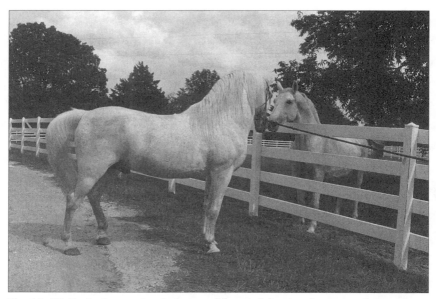
Fig. 14–27. Testosterone promotes sex drive and the development of secondary sex characteristics.

The *root* of the penis is attached to the ischial arch of the pelvis by two crura (literally meaning, "legs").

Erection is achieved when more blood flows into the penis than is allowed out. Muscle contractions of the penis constrict the veins, slowing the outflow of blood. The increased blood volume swells the erectile tissue, hardening and enlarging the penis. The length of the penis increases by about 50%, but the diameter does not increase by much. After ejaculation, the muscles relax and allow blood to flow back into the general circulation. Then the penis relaxes and shrinks back to its resting size.

Muscles acting on the penis include the *retractor penis muscle* from the coccygeal vertebrae, the two *ischiocavernosus muscles* attaching at the crura, and the *bulbospongiosus muscle* which is a continuation of the urethralis muscle surrounding the urethra.

Blood is supplied to the penis through the *internal* and *external pudendal arteries* and *obturator artery.* Nerve supply is accomplished by the pudendal nerve and pelvic plexus.

Prepuce

Surrounding the penis is a double fold of skin called the *prepuce* or sheath. It functions to protect the sensitive penis. Its outer surface looks like skin, but the interior has a preputial and a penile layer. These layers are hairless and are supplied with large amounts of sebaceous glands. The glands continually secrete a fatty, foul-smelling material called smegma. This material should be removed with mild soap and water every few weeks.

Testosterone

Testosterone promotes sex drive and the development and functioning of the accessory sex glands. Testosterone is responsible for the secondary sex characteristics of the stallion. Examples include development of a crest (varied in size according to breed), less fat storage, and suppressed mammary development.

APPENDIX

DIRECTIONAL TERMS

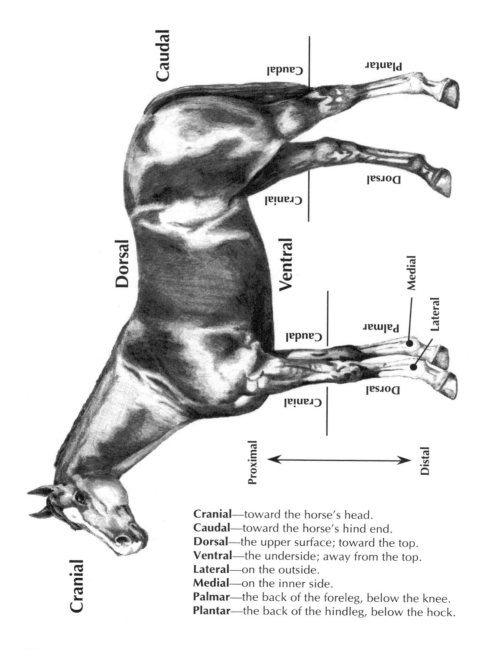

Cranial—toward the horse's head.
Caudal—toward the horse's hind end.
Dorsal—the upper surface; toward the top.
Ventral—the underside; away from the top.
Lateral—on the outside.
Medial—on the inner side.
Palmar—the back of the foreleg, below the knee.
Plantar—the back of the hindleg, below the hock.

ALTERNATE ANATOMIC TERMS

Structure

Bones

Alternate Terms

Structure	Alternate Terms
atlas	first cervical vertebra, C1
axis	second cervical vertebra, C2
calcaneus	calcaneum, fibular tarsal bone, heel bone
cannon bone	third metacarpal bone (foreleg), MCIII third metatarsal bone (hindleg), MTIII
coccygeal vertebrae	caudal vertebrae
coffin bone	distal phalanx, third phalanx, pedal bone, P_3
femur	roundbone, thigh bone
hock bones	tarsal bones
humerus	arm bone, clod bone
hyoid bone	hyoid apparatus
ilium	haunch bone, hook bone
incus	anvil
ischium	pin bone
knee bones	carpal bones
long pastern bone	first pastern bone, first phalanx, proximal phalanx, P_1
malleus	hammer
maxilla	upper jawbone
navicular bone	distal sesamoid bone
os coxae	hip bone, aitch-bone, innomiate bone
patella	kneecap
sacrum	sacral vertebrae, holy bone
scapula	shoulder blade
sesamoid bones	proximal sesamoid bones
short pastern bone	second pastern bone, middle pastern bone, middle phalanx, second phalanx, P_2
splint bones	second (medial) or fourth (lateral), metacarpal bones (foreleg), MCII or MCIV, second or fourth metatarsal bones (hindleg), MTII or MTIV
stapes	stirrup
sternum	breastbone
tuber coxae	hook bone
tuber ischii	ischiatic tuberosity, pin bone
tuber sacrale	sacral tubers

Structure	Alternate Terms
Joints	
atlantoaxial joint	"No" joint
atlanto-occipital joint	"Yes" joint
coffin joint	distal interphalangeal joint
fetlock joint	ankle, metacarpophalangeal joint (foreleg)
	metatarsophalangeal joint (hindleg)
hip joint	coxofemoral joint
intercarpal joint	midcarpal joint
pastern joint	proximal interphalangeal joint
radiocarpal joint	antebrachiocarpal joint
tibiotarsal joint	tarsocrural joint
shoulder joint	scapulo-humeral joint
Muscles	
ascending pectoral	caudal deep pectoral, pectoralis profundus, pectoralis ascendens
bulbospongiosus	bulbocavernosus
caudal tibial	tibialis caudalis
cranial tibial	tibialis cranialis
common digital extensor	extensor digitorum communis
corrugator supercilii	levator of the medial angle of the eye
deep digital flexor	flexor digitorum profundus, flexor perforans
deep gluteal	gluteus profundus
descending pectoral	cranial superficial pectoral, pectoralis descendens
external abdominal oblique	obliquus externus abdominis
external anal sphincter	sphincter ani externus
external intercostals	intercostales externi
external obturator	obturatorius externus
hamstrings	biceps femoris, semitendinosus, semimembranosus combined
internal abdominal oblique	obliquus internus abdominis
internal intercostals	intercostales interni
internal obturator	obturatorius internus
lateral digital extensor	extensor digitorum lateralis
lateral digital flexor	flexor digitorum lateralis, flexor hallucis longus
levator ani	medial coccygeus
levator labii superioris	levator of the upper lip

Structure	Alternate Terms
levator palpabrae superioris	levator of the upper eyelid
longus capitis	long muscle of the head, rectus capitis ventralis major
longissimus capitis	longest muscle of the head
longissimus dorsi	eye muscle, long dorsi
medial digital flexor	flexor digitorum medialis, long digital flexor
middle gluteal	gluteus medius
peroneus tertius	fibularis tertius
radial carpal extensor	extensor carpi radialis
radial carpal flexor	flexor carpi radialis
rectus capitis dorsalis major/minor	dorsal straight muscle of the head
sacrospinal	erector of spine, erector spinae
sartorius	tailor's muscle
semispinalis capitis	biventer and complexus muscles combined
serratus dorsalis	dorsal serrate
serratus ventralis	ventral serrate
subclavius	cranial deep pectoral
superficial digital flexor	flexor digitorum superficialis, flexor perforatus
superficial gluteal	gluteus superficialis, gluteus maximus (human)
transverse pectoral	caudal superficial pectoral, pectoralis transversus
trapezius	cucullaris
ulnar carpal extensor	extensor carpi ulnaris, ulnaris lateralis
ulnar carpal flexor	flexor carpi ulnaris
vestibular constrictor (of vulva)	constrictor vestibuli
vulvar constrictor	constrictor vulvae

Tendons & Ligaments

Achilles tendon	common calcanean tendon
distal sesamoidean ligaments	XYZ ligaments
inferior check ligament	carpal check ligament (foreleg), tarsal check ligament (hindleg)
nuchal ligament	ligamentum nuchae, back-strap
round ligament	ligament of the femoral head
superior check ligament	radial check ligament
suspensory ligament	interosseus muscle

BIBLIOGRAPHY

Bennett, Deb. *Principles of Conformation Analysis.* Volumes I – III. Fleet Street
Publishing Corporation, Gaithersberg, MD, 1988.

Bromiley, M. *Equine Injury, Therapy and Rehabilitation.* Blackwell Science Ltd,
Oxford, England, 1993.

Clayton, H.M. *Conditioning Sport Horses.* Sport Horse Publications, Saskatoon,
Saskatchewan, Canada, 1991.

DeMouthe Smith, Jean F. *Horse Markings and Coloration.* A.S. Barnes and
Company, New York, NY, 1977.

Evans, J. Warren et al. *The Horse.* WH Freeman and Company, New York, NY, 1990.

Foster, Carol. *The Athletic Horse: His Selection, Work and Management.* Howell
Book House, Inc., New York, NY, 1986.

Frandson, R.D. *Anatomy and Physiology of Farm Animals.* Lea & Febiger, Philadelphia, PA, 1965.

Goody, Peter C. *Horse Anatomy.* JA Allen and Company, Ltd., London, England,
1983.

Harris, S.E. *Horse Gaits, Balance and Movement.* Howell Book House, New York,
NY, 1993.

Hayes, M. Horace and Peter D. Rossdale, Ed. *Veterinary Notes for Horse Owners.*
Simon & Schuster, New York, NY, 1987.

Hodges, Jo and Sarah Pilliner. *The Equine Athlete.* Blackwell Science Ltd, Oxford,
England, 1991.

Kainer, Robert A. and Thomas O. McCraken. *The Coloring Atlas of Horse Anatomy.*
Alpine Publications, Loveland, CO, 1994.

King, Christine M. and Richard A. Mansmann. *Equine Lameness.* Equine Research, Inc. Tyler, TX, 1997.

Loving, Nancy S. *Veterinary Manual for the Performance Horse.* Equine Research,
Inc., Tyler, TX, 1993.

McBane, Susan. *The Illustrated Encyclopedia of Horse Breeds.* Wellfleet, Edison,
NJ, 1997.

Oliver, Robert and Bob Langrish. *A Photographic Guide to Conformation.* JA Allen
and Company, Ltd, London, England, 1991.

Smythe, RH, revised by Peter Gray. *Horse Structure & Movement.* Third Edition. JA
Allen and Company, Ltd, 1993.

Stashak, T.S. *Adams' Lameness in Horses.* Fourth Edition. Lea and Febiger,
Philadelphia, PA, 1987.

Wagoner, Don, Ed. *Breeding Management & Foal Development.* Equine Research,
Inc., Tyler, TX, 1985.

Wagoner, Don, Ed. *Equine Genetics & Selection Procedures.* Equine Research, Inc.,
Tyler, TX, 1978.

Wagoner, Don, Ed. *The Illustrated Veterinary Encyclopedia for Horsemen.* Equine
Research, Inc., Tyler, TX, 1977.

Wagoner, Don, Ed. *Conditioning to Win.* Equine Research, Inc., Tyler, TX, 1975.

Way, Robert F. and Donald G. Lee. *The Anatomy of the Horse.* Breakthrough
Publications, Millwood, NY, 1983.

FIGURE CREDITS

All Artwork by *Sherrie Engler.*

The staff of Equine Research, Inc. would like to thank the following people for their essential contributions in research and skill to the photographs in this book:

Ruth Ellen, AQHA Judge
Peri Hughes, Photographer
Barbara Ann Giove, Photographer
Monica Thors, Photographer
Babs Bashore, Photographer
Theresa and Dave Jones, Photographers and Editors for Chapter 9, *Feet*
James C. Hunt, DVM
Chris Brown, Equine Dentist
Joseph Sparado, New York State Thoroughbred Breeding & Development Fund

All photos are property of Equine Research, Inc. except the following:

Cover Photo by *Serita Hult.*

Figure 1–1. J P Hamer Courtesy of Justice Farm, Inc. Photo by Bill Straus.
Figure 1–2. Barbara Livingston.
Figure 1–3. Courtesy of Arabian Horse Trust. Photo by Jerry Sparagowski.
Figure 1–4. Monica Thors.
Figure 1–5. Courtesy of the American Quarter Horse Association. Painting by Orren Mixer.
Figure 1–12. Courtesy of Dave and Theresa Jones.
Figure 1–13. Don Trout.
Figure 1–14. Courtesy of the Unites States Trotting Association.
Figure 1–18. Courtesy of the American Morgan Horse Association. Photo by Quince Tree Photography.
Figure 1–21. Laurel Taylor.
Figure 1–28. Jerry Sparagowski. Used with permission by Mandolyn Hill Farm.
Figure 2–1. Babs Bashore.
Figure 2–2. Cappy Jackson.
Figure 2–5. Barbara Ann Giove.
Figure 2–8. Barbara Livingston.
Figure 2–9. Babs Bashore.
Figure 2–10. Courtesy of the International Arabian Horse Association.
Figure 2–11. Courtesy of the United States Trotting Association. Photo by Ed Keys.
Figure 2–12. Courtesy of Oak Hill Ranch.
Figure 2–13. Sheri Cook.
Figure 2–14. Courtesy of the Norwegian Fjord Horse Association and Anne Karns Crandall.
Figure 2–15. Susan Lustig McPeek.
Figure 2–19. Patty Lambert.
Figure 2–20. Susan Lustig McPeek.
Figure 2–26. Laurel Taylor.
Figure 2–27. Monica Thors.
Figure 2–28. Barbara Ann Giove.

Figure 2–29. Courtesy of Dave and Theresa Jones.
Figure 2–30. Carol Simons.
Figure 2–33. Barbara Ann Giove.
Figure 2–36. Peri Hughes.
Figure 2–37. Barbara Livingston.
Figure 2–39. Laurel Taylor.
Figure 2–40. Tish Quirk.
Figure 2–49. Genie Stewart-Spears.
Figure 2–53. Barbara Ann Giove.
Figure 3–1. Courtesy of Pin Oak Stud. Photo by Tony Leonard.
Figure 3–2. Susan Lustig McPeek.
Figure 3–5. Tish Quirk.
Figure 3–6. Nancy O. Bold Fletcher.
Figure 3–12. Mark Wyville.
Figure 3–16. Genie Stewart-Spears.
Figure 4–1. Tish Quirk.
Figure 4–6. Woods' Photography.
Figure 4–9. Don Trout.
Figure 5–1. Don Trout.
Figure 5–8. Don Trout.
Figure 6–1. Joseph V. DiOrio.
Figure 6–4. Barbara Livingston.
Figure 6–8. Tish Quirk.
Figure 6–9. Courtesy of Dave and Theresa Jones.
Figure 6–11. Amy Toner.
Figure 6–26. Courtesy of Dave and Theresa Jones.
Figure 6–27. Courtesy of Dave and Theresa Jones.
Figure 6–34. Barbara Ann Giove.
Figure 6–37. Tish Quirk.
Figure 6–38. Barbara Ann Giove.
Figure 6–40. Courtesy of Dave and Theresa Jones.
Figure 6–42. Susan Lustig McPeek.
Figure 6–45. Courtesy of *Quarter Racing Journal*. Photo by Scott Martinez.
Figure 6–47. Joseph V. DiOrio.
Figure 6–48. Joseph V. DiOrio.
Figure 6–49. Patty Lambert.
Figure 6–52. Genie Stewart-Spears.
Figure 6–66. Al Brodsky.
Figure 6–79. Nancy O. Bold Fletcher.
Figure 7–1. Barbara Livingston.
Figure 7–2. Don Trout.
Figure 7–3. Susan Lustig McPeek.
Figure 7–4. Courtesy of Arabian Horse Trust. Photo by Jerry Sparagowski.
Figure 7–5. Don Trout.
Figure 7–11. Courtesy of Dave and Theresa Jones.
Figure 7–14. Don Trout.
Figure 7–15. Peri Hughes.
Figure 7–16. Susan Lustig McPeek.
Figure 7–35. Monica Thors.
Figure 8–1. Carol Simons.
Figure 8–3. Susan Lustig McPeek.
Figure 8–4. Susan Lustig McPeek.
Figure 8–5. Maureen Gallatin.

Figure 8–14. Courtesy of Dave and Theresa Jones.
Figure 8–25. Monica Thors.
Figure 8–31. Babs Bashore.
Figure 8–32. Babs Bashore.
Figure 8–34. Courtesy of Dave and Theresa Jones.
Figure 8–35. Maureen Gallatin.
Figure 8–37. Courtesy of Cliff Honnas, DVM, Texas A&M University.
Figure 8–39. Courtesy of Overbrook Farm. Photo by Tony Leonard.
Figure 8–43. Barbara Ann Giove.
Figure 8–48. Don Trout.
Figure 8–50. Don Trout.
Figure 8–65. Genie Stewart-Spears.
Figure 8–77. Genie Stewart-Spears.
Figure 8–78. Carolyn Carnes.
Figure 9–1. Tish Quirk.
Figure 9–3. Courtesy of Dave and Theresa Jones.
Figure 9–4. Courtesy of Dave and Theresa Jones.
Figure 9–10. Courtesy of Dave and Theresa Jones.
Figure 9–13. Courtesy of Dave and Theresa Jones.
Figure 9–19. Courtesy of Dave and Theresa Jones.
Figure 9–21. Courtesy of Dave and Theresa Jones.
Figure 9–25. Courtesy of Dave and Theresa Jones.
Figure 9–26. Courtesy of Dave and Theresa Jones.
Figure 9–30. Tish Quirk.
Figure 9–43. Genie Stewart-Spears.
Figure 9–48. Genie Stewart-Spears.
Figure 10–1. Peri Hughes.
Figure 10–2. Courtesy of Vinery Kentucky. Photo by Tony Leonard.
Figure 10–3. Courtesy of McReynolds Farm.
Figure 10–4. Al Brodsky.
Figure 10–5. Courtesy of the American White and American Creme Horse Registry.
Figure 10–6. Courtesy of Canadale Dales Pony Stud.
Figure 10–7. Tish Quirk.
Figure 10–8. Carolyn Carnes.
Figure 10–12. Courtesy of the International Colored Appaloosa Association. Photo by Mark Linton.
Figure 10–15. Courtesy of the American Paint Horse Association.
Figure 10–16. Courtesy of the American Paint Horse Association.
Figure 10–18. Courtesy of the Palomino Horse Association. Photo by John Schively.
Figure 10–19. Courtesy of Nancy Stolz Petterson and Airlie Farm.
Figure 10–20B. Barbara Ann Giove. Courtesy of the Red Barn.
Figure 10–21A. Carolyn Carnes.
Figure 10–21B. Laurel Taylor.
Figure 10–21C. Woods' Photography.
Figure 10–21D. Susan Lustig McPeek.
Figure 10–21E. Babs Bashore.
Figure 10–21F. Babs Bashore.
Figure 10–22B. Susan Lustig McPeek.
Figure 10–22C. Courtesy of the Palomino Horse Association. Photo by John Schively.
Figure 10–22D. Susan Lustig McPeek.
Figure 10–22E. Susan Lustig McPeek.
Figure 10–23C. Sheri Cook.

Figure 11–1. Don Trout.
Figure 11–2. Courtesy of the International Arabian Horse Association.
Figure 11–3. Joseph V. DiOrio.
Figure 11–4. Don Trout.
Figure 11–5. Courtesy of the United States Trotting Association. Photo by Ed Keys.
Figure 11–6. Courtesy of the American Morgan Horse Association. Photo by Waltenberry.
Figure 11–7. Sheri Cook.
Figure 11–8. Courtesy of the Lipizzan Association of North America.
Figure 11–9. Courtesy of the Appaloosa Horse Club. Photo by Debby Chesna.
Figure 11–10. Amy Toner.
Figure 11–11. Courtesy of the International Buckskin Horse Association.
Figure 11–12. Courtesy of Ward Quarter Horses. Photo by Robyn Ward.
Figure 11–13. Courtesy of the American Saddlebred Horse Association. Photo by Jamie Donaldson.
Figure 11–14. Courtesy of the Tennessee Walking Horse Breeders' and Exhibitors' Association. Photo by Stuart Vesty.
Figure 11–15. Courtesy of LTO Farms, Mark A. Landers, and Everett Clamp.
Figure 11–16. Courtesy of the Paso Fino Horse Association. Photo by Darlene Wohlart.
Figure 11–17. Courtesy of Oak Hill Ranch.
Figure 11–18. Courtesy of the American Warmblood and Sporthorse Guild.
Figure 11–19. Courtesy of Hilltop Farm, Inc. Photo by Micki Dobson.
Figure 11–20. Courtesy of the Oldenburg Registry of North America.
Figure 11–21. Courtesy of the Swedish Warmblood Association and Los Alamos Dressage Center.
Figure 11–22. Courtesy of the American Trakhener Association. Photo by Pat Goodman.
Figure 11–23. Courtesy of Hilltop Farm, Inc. Photo by Micki Dobson.
Figure 11–24. Courtesy of Mulberry Lane Farms.
Figure 11–25. Sheri Cook.
Figure 11–26. Courtesy of the Percheron Horse Association of America. Photo by Brian K. Richman.
Figure 11–27. Courtesy of the American Shire Horse Association. Photo by Sharon McLin.
Figure 11–28. Courtesy of the Clydesdale Breeders of the United States. Photo by Brian K. Richman.
Figure 11–29. Courtesy of the American Suffolk Horse Association.
Figure 11–30. Courtesy of the National Chincoteague Pony Association. Photo by Gale P. Frederick.
Figure 11–31. Courtesy of the American Dartmoor Pony Association and Coopermill Pony Farm. Photo by Chris Lucas.
Figure 11–32. Courtesy of Marlyn Exmoors. Photo by Ann Holmes MRCVS.
Figure 11–33. Courtesy of New Farm.
Figure 11–34. Courtesy of the Norwegian Fjord Horse Association and Anne Karnes Crandall.
Figure 11–35. Courtesy of the Galiceno Horse Breeders Association and Linda Kelley.
Figure 11–36. Courtesy of the Swedish Gotland Association and Kokovoko Breeding Farm.
Figure 11–37. Courtesy of the American Hackney Horse Society.
Figure 11–38. Courtesy of the New Forest Pony Association.
Figure 11–39. Courtesy of the Pony of the Americas Club, Inc. Photo by Jeff Kirkbride.
Figure 11–41. Courtesy of Smoke Tree and Kathy Reese. Photo by Arthur Thomson.
Figure 11–42. Courtesy of Smoke Tree and Kathy Reese. Photo by Arthur Thomson.
Figure 11–43. Amy Toner.
Figure 12–1. Doug Prather.
Figure 12–2. Courtesy of the International Buckskin Horse Association.
Figure 12–3. Joseph V. DiOrio.

GLOSSARY

abdomen Area between the diaphragm and pelvis; belly.

abdominal Pertaining to the abdomen.

abduction Moving a part away from the midline of the body.

abscess Localized collection of pus in a cavity formed by tissue breakdown.

acetabulum Socket in the lower side of the os coxae; forms the hip joint with the head of the femur.

Achilles tendon Gastrocnemius and soleus tendons that run down the back of the gaskin and attach onto the point of the hock; part of the common calcaneal tendon.

acquired Develops after birth as a result of injury, malnutrition, or diease.

action Style and height of the horse's legs during locomotion.

adduction Moving a part toward the midline of the body.

adrenal gland Pair of glands located near the kidneys that produce, among other hormones, adrenaline.

adrenaline Stress hormone produced by the adrenal glands.

albino Congenital lack of pigmentation in the skin, hair, or eyes.

alveoli Tiny air saccules in the lungs where gas exchange takes place.

amble Four-beat gait resembling the pace but without suspension.

ampulla Bell-shaped enlargement at one end of a tubular structure.

anatomy Science of the form and structure of a living organism.

anesthetic Drug that eliminates sensation, especially pain.

annular ligament Ligament that wraps around a structure, e.g. the back of the fetlock and knee.

antebrachial Pertaining to the forearm.

anterior Directional term meaning toward the front.

antibodies Immune system products designed to respond to a specific threat.

anus Exterior opening of the rectum.

apex Tip; narrow end.

aponeurosis Broad, flat tendon.

Appaloosa Breed of horses characterized by varying patterns of spots on a white coat.

apron face White face marking that covers the forehead to the muzzle and includes the upper and lower lips.

arch Convex or bowed structure, as of the top of a vertebra below the dorsal spinous process.

arterial Pertaining to an artery.

arteriole Tiny branch of an artery.

artery Vessel through which oxygen-enriched blood passes from the heart toward the body tissues.

arthritis Inflammation of a joint; generally reserved for severe joint disease.

articular Pertaining to a joint.

articular cartilage Thin layer of cartilage on the bone surfaces within a joint; joint cartilage.

articulation See joint.

asternal Not joined to the sternum.

atlas First cervical vertebra.

atrium One of two upper chambers of the heart that receives blood and passes it on to the corresponding ventricle.

atrophy Wasting away of tissue.

auditory Pertaining to the ear or sense of hearing.

auricle Projecting, external part of the ear; pinna.

autonomic nervous system Involuntary control system for heartrate, blood vessels, body temperature, digestive functions, and respiration; division of the peripheral nervous system.

axillary Pertaining to the armpit.

axis Second cervical vertebra.

back Topline area between the withers and the point of the croup.

bacterial fermentation Process by which bacteria in the cecum convert carbohydrates to volatile fatty acids, producing energy.

balance Good conformation where each part of the horse is proportional to all the others.

bald face White face marking that covers the forehead, eyes, nostrils, and upper lip.

ball and socket joint Joint where the rounded end of one bone fits into the cup-shaped end of another.

barrel Thorax and abdomen.

barrel racing Timed rodeo competition where the horse and rider circle three barrels in a cloverleaf pattern.

bars Structures on the bottom of the foot on each side of the frog; formed by the hoof wall as it turns forward and inward at the heels.

base narrow Conformational fault where the distance between the forearms or gaskins is greater than the distance between the feet.

base wide Conformational fault where the distance between the forearms or gaskins is smaller than the distance between the feet.

bench knee Conformational fault where the cannon bone is offset to the outside of the knee; offset knees.

bicipital Pertaining to a biceps muscle, which has two heads.

bile Clear yellow or orange fluid produced by the liver that aids digestion.

birth canal Structures of the mare's reproductive tract through which the foal passes during delivery.

bladder See urinary bladder.

blood vessel Hollow tubes, i.e. arteries and veins, that carry blood.

bloodstream Blood coursing the circulatory system as a whole.

body 1) Trunk of the horse, containing the internal organs and excluding the head, neck, and legs. 2) Largest and most essential part of a structure.

bog spavin Fluid-filled swelling low and inside on the hock.

bone Hard, rigid structures making up most of the skeleton.

bone chip See chip.

bone density See bone mineral content.

bone marrow Jelly-like substance in the center of the long bones; produces red blood cells and some white blood cells.

bone mineral content Amount of mineral deposited in the bone.

bone spavin Osteoarthritis in the lower hock joints; causes bone spurs and narrowing of the affected joint space(s).

bow legs Conformational fault where the knees or hocks deviate away from each other.

bowed tendon Fiber damage and inflammation in one of the flexor tendons; the swelling gives it a bowed-out appearance.

brachial Pertaining to the arm.

brainstem See medulla oblongata.

breakover Act of rolling the hoof forward—lifting the foot from the ground heel first, as the horse moves ahead.

breast See chest.

breastbone See sternum.

broad ligament Ligament that runs from the roof of the abdominal cavity to the ovaries and uterus, suspending it within the abdomen.

bronchi Any of the large air passages, especially the two main branches of the trachea conducting air to each lung.

bronchioles Progressively smaller airways within the lungs into which the bronchi divide.

bucked knees Conformational fault where the knee arcs forward; sprung knees, over at the knee.

bucked shins Pain and new bone production at the front of the cannon bones on the forelegs of young racehorses; shin soreness.

buckskin Coat color where the body is yellow-brown and the points are dark, with a dorsal stripe; shoulder stripe and zebra stripes on the withers and lower legs may occur.

bull head Conformational feature where the horse's forehead bulges outward.

bulldog mouth When the bottom teeth jut out beyond the top teeth; undershot jaw, underbite.

bursa Small sac of fluid between a bone and a tendon or ligament; minimizes friction and pressure between the two structures. Plural = bursae.

calcaneus Large bone at the back of the hock, part of which projects upward and backward to form the point of the hock (tuber calcis).

calcification; calcified Replacement of cartilage or soft tissue with mineral deposits, mostly calcium.

calcium Dietary mineral essential for strong bones and normal muscle function.

calf knee Conformational fault where the knee bends back slightly when viewed from the side; back at the knee.

camped out behind Conformational fault where the hindlegs are angled too far out behind the body.

camped out in front Conformational fault where the forelegs are too far out in front of the body.

camped under behind Conformational fault where the hindlegs angle too far underneath the body.

camped under in front Conformational fault where the forelegs angle too far underneath the body.

cancellous bone Lattice-like, softer bone beneath the dense, outer cortex; spongy bone.

canine teeth Four small pointed teeth located between the incisors and premolars; tush.

cannon Area between the knee or hock and fetlock.

cannon bone Underlying bone of the cannon; large metacarpal/metatarsal, third metacarpal/metatarsal.

capillary Smallest of the blood vessels—thin layers of endothelial cells through which may pass water, nutrients, dissolved gases, and wastes.

capped elbow Inflammation and swelling of the bursa over the point of the elbow; shoe boil.

capped hock Inflammation and swelling of the bursa over the point of the hock.

carotid artery One of two major arteries on each side of the neck, conducting blood to the brain.

carpal Pertaining to the knee.

carpal canal Channel behind the knee that provides passage for the lateral digital extensor muscle and its synovial sheath.

carpometacarpal joint Immobile lower knee joint, between the lower row of carpal bones and the top of the cannon and splint bones.

carpus Knee joint; wrist in humans.

cartilage Special type of firm, non-bony connective tissue; sometimes a precursor to bone.

cartilaginous Made of, or resembling cartilage.

caruncle Small fleshy eminence, e.g. at the inner corner of the eye.

caudal Directional term meaning toward the horse's hind end.

cellulose Carbohydrate forming the skeleton of most plants.

cement Bone-like layer covering a tooth.

center of gravity Point of perfect balance in the body around which the mass of the body is centered.

central nervous system Brain and spinal cord.

cephalic Pertaining to the head.

cerebellum Smaller, posterior part of the brain, controlling muscle coordination and balance.

cerebrum Larger, anterior part of the brain, controlling intelligence, memory, emotion, and the senses.

cervical Pertaining to the neck, or to the neck of any organ or structure, such as the cervix of the uterus.

cervix Neck; usually the muscular, neck-like structure that separates the vagina from the uterus.

check ligament Ligament that connects a bone to a tendon and limits the tendon's action; accessory ligament.

cheek teeth Premolars and molars located in the cheek area of the mouth.

chest Front of the horse from the base of the neck to the tops of the forelegs; breast.

chestnut 1) Small mass of horn on the inside of the forearm just above the knee. 2) Coat color where the body is any shade of red or brown and the points echo the body color; sorrel.

chip Small piece of bone or cartilage that has been chipped off the main bone.

chronic Long-term or recurring over a long time.

chyme Semi-digested food.

cilia Hair-like processes extending from a cell surface that move rhythmically to transport mucus over a surface.

circulatory system Heart, blood, blood vessels, and their controlling mechanisms, responsible for the movement of blood and lymph.

circumduction Circular movement of a leg.

club foot Abnormal foot shape in which the heels grow very long, and the front of the hoof wall is nearly vertical.

coarseness Lacking quality or refinement; thick.

cob Type of heavy, muscular horse or pony with a short neck, round barrel, short coupling, and short legs, usually not more than 15.3 hands.

coccygeal Pertaining to the tail.

cochlea Shell-like tube of the inner ear that is the primary organ of hearing.

coffin bone Largest bone within the foot between the short pastern bone and sole; third phalanx, pedal bone.

coffin joint Joint between the short pastern bone, navicular bone, and coffin bone in the foot.

coldblood Heavy horses with even dispositions, without Arabian blood, usually from Northern Europe.

collagen Microscopic fibers that give tissues, such as skin, tendons, ligaments, and joint cartilage their strength and resilience.

collateral ligaments Short, strong ligaments on either side of a joint that help support it.

collection Trained posture involving lightening the forehand, elevating the back, and engaging the hindquarters; self-carriage.

color breed Breed of horse based primarily on coat color and markings.

combined driving Driving competition accomplished in four phases: presentation, dressage, marathon, and obstacle.

common calcaneal tendon Aggregate tendons of the superficial digital flexor, biceps femoris, semitendinosus, and Achilles tendon.

competitive trail Long distance race of 25 – 100 miles, over varying terrain and weather; the horse in the best condition at the end of the race wins.

concave profile Conformational feature where the horse's face curves slightly inward; dished face.

concussion Violent jar; compression stresses caused by impact.

condyle Rounded portion of bone at a joint surface; knuckle.

conformation Alignment of the parts of the horse's body.

congenital Present at birth; may be hereditary or caused by conditions during pregnancy.

connective tissue Supportive fibers containing collagen that form fascia, tendons, and ligaments.

contracted heels Condition where the heels are narrowed, with the bars nearly parallel and the frog unnaturally small.

convex profile Conformational feature where the horse's face arches slightly outward; Roman nose.

corium Specialized vascular tissue lining the inside of the hoof; produces horn.

cornea Transparent, colorless, exposed front part of the eye.

coronary Encircling like a crown, as applied to blood vessels, ligaments, or nerves; the coronary corium encircles the hoof.

coronary corium Cells beneath the coronet that produce the horn tubules making up the hoof wall, and also insensitive laminae.

coronet 1) Area of the leg where the hair stops and the hoof wall begins. 2) White leg marking consisting of a small strip around the coronet area.

coronoid process Upper extension of the mandible that projects into the temporal fossa of the skull.

costal Pertaining to the ribs.

coupling Muscularity and length of the loin, where the hindquarter muscles connect to the spinal column.

cow hocks Conformational fault where the hocks angle in and the feet angle out when viewed from the rear.

cow sense Inherent ability of a stock horse to predict a cow's movements and react accordingly.

cranial Pertaining to the cranium; also directional term meaning toward the horse's head.

cranial nerve Nerve that leaves the base of the brain and supplies structures in the head and neck.

cranium Collectively, the bones that enclose the brain and form part of the cavities for the eyes and nasal passages.

crest Uppermost part of the neck; larger in the stallion.

cribbing Noisy stable vice in which the horse grasps the fence or other object with the incisor teeth, arches the neck, and swallows air.

croup Topline from the loins to the tail base.

crown Top of a tooth.

cruciate Criss-crossing.

crural Pertaining to a leg.

cuboidal bones Block-shaped bones in the knee and hock.

cup Pits in the center of the teeth that blacken with feed, but smooth out with age.

curb Inflammation and thickening of the plantar tarsal ligament.

cutaneous Pertaining to the skin.

cutting Rodeo competition in which a horse and rider team separate one cow from a herd and prevent it from returning within a sepcified time period.

dam Female parent.

deep Directional term meaning away from the surface; more internal.

defecation Passing manure; bowel movement.

degenerative joint disease Chronic joint disease involving cartilage damage and joint capsule thickening; DJD, arthritis.

dens Odontoid process of the axis; hooks under the atlas.

dental star End of the pulp cavity in a tooth, covered with secondary dentine.

dentine Inner, hard layer of a tooth that surrounds the pulp cavity and consitutes much of the tooth's bulk.

depressor Muscle that pulls a body part downward.

diaphragm Thin, dome-shaped sheet of muscle that separates the thorax and abdomen; when it contracts air is drawn into the lungs.

digestion Process of breaking down food into useful nutrients and absorbing them into the blood.

digestive system Organs responsible for the ingestion, processing, and expulsion of food, as nutrients are absorbed.

digit Fetlock, pastern, and coffin joints.

digital Pertaining to the digit.

digital cushion Dense, spongy tissue in the back half of the foot, between the frog and the deeper structures.

distal Directional term meaning away from the body; part furthest from the body.

distal sesamoid bone See navicular bone.

dock Top part of the tail that contains the coccygeal vertebrae.

dorsal Directional term meaning the upper surface; toward the top.

dorsal spinous processes Ridges of bone projecting upward from the tops of the vertebrae.

dorsal stripe Dark stripe that runs along the spine from mane to tail head.

double-rumped Conformational characteristic where the horse has a groove down the spine.

draft horse Heavy horse used for pulling vehicles.

dressage Popularly, schooling horse and rider to be in harmony where the horse willingly and without apparant aid performs a set pattern of movements at certain locations within the arena.

dropped sole Sole that bulges toward the ground surface, instead of being slightly concave or level.

duct Tubular passage that conveys fluids.

ductus deferens Excretory duct of the testicle, passing from the testicle to the ejaculatory duct; vas deferens.

dun Coat color where the body is dark yellow-brown and the points are dark.

eardrum Thin membrane stretched across the ear canal between the external ear and the middle ear.

elbow 1) Joint between the lower end of the humerus and the upper ends of the radius and ulna.   2) Area of the foreleg between the upper arm and forearm.

enamel White, porcelain-like covering of a tooth crown.

endurance race Long distance race of 25 – 100 miles over varying terrain and weather; the first horse in good condition to cross the finish line wins.

engagement Pulling the hindquarters under the body for self carriage, sudden turns, or quick stops.

enzyme Protein that accelerates specific chemical reactions but does not change during the reaction.

epididymis U-shaped tube for storing and transporting sperm, attached lengthwise to each testicle and having a head, body, and tail.

epiglottis Small cartilage at the entrance to the larynx that prevents food from entering the larynx and trachea while swallowing.

epithelium Layer of cells covering the external or internal body surfaces; e.g. skin.

equids Members of the family Equidae, including horses, donkeys, and zebras.

erectile tissue Tissue containing vascular spaces that become engorged with blood.

ergot Small mass of horn under the bottom curve of the fetlock.

esophagus Muscular tube extending from the pharynx to the stomach.

estrous cycle Female reproductive cycle; heat cycle.

eustachian tube Tube between the middle ear and pharynx; serves to equalize air pressure on both sides of the eardrum.

eventing Competition consisting of three phases: dressage, show jumping, and endurance; performed over one, two, or three days.

excretion Eliminating the body's waste materials.

extension Opening the angle of the joint by pulling the bones on either side away from each other; straightening.

extensor muscle Muscle that straightens a joint.

extensor process Bony protrusion at the top of the coffin bone.

extracellular Between the cells.

facial crest Ridge of bone on the face from the orbit to about the cheek teeth.

Fallopian tube See oviduct.

false rib Asternal rib that does not connect directly to the sterum.

farrier Professional who trims horses' feet and fits them with horseshoes; horseshoer, blacksmith.

fascia Sheets or bands of strong, fibrous, connective tissue located between muscles or beneath the skin.

fatty acids Key components of fat and an important muscle fuel.

feathering Long hair on the back of the fetlocks of coldbloods.

femoral Pertaining to the femur of the thigh.

femoral head Rounded top of the femur that fits into the acetabulum to form the hip joint.

femur Underlying bone of the thigh, between the hip and stifle.

fetlock 1) Joint between the cannon bone and long pastern bone. 2) Area between the cannon and pastern.

fetus Unborn foal.

fever rings Hoof rings caused by severe stress or illness, especially when it includes a fever.

fibrocartilage Cartilage made of thick collagen bundles and cartilage cells.

fibrous Containing fibers: fibrous tissue is scar tissue.

fibula Small bone attached to the top and outside of the tibia.

flank Area of the abdomen below the loin and between the ribs and hip.

flat-footed Feet with soles that are flat or dropped, instead of curving away from the ground surface.

flehmen Body position in which the head and neck are outstretched and the upper lip curled upward.

flexion Closing the angle of the joint by bringing the bones on either side toward each other; bending.

flexor muscle Muscle that causes joint flexion when it contracts.

float File the teeth with a rasp to remove sharp ridges.

floating ribs Last one or two asternal ribs that do not join the other asternal ribs via the costal arch.

foaling paralysis Temporary hindleg paralysis experienced by mares when the foal puts pressure on the obturator nerve during delivery.

follicle Small sac or cavity, such as in the ovary from which an ovum is released.

foot flight Path the foot travels during a step.

foramen Opening or passageway, usually through a bone.

forearm Area of the foreleg between the elbow and knee.

forehand Head, neck, shoulders, and forelegs.

forelock Part of the mane that falls onto the forehead.

fossa Depression or hollow on a bone. Plural = fossae.

founder See laminitis.

founder rings Hoof rings caused by laminitis or other foot inflammation.

four beat gait Gait where at least one foot is always on the ground.

fox trot Slow four-beat gait wherein the horse walks with the front feet and trots with the hind feet, and the hind feet slide into place.

frog V-shaped cushion of soft keratinized tissue between the bars of the foot.

frog corium Layer of cells above the frog that produces the horn of the frog.

gait Manner of locomotion; movement of the feet and legs in a certain rhythm or pattern.

gaited horse Horse or breed of horses that perform a gait other than the walk, trot, or canter.

Galvayne's groove Furrow that appears in the upper corner incisors at about age 10, and disappears by age 30.

gaskin Area of the hindleg between the stifle and hock.

gastric Pertaining to the stomach.

genetic Inherited; a trait passed down from parent to offspring.

girth Area encircling the thorax just behind the elbow, where the girth of a saddle runs; heartgirth.

gland Organ that secretes materials not needed for its own processes.

glans Small, round mass or glandlike structure; specifically, the cap-shaped expansion at the end of the penis.

glass eye Eye that lacks any pigmentation in the iris and appears white.

gluteal Pertaining to the buttocks.

good bone When measuring the circumference of the cannon bone, at least 7 inches of bone per 1,000 pounds of body weight.

goose-rumped Conformational fault where the point of the buttock is too low and the croup is angled severely.

greater trochanter of the femur Prominence rising above the head of the femur.

greater tuberosity of the humerus Knob on the front of the humerus that forms the point of the shoulder.

groin Area where the abdomen meets the thigh.

growth cartilage Specialized cartilage at the ends of the long bones that changes into bone.

grulla Color coat where the body is slate, smoky blue, or mousy with dark points; dorsal stripe, shoulder stripe, and zebra markings on the withers and lower legs may occur.

gutteral pouch Air-filled blind sac, accessory to the eustacian tube, located on each side of the head above the pharynx.

gymkhana Competition of mounted games for children designed to improve riding skills.

hamstrings Biceps femoris, semitendinosus, and semimembranosus muscles.

hand Unit of measure of the horse's height; one hand is equal to four inches.

hard palate Roof of the mouth; supported by bone.

harness racing Race where a trotter or pacer is driven by a driver in a sulky.

head of the femur Ball-shaped knob on the top end of the femur; inserts into the acetabulum to form the hip joint.

header 1) Person who ropes the calf's horns during a team roping competition. 2) Horse on which that person is mounted.

heart Hollow muscular organ in the center of the thorax that forces blood through the blood vessels by contracting rhythmically.

heart rate Number of times the heart beats in one minute.

heartgirth Area encircling the thorax just behind the elbow, where the girth of a saddle runs; girth area.

heavy hunter Hunter that has many physical characteristics of a draft horse.

heel bulbs Two round sections of the heel above the coronet.

heeler 1) Person who ropes the calf's hind feet during a team roping competition. 2) Horse on which that person is mounted.

hernia Abnormal protrusion of part of organ through the structures normally containing it.

high hocks Conformational characteristic where the hocks are higher than halfway between the stifle and the ground.

high white rule Rule of some breed registries (such as AQHA) eliminating any horse whose white leg markings extend above the knee or hock.

hindquarters Upper part of the hindleg, including the croup, pelvis, and thigh.

hinge joint Joint that is only capable of flexion and extension.

hip joint Joint between the os coxae and femur.

hock Area or joint between the gaskin and cannon of the hindleg.

hoof crack Narrow, vertical or horizontal fault in the hoof wall.

hoof rings Horizontal disfigurement in the hoof wall extending the entire circumference of the foot.

hoof wall Visible, horny outer covering of the horse's foot.

hoof wall angle Angle of the front of the hoof wall in relation to the ground.

hoof wall–coffin bone bond Tight connection between the sensitive and insensitive laminae, which holds the hoof wall and coffin bone together.

hoof-pastern angle Relationship between the hoof wall angle and pastern angle.

hormone Chemical produced in the body by a gland or organ that travels in the blood or lymphatic system to a distant specific organ, to regulate its activity.

horn Hard substance of which the hoof wall and sole are made; mostly consists of hair-like tubules of keratin.

horn tubules Hollow tubes made of keratin that together make up the hoof wall.

hotblood Spirited, high-strung horse, usually of Arabian or Thoroughbred decent.

humerus Upper arm bone between the scapula and radius/ulna.

hunter 1) Horse that carries a rider on a hunt: chasing a stag, hare, fox, or drag line behind a pack of hounds. 2) Show horse participating in hunt classes, judged on attitude, conformation, and performance on an artificial hunt course.

hyoid bone Set of bones that attach the larynx to the base of the skull.

hyperextension Extension of a leg far beyond the norm, except in the fetlock where it is normal.

hyperflexion Flexion of a leg far beyond the norm.

ilium Cranial part of the os coxae (pelvic bone; hip bone); hook bone.

immune system Organs responsible for defending the body against invading microorganisms; major components are white blood cells and antibodies.

impaction colic Abdominal pain due to a blockage in the intestines.

impulsion Energy and drive of the horse in motion, powered by the hindquarters.

incisor teeth Set of twelve front teeth of the horse used for cutting.

infraspinatus Beneath (caudal to) the scapular spine.

inguinal ligament Caudal part of the aponeurosis of the external abdominal oblique muscle, connecting the prepubic tendon to the os coxae.

insensitive laminae Tiny corrugations on the inside of the hoof wall.

insertion Point where a muscle ends.

insulin Chemical produced by the pancreas that moves blood glucose (a sugar) into muscle cells to be stored as glycogen; regulates sugar and fat metabolism.

intercarpal Between the bones of the knee.

intercostal Between the ribs.

interference Hitting one leg with the hoof of the opposite leg or the leg in front.

interosseous ligament Connective tissue between bones, as between the splint bones and cannon bones.

intersesamoidean Between the sesamoid bones.

intervertebral Between the vertebrae.

intestinal Pertaining to the large and small intestines.

intra-articular Within a joint.

iris Round, colored membrane behind the cornea of the eye; contains layers of muscle fibers that dilate or contract the pupil.

ischium Caudal, dorsal part of the os coxae; pin bone.

joint Union between two or more bones; articulation.

joint capsule Fibrous enclosure around the ends of the bones in a joint. Lined with the synovium.

joint fluid See synovial fluid.

jowl Part of the head that lies within the branches (rami) of the mandible.

jugular groove Groove on each side of the neck beneath which the jugular vein is located; jugular furrow.

jugular vein One of the two major veins on each side of the neck, returning blood to the heart.

keratin Dense protein that makes up the horn of the hoof wall, the outer layer of the skin, and hair.

kidneys Paired organs in the upper abdomen that filter the blood, extracting fluid wastes from the body and producing urine.

knee 1) Joint between the radius and cannon bone; carpus. 2) Area between the forearm and cannon in the foreleg.

knock knees Conformational fault where the legs deviate outward from the knees down; in at the knees.

labia External vulval lips on either side of the vaginal opening.

lacrimal Pertaining to tears.

laminae Layers or folds of tissue; e.g. the tiny corrugations on the inside of the hoof wall.

laminar corium Layer of cells between the surface of the coffin bone and the hoof wall that produce the sensitive laminae.

laminitis Painful foot condition in which the blood supply to the hoof wall is interrupted, and the hoof wall–coffin bone bond breaks down; founder.

larynx Structure composed of nine cartilages located between the pharynx and trachea; voice box.

lateral Directional term meaning on the outside.

lateral cartilages Firm pieces of cartilage protruding up and back from the wings of the coffin bone.

lateral gait Gait where both right feet move, followed by both left feet.

levator Muscle that pulls a body part upward.

ligament Band of strong, fibrous tissue that connects bones and cartilage, and supports joints.

light horse Lean-legged athletic breeds built for speed and agility; not pony or draft types.

liver Largest gland in the body responsible for manufacturing and secreting bile, and processing and storing digested nutrients.

loaded shoulders Shoulders that are overly thick, either due to fat or muscling.

loin Area of the back between the last rib and hip.

long bone Long, thick bone shaped roughly like a cylinder, with a medullary cavity in the center; e.g. ribs, humerus, femur, radius, tibia, and cannon bones.

long pastern bone Larger of the two bones of the pastern between the cannon bone and short pastern bone; first phalanx, first pastern bone.

long toe–low heel Abnormal foot shape in which the heels are low and the hoof wall grows longer at the toe; the hoof wall angle is lower than normal.

low-set hocks Conformational characteristic where the hocks are lower than halfway from the stifle to the ground.

lumbar Pertaining to the loins.

lumbodorsal fascia Sheet of strong tissue draped over the horse's back and loins.

lumbosacral joint Junction between the last lumbar vertebra and the sacrum.

lumbosacral plexus Last five lumbar spinal nerves and the sacral spinal nerves; supplies the hindleg with sensation and motion.

lungs Large, paired, sack-like respiratory organs located in the thorax on either side of the heart.

lymph node Masses scattered throughout the body that filter foreign bodies from lymph fluid and produce immune system cells.

lymphatic system System complementary to the circulatory system that collects lymph from the tissues and returns it to the general circulation.

mandible Jawbone, consisting of a body and ramus on each side.

mandibular Pertaining to the jaw, located near the jaw.

manubrium Uppermost tip of the sternum.

mealy Coat color resembling meal; a light yellow-tan color.

medial Directional term meaning on the inner side.

median Located in the middle of a structure or body.

medulla oblongata Base of the brain; responsible for awareness or consciousness and involuntary actions of the heartbeat and respiration; brainstem.

medullary cavity Relatively hollow center of the long bones; called the bone marrow cavity because it contains bone marrow.

membrane Thin layer of tissue that covers a surface, lines a cavity, or divides a space or organ.

meniscus Thick, C-shaped cartilage within the stifle joint, between the femur and tibia; plural = menisci.

mesentery Wide sheet of tissue that supports an organ, such as that which supports the small intestine.

metacarpal bones/metatarsal bones Cannon and splint bones in the foreleg and hindleg, respectively.

metacarpal groove Furrow created by the cannon and splint bones.

midline Imaginary dividing line between the left and right sides of the body.

milk cistern Resevoirs in the udder that store the milk produced by the mammary glands.

milk teeth See temporary teeth.

minerals Elements that are required by the body; e.g. calcium, phosphorus, magnesium, and copper.

molars Twelve permanent teeth located in the cheek area behind the premolars; used for grinding.

motor nerve Nerve responsible for stimulating a muscle to contract, creating movement.

mottled Skin or coat that is speckled with small dark spots.

mucous membrane Pink membrane that lines the mouth, nasal passages, eyelids, vulva, etc.

mucus Clear, viscous, liquid secretion of the mucous membranes.

muscle Elastic organ that contracts and relaxes to create movement.

musculocutaneous Pertaining to muscle and skin.

musculoskeletal system Bones, cartilage, joints, muscles, tendons, and ligaments of the spinal column and legs.

mutton withered Conformational fault where the withers are too low and flat.

nasal Pertaining to the nose.

nasal passages Pathways in the head conducting outside air to the throat.

nasal septum Strip of cartilage separating the left and right nasal passages.

nasogastric tube Long tube that is passed through the nostril, down the esophagus, and into the stomach; stomach tube.

navicular bone Smallest bone in the foot at the back of the coffin joint.

navicular syndrome Degenerative condition of the navicular bone and/or supporting structures.

nerve Cord-like structure made of nerve fibers that convey impulses between the central nervous system and a body part.

nerve root Nerve bundle that emerges from the spinal canal; consists of several nerves that branch off to specific tissues.

nervous system Brain, spinal cord, and nerves; responsible for internal communication between the brain and body tissues.

nuchal crest Highest point of the occipital bone in the skull; forms the poll.

nuchal ligament Broad, thick ligament that runs from the poll to the withers, beneath the mane.

oblique At an angle.

obturator foramen Large opening in the os coxae between the pubis and ischium.

offset knee See bench knee.

olecranon Projecting part of the ulna forming the point of the elbow.

olfactory Pertaining to the sense of smell.

optic Pertaining to the eye.

oral Pertaining to the mouth.

orbit Round cavity in the skull where the eyeball lies.

organ Semi-independent part of the body that performs a special function(s).

orifice External opening of the body.

origin Point where a muscle begins.

os coxae Three pairs of fused bones forming the pelvis; hip bone.

osselets Arthritis and new bone formation at the fetlock joint.

ossify Change into bone through the addition of minerals.

ovarian Pertaining to the ovaries or activity of the ovaries.

ovary One of two glands in the mare that contain ova (eggs).

over-reaching Interference where the toe of the hind foot strikes the heel of the forefoot.

overdorsiflexion Bending toward the rear; fatigue allows the horse's fetlocks to droop, overdorsiflexing them, resulting in injury.

overextension Excessive extension, or straightening, of a joint.

overo Pinto coat pattern where the markings extend from under the belly, but rarely over the back; their edges are feathery and uneven.

oviduct One of two passageways from an ovary to the uterus and the site of fertilization of the ovum; Fallopian tube.

ovulation Release of an ovum from a mature follicle of the ovary.

ovum Female reproductive cell; egg.

oxygenation Saturate with oxygen.

pacer Harness racehorse that performs at the pace.

paddling Gait abnormality where the front foot travels outward during flight; common in horses that toe in.

Paint Breed of horse with pinto markings registerable by the American Paint Horse Association.

palmar Directional term meaning the area at the back of the foreleg, below the knee.

palomino Coat color and breed of horse where the body is golden and the mane and tail are light.

pancreas Organ located at the top of the abdomen in front of the kidneys that manufactures and secretes digestive enzymes and insulin.

papillae Small, nipple-shaped projection.

parotid Located near the ear.

parrot mouth Conformational fault in which the upper jaw is longer than the lower jaw; overshot jaw, overbite.

parti-colored Coat, mane, or tail with more than one color in distinctive areas.

paso Smooth, lateral, four-beat gait of varying speeds, resembling a broken pace: the hind foot lands just before the forefoot on the same side.

passage Dressage movement in which the horse trots slowly in extreme collection and with high action..

pastern 1) Area between the fetlock and coronet. 2) White leg marking extending from the coronet to just below the fetlock; half sock.

pastern joint Joint between the long and short pastern bones.

patella Small, pyramid-shaped bone located in the stifle joint; kneecap.

peak of the withers Highest point of the withers.

pectoral Pertaining to the chest.

pedal Pertaining to the foot.

pelvic cavity Basin-like area formed by the os coxae, pelvic ligaments, sacrum, and first few coccygeal vertebrae.

pelvic flexure Sharp, narrow turn of the large intestine located on the left side of the abdomen.

pelvic girdle See pelvic cavity.

pelvic limb Hindleg.

pelvis 1) Area enclosed by the os coxae, pelvic ligaments, sacrum, and first few coccygeal vertebrae. 2) Common term for the os coxae (hipbone).

penis Male organ of copulation.

periople Thin, cuticle-like layer of cells that covers the top part of the hoof wall, just below the coronet.

perioplic corium Layer of cells above the coronet that produce the periople.

periosteum Thin outer covering of a bone.

peripheral Directional term meaning at or near the outer edge.

peripheral nervous system Nerves outside the central nervous system that supply the tissues.

peristalsis Wormlike movement by which the digestive tract propels its contents.

peritoneum Membrane lining the abdominal cavity.

permanent teeth Adult teeth that are not shed except perhaps in old age.

pharynx Cavity connecting the nasal passages and mouth to the larynx and esophagus.

physis Area of specialized cartilage near the ends of the bones in young horses; called the growth plate because it is responsible for bone growth.

physitis Inflammation or abnormal cell activity in a physis; causes painful swelling.

piaffe Dressage movement in which the horse trots rhythmically in place.

piebald Coat color where a black horse has large, defined white patches.

pigeon-toed See toed-in.

pigmented skin Dark-colored skin; contains many pigment cells.

pinto Coat color and breed of horse where the entire body has large, assymetrical white and dark patches.

pirouette Dressage movement in which the horse turns 360 degrees on the inside hindleg.

plantar Directional term meaning the back of the hindleg, below the hock.

plexus Network of veins or nerves.

point of the buttock Bony point formed by the tuber ischii of the os coxae.

point of the croup Bony point formed by the tuber sacrale of the os coxae.

point of the elbow Bony point formed by the olecranon process of the ulna.

point of the hip Bony point formed by the tuber coxae of the os coxae.

point of the hock Bony point formed by the tuber calcis of the calcaneus.

point of the shoulder Bony point formed by the greater tuberosity of the humerus.

points 1) Bony prominences on the outside of the horse that indicate certain skeletal landmarks. 2) Mane, ear rims, tail, and lower legs.

poll Uppermost point of the head, between the ears.

polo Game played by two teams of four riders; goals are scored when a player hits the ball using the polo mallet through the .opposing team's goal posts.

polocrosse Mounted game of lacrosse; goals are scored when a rider scoops up a ball in a net and carries or throws it through the opposing team's goal posts.

pony Any horse shorter than 14.2 hands (58 inches) at the withers.

popped knee Inflamed and enlarged knee joint.

posterior Directional term meaning toward the rear.

premolar Twelve permanent teeth located in the cheek area in front of the molars; used for grinding.

prepubic tendon Tendon of insertion of the rectus abdominis muscle.

prepuce Fold of skin surrounding the penis; sheath.

process Projection of bone.

proximal Directional term meaning toward the body; part closest to the body.

proximal sesamoid bones See sesamoid bones.

Przewalski's horse Ancient breed of wild, dun-colored horses with dark manes, no forelock, and half tails, those being different characteristics of the horse and donkey; now exists only in captivity.

pubis Cranial, ventral bone of the os coxae.

pulse Rhythmic throbbing of a blood vessel that may be felt with the finger.

pupil Opening in the center of the iris that regulates the amount of light reaching the retina of the eye.

quarter Part of the hoof from the widest point back to the heels.

rack Fast, flashy, four-beat gait where each foot lands separately; single-foot.

radial Pertaining to the radius.

radius Major underlying bone of the forearm.

ramus Vertical extension of each half of the mandible; plural = rami.

reciprocal apparatus System of muscles and tendons that tie the stifle and hock together: the stifle cannot flex without also flexing the hock and vice versa.

red blood cells Blood cells that carry hemoglobin which transport oxygen.

reining Rodeo and Olympic competition where the horse is ridden on a loose rein in one of nine patterns at speed.

renal Pertaining to the kidney.

reproductive system Organs and glands responsible for reproduction.

respiratory rate Number of times the horse breathes in one minute.

respiratory system Organs responsible for the intake of air, exchanging oxygen for carbon dioxide, and exhaling air.

ribs Eighteen (usually) paired, curved bones extending from the thoracic vertebrae to the bottom of the barrel.

ringbone Bony growth in the pastern or coffin joints due to degenerative joint disease.

roach back Conformational fault where the back is hunched, or bowed up slightly with a concave arch along the topline.

road founder Laminitis caused by concussion on the feet due to hard surfaces.

roaring Collapse of the arytenoid cartilages in the larynx due to nerve damage and causes a "roaring" noise during inhalation; laryngeal hemiplegia.

rollback Turn of 180 degrees with the hind feet planted and the forehand elevated, then the horse gallops in the opposite direction; set and turn.

Roman nose See convex profile.

roping Timed rodeo competition in which a calf or steer is roped from horseback, thrown to the ground, and tied; may be calf roping, team roping, or steer roping.

rotation Twisting around the axis.

running walk Medium fast, walking, four-beat gait in which the hind foot oversteps the forefoot by 12 inches or more.

sacral vertebrae See sacrum.

sacro-iliac joints Pair of joints between the sacrum and ilium; located several inches below the tuber sacrale.

sacro-iliac subluxation Partial dislocation of the sacro-iliac joint(s) due to tearing of the sacro-iliac ligaments.

sacrum Part of the spinal column along the croup, consisting of five fused sacral vertebrae.

saliva Clear, enzyme-containing secretion of the salivary glands of the mouth.

salivary glands Any of the glands around the mouth that secrete saliva.

scapula Shoulder blade.

scapular Pertaining to the scapula.

sclera "White" of the eye.

scope Degree of extension and flexion of the legs and body while the horse is in motion.

scrotum Pouch of skin that contains the testicles.

sebaceous glands Glands in the skin that secrete an oily stubstance through the hair follicles.

second thigh See gaskin.

seedy toe See white line disease.

semen Fluid comprised of sperm cells and secretions of the testicles, seminal vesicles, prostate gland, and bulbourethral glands.

semilunar Shaped like a half-moon.

seminal Pertaining to semen.

sensitive laminae Tiny corrugations in the laminar corium of the hoof wall.

sensory nerve Nerve that transmits signals of sensation, such as pain, temperature, pressure, and tension, from the tissues to the brain.

sesamoid bone Small nodular bone embedded in a tendon or joint capsule, e.g. the paired proximal sesamoid bones at the back of the fetlock joint.

sesamoidean Pertaining to the sesamoid bones.

sesamoiditis Inflammation and subsequent bony reaction of the sesamoid bones at the back of the fetlock.

sheared heels Abnormal foot conformation where one heel bulb is higher than the other and the tissue between them is torn.

sheath See prepuce.

short pastern bone Smaller of the two bones of the pastern between the long pastern bone and coffin bone; second phalanx, second pastern bone.

shoulder girdle Group of large muscles that support the shoulder joint.

shoulder joint Shallow ball and socket joint between the bottom of the scapula and the top of the humerus.

show class Competition in which horses are judged according to conformation, physical condition, and/or adherence to breed standards.

show jumping Jumping competition where the horse and rider perform in a defined area over a series of artificial obstacles in a certain order and within a certain time period.

sickle hocks Conformational fault where the cannons in the hindlegs angle forward as viewed from the side.

sidebone Calcification and hardening of the lateral cartilages in the foot.

sinuses Air-filled cavities beneath the facial bones; open into the nasal passages.

sire Male parent.

skewbald Coat color where a brown horse has large, defined patches of white.

slab-sided Conformational fault where the ribs are short, flat, or upright.

sliding stop Manuever where the horse sets its hindlegs and "sits down," coming to an sudden halt from the gallop.

slow pace Slow, four-beat gait similar to the pace and rack but with a hesitation inserted between the left and right sides.

smegma Cheesy material, principally composed of dead skin cells, found beneath the prepuce.

soft palate Sheet of pliable tissue at the back of the hard palate.

soft tissue Tissue other than bone, teeth, hooves, and abnormal mineral deposits; e.g. skin, subcutaneous tissue, tendons, ligaments, and muscles.

solar surface Lower edge of the coffin bone, facing the sole.

sole Horn and sensitive tissue on the underside of the foot, between the hoof wall and the frog.

sole corium Layer of cells lining the solar surface of the coffin bone that produce the sole.

sperm Male reproductive cell.

spermatic cord Structure extending from the deep inguinal ring to the testicle, contains the ductus deferens, cremaster muscle, blood vessels, and nerve supply.

sphincter Ring-like muscle fibers or specially arranged oblique fibers that reduce the opening of a tube or the interior of an organ.

spin Maneuver where the horse plants one hind leg and whirls 360 degrees.

spinal canal Tunnel in the vertebrae through that the spinal cord runs.

spinal column Series of vertebrae that surround the spinal cord; backbone, spine, vertebral column.

spinal cord Cord-like part of the central nervous system traveling within the spinal column from the foramen magnum to the cauda equina.

spinal nerves Nerves emerging from between the vertebrae to supply the tissues.

spine See spinal column.

spine of the ischium Ridge where the left and right halves of the ischium fuse together.

spinous process Projection of bone from a vertebra.

splay-footed See toed-out.

spleen Large hemyl node located in front of the stomach in the abdomen; stores and filters blood.

splint Bony swelling on the side of the cannon bone or splint bone, caused by trauma or concussion.

splint bone Either of the two small bones on each side of the cannon bone.

sport horse Warmblood horse used for sporting events such as show jumping, eventing, and dressage.

sprinter Racehorse that performs well over short distances, i.e. less than one mile.

square up Getting the horse to stand straight with the fore and hindlegs even with each other, and weight evenly distributed on all four legs.

stance Manner in which the horse chooses to stand.

standing under See camped under behind or camped under in front.

star-gazing Traveling with the head too high.

stay apparatus System of muscles, tendons, and ligaments in the leg that allow the horse to stand with little or no muscle effort.

stayer Racehorse that performs well over long distances, i.e. one mile or more.

steeplechase Cross-country, timed race over natural obstacles, including water jumps.

sternal Pertaining to or toward the sternum.

sternebrae Eight joined segments of the sternum.

sternum Bone that runs between the forelegs and connects the lower ends of the ribs together; breastbone.

stifle Area or joint between the thigh and gaskin of the hindleg.

stock horse Horse that is used to work and herd livestock.

stocking up Harmless fluid buildup in the lower legs, usually caused by inactivity.

straight behind Overly straight hindlegs caused by too little angulation of the stifle, hock, and pastern joints, as viewed from the side; post-legged.

strangles Infection of the lymph nodes of the upper respiratory tract with *Streptococcus equi*; causes fever, runny nose, and abcessing of the lymph nodes; equine distemper.

stride length Distance that a foot travels with each step.

subcutaneous Beneath the skin.

sublingual Beneath the tongue.

subscapular Below the scapula.

sulcus Groove or crevice; e.g. the grooves on either side, and down the center of the frog. Plural = sulci.

superficial On or near the surface.

supraorbital Above the orbit.

suprascapular Above the scapula.

supraspinatus Above the scapular spine.

supraspinous Above the spine or a spinous process.

suspensory apparatus Structures that support the fetlock, including the suspensory ligament, flexor tendons and their check ligaments, and the distal sesamoidean ligaments.

suspensory ligament Ligament that holds up a part, e.g. suspensory ligament of the fetlock or suspensory ligament of the navicular bone.

suture Union between the skull bones that is composed of fibrous tissue.

sweeney Damage to the suprascapular nerve at the front of the shoulder blade, causing atrophy of the shoulder muscles and instability of the shoulder joint.

synovial fluid Viscous, transparent fluid that fills a joint space, tendon sheath, or bursa.

synovium Membrane that lines the joint capsule, tendon sheath, or bursa, and produces synovial fluid; synovial membrane.

table Chewing surface of a tooth.

tail base Where the tail joins the rump.

tail carriage Height at which the horse carries its tail.

talus Large hock bone that forms the tibiotarsal joint with the tibia.

tarsal Pertaining to the hock.

team roping Timed, mounted rodeo competition in which a calf's horns are roped by the header and its hind feet by the heeler, then held motionless between them.

temporal fossa Rounded hollow above the horse's eye.

temporary teeth Teeth of a young horse that are shed at various ages to be followed by permanent teeth.

tendinous Pertaining to or resembling a tendon, containing tendon fibers.

tendon Bundle of collagen fibers that connects muscle to bone and transmits the contractile force of the muscle to the bone.

tendon sheath Thin sheath that surrounds and protects a tendon as it runs over a joint or irregular bony surface.

testicle One of two male reproductive glands inside the scrotum that produces sperm cells and testosterone.

thigh Area of the hindleg between the hip and stifle.

thoracic Pertaining to the thorax.

thoracic limb Foreleg.

thorax Part of the body between the neck and diaphragm, encased by the ribs.

thoroughpin Non-painful, fluidy swelling at the back of the hindleg, just above the point of the hock.

throatlatch Area of the neck immediately behind the head, where the throat-latch strap of a bridle runs.

tibia Major bone of the gaskin, between the hock and stifle.

tibial Pertaining to the tibia.

tibial crest Ridge of bone along the front of the tibia, just below the stifle.

tibial spine Narrow peak of bone on the top of the tibia.

tied in at the knee Conformational fault where the flexor tendons appear to be too close to the cannon bone just below the knee.

tobiano Pinto coat pattern where the markings extend from the head, chest, belly, and buttocks, and often over the back; their edges are clearly defined.

toed-in Conformational fault in which the toe(s) points slightly inward; pigeon-toed.

toed-out Conformational fault in which the toe(s) points slightly outward; splay-footed.

tonsils Lymph nodes in the throat that are a first line of defense against foreign invaders.

topline Uppermost line of the horse's neck, back, and croup.

trachea "Windpipe" from the larynx to the bronchi of the lungs.

transverse Extending from side to side; perpendicular to the long axis.

trekking Packing trip over several days.

trochanter One of three tuberosities on the femur: greater trochanter, lesser trochanter, and third trochanter.

trochlear groove Shallow channel at the lower end of the femur; the patella slides up and down this groove at the front of the stifle.

trotter Harness racehorse that performs at the trot.

true ribs Sternal ribs that connect directly to the sternum via their costal cartilage.

tuber calcis Bony point at the back of the hock; point of the hock.

tuber coxae Bony point at the side of the pelvis, just behind the flank; point of the hip.

tuber ischii Bony point at the back of the pelvis, a few inches below the tail base; point of the buttock.

tuber sacrale Bony point at the top of the pelvis; point of the croup.

tubercle Small bump on a bone.

tuberosity Large knob or protuberance on a bone.

udder See mammary glands.

ulna Small bone on the back of the forearm next to the radius.

ulnar Pertaining to the ulna.

under-run heels Abnormal foot shape in which the heels are lower than normal and are at a lower angle than the front of the hoof wall.

underline Lower line of the horse's neck, belly, and groin.

unpigmented skin Pink skin, with few or no pigment cells.

upward fixation of the patella When the medial patellar ligament becomes hooked over the medial condyle of the femur, locking the stifle in an extended position.

ureter One of two tubes between each kidney and the urinary bladder.

urethra Tube that carries urine from the urinary bladder to the body's exterior; also carries semen in the stallion.

urinary bladder Hollow organ responsible for storing urine until it is passed out of the body.

urinary system Organs responsible for extracting and processing fluid waste, and excreting it as urine.

urine Fluid excreted by the kidneys and stored in the bladder until it is passed out through the urethra.

uterine horn Two long, narrow parts of the uterus located between the uterine body and the ovaries.

uterus Hollow, muscular organ in the mare where the fetus develops; womb.

vagina Passage from the cervix to the vulva.

varnish marks Coat pattern of dark areas over the bony points of the horse.

vas deferens See ductus deferens.

vascular Full of blood vessels.

vasodilation Increase in the diameter of a blood vessel.

vein Wide, thin-walled vessel that carries de-oxygenated blood from the body tissues back to the heart.

venous Pertaining to the veins.

ventral Directional term meaning the underside; away from the top.

ventricle One of the two lower chambers of the heart that receives blood from the corresponding atrium.

venule Tiny branch of a vein.

vertebra Bone of the spinal column. Plural = vertebrae.

vertebral Pertaining to or toward a vertebra.

vessel Any channel for carrying a fluid.

vestigial Remaining from a previous stage of species development, having no modern function.

villi Hair-like projections on certain mucous membranes.

vocal cords Thin bands stretched across the larynx that vibrate to create vocal sounds.

volar See palmar.

vulva External opening of the reproductive and urinary systems in the mare.

Warmblood Cross between a hotblooded breed and a coldblooded breed; specifically, sport horses popular in Olympic equestrian events.

weight-bearing Load on the legs from the horse's body weight; increases with speed, and with a rider.

well-sprung ribs Ribs that arch out from the spine at the top and then project slightly backward.

white blood cells Immune system cells that respond to tissue damage and infection.

white line Pale inner layer of the hoof wall, visible at the ground surface of the hoof, between the main part of the wall and the sole.

white line disease Infection in a crevice between the hoof wall and sole that begins at the ground surface and may spread up or around the hoof wall; seedy toe.

windpuff, wind gall Small fluid-filled swelling around the fetlock; may be related to the fetlock joint or the flexor tendon sheath.

wing of the ilium Part of the pelvis that curves up from the point of the hip to the tuber sacrale.

withers Prominent meeting point of the neck, shoulder, and back.

wolf tooth Small, vestigial premolar that may erupt in the upper jaw in front of the cheek teeth.

wood chewing Stable vice where a horse chews on wooden surfaces: stall doors, feed box, windowsill, etc.; crib-biting.

xiphoid cartilage Sword-shaped rearmost tip of the sternum, located in the girth area at the dorsal midline.

yearling Young horse that is between the ages of one and two years.

Index

Numbers in *italics* indicate illustrations.

muscle(s)
  popliteus   *29, 222, 223,* 232, *234*
  psoas major   184, *186,* 221
  psoas minor   184, *186,* 221,
    222, 223
  quadratus femoris   *29,* 220, *221*
  quadriceps femoris   *29, 222, 223,*
    225, 229, 231–232, *250,* 251–252
  radial carpal extensor   *28, 32,*
    133, 140, 147, 159
  radial carpal flexor   *28, 133, 140,*
    147, 148
  rectus abdominis   *184, 185,* 186
  rectus capitis dorsalis   *56,* 57, 84
  rectus capitis ventralis major   83
  rectus femoris   231–232
  respiratory   188
  retractor penis   *426, 427,* 428
  rhomboideus   *28, 29, 31,* 79, *80,*
    81, 92, 93, 128, 133
  sartorius   221–224, *222*
  scalene   *29, 80,* 81
  scutularis   *30*
  semimembranosus   *29, 33, 216,*
    219, *221, 223,* 232
  semispinalis capitis   83
  semitendinosus   *28, 29, 30, 31,*
    33, 216, 219, *220, 221, 222, 223,*
    232, *234,* 236
  serratus dorsalis   *30, 92*
  serratus ventralis   *28, 29, 30, 31,*
    80, 81, 92, 93, 94, 128, 130–
    131, *132,* 158, *159*
  shoulder   126–134, *128, 132, 133*
  soleus   *29, 33, 216, 221,* 236, 240–
    243, *242*
  spinalis et semispinalis   *31, 93*
  splenius   *28, 30, 80,* 81–
    83, *92, 93, 94*
  sternocephalic   *80, 81,* 84
  sternomandibular   *28, 32*
  sternothyrohyoid   *29, 32*
  stifle   231–233
  subclavius   *28, 29, 31, 32, 93,*
    99, 100, *133*
  subscapularis   132, *133*
  superficial digital flexor   141, 232,

    235, 236, 243, *244, 250*
  superior labial levator   58
  supraspinatus   *29, 31, 32, 81,*
    92, 93, 131–132, *132, 133,* 136
  supraspinous   *92*
  taeniae coli   415
  tail   227–228, *228*
  temporal   *29*
  tensor fascia antebrachii   *133*
  tensor fascia latae   *28, 220,* 221,
    222, 223, 250, 251–252
  teres major   132, *133*
  teres minor   132
  thorax   183–188
  transverse
    abdominis   *29, 31, 185,* 186
  transverse nasal   *32*
  trapezius   *28, 30, 32,* 79, *80,*
    93, 94, 128
  triceps   *28, 29, 30, 31, 32, 93*
    lateral head   *132,* 137
    long head   *128, 132,* 133,
      158, *159*
    medial head   *133,* 137
  ulnar carpal extensor   *28*
  ulnar carpal flexor   *28, 133,*
    140, 147, 148
  upper arm   107–108, *108,* 126–
    134, *128, 132, 133*
  urethralis   418, 425, 428
  ventral sacrococcygeal   *422*
  vestibular constrictor   422
  voluntary   27
  vulvar constrictor   422
  withers   *92,* 92–94, *93, 94*
  zygomatic   *58*
musculoskeletal system   15–34
mushroom-foot   259–260
muzzle   *4, 41,* 48–49

N

nasal passages   16, *54,* 55–
  56, *56, 395*
nasal septum   56
nasolacrimal apparatus   *60*
navicular bone.   *See bone(s): navicular*

stocking *306*
stomach *411*, 412–413, *413*
straight behind 12, 192, *193*, 204–206, *207*
stride length 109, 111, 204
strip *304*
subcutaneous tissue 23
Suffolk pony *337*, 337–338
suspensory apparatus 157–158, 251
swan neck 72, *74*
sway back *170*, 171, 177
Swedish Gotland pony 343–344, *344*
Swedish Warmblood 328, *329*
sweeney 136
synovial fluid 22, 26

T

tail
  anatomy 227–228
  conformation *198*
tarsus. *See hock*
teat cisterns *423*
teeth
  canine *53*, 54, *376*, 379, *381*
  cheek 47–48, *53*, 57, 62, 375. *See also herein molar; premolar*
  incisor *20*, 47, *53*, 54, 61–62, 375–376, *376*, *377*, 379
  milk. *See herein temporary*
  molar 375, *376*, 379
  permanent *379–391*
  premolar 375, *376*, 379
  temporary 377–378
  wolf *376*, 379
tendon sheath 26
tendon(s) 26. *See also muscle(s)*
  Achilles *28*, *33*, 202, *234*, 236, *242*
  biceps brachii *134*, 158, *159*
  biceps femoris *230*
  calcaneal. *See herein Achilles*
  cannon *150*, 247
  common calcaneal *234*, 236
  common digital extensor *32*, *140*, *150*, *155*, 158, *159*, *161*, *162*, 247, *250*, 251–252, 273, 275, *276*, 278

cranial tibial *243*
cunean 244, 246
tendon(s)
  deep digital flexor *119*, *140*, 146, *150*, *154*, 155, 157–158, *159*, 161, *162*, 247, 251–252, 262, 273, 275, *276*, 277, *279*
  external abdominal oblique *184*
  fetlock *154*, 154–157
  fibularis tertius. *See herein peroneus tertius*
  foot 275, *276*, *278*, *279*
  forearm *140*
  foreleg *140*
  gaskin *234*, 236, *243*
  gastrocnemius *250*
  hindleg *234*
  hock 240–244, *243*
  internal abdominal oblique *185*
  lacertus fibrosis 158, *159*
  lateral digital extensor *28*, *140*, *150*, *161*, 247
  long digital extensor *230*, *243*, 247
  oblique carpal extensor *32*, *140*, *147*
  pastern *161*, *162*
  peroneus tertius *223*, *231*, 236, *243*, *244*, *250*, 251–252
  prepubic 186, 214
  quadriceps femoris *230*
  radial carpal extensor 158
  radial carpal flexor 146
  superficial digital flexor *29*, *33*, *119*, *140*, 146, *150*, *154*, 154–155, 157–158, *159*, 222, 223, 242, 247, 251–252, 275, *276*, *279*
Tennessee Walking Horse 199, 204, 308, 321–322, *322*
testicle *424*, 424–425, *425*
testicular septa *424*
testosterone *424*, 429
thalamus *403*
thigh *4*, *192*
  anatomy 210–227
  conformation 200